Atlas of Organ Transplantation

Abhinav Humar, Arthur J. Matas and
William D. Payne

Atlas of Organ Transplantation

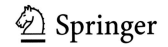 Springer

Abhinav Humar, MD,
    FRCS
Department of Surgery
Division of
    Transplantation
University of Minnesota
Minneapolis, MN
USA

Arthur J. Matas, MD,
    FACS
Department of Surgery
Division of
    Transplantation
University of Minnesota
Minneapolis, MN
USA

William D. Payne, MD,
    FACS
Department of Surgery
Division of
    Transplantation
University of Minnesota
Minneapolis, MN
USA

Cover photograph by author.

British Library Cataloguing in Publication Data

Atlas of organ transplantation
    1. Transplantation of organs, tissues, etc. – Atlases
    I. Humar, Abhinav   II. Matas, Arthur J.   III. Payne, William D.
    617.9′54

    ISBN-13: 9781846283147
    ISBN-10: 1846283140

Library of Congress Control Number: 2005938494

ISBN-10: 1-84628-314-0   e-ISBN 1-84628-316-7   Printed on acid-free paper
ISBN-13: 978-1-84628-314-7

Printed in Singapore.

9 8 7 6 5 4 3 2

Springer Science+Business Media
springer.com

Preface

The field of organ transplantation has undergone remarkable changes in the last decade. The growing numbers of agents available for immunosuppression have played a significant role in the advancement of this field. However, just as important has been the development of surgical innovations in the field. This includes not only the development of new surgical procedures, but also modifications of the existing ones. This has involved all areas of organ transplantation including deceased-donor procurement techniques, living-donor transplantation, and transplantation of the individual organs including kidney, liver, pancreas, and intestine. Examples include procurement from non–heart-beating donors; living-donor transplants involving the liver, pancreas, or intestine; laparoscopic donor nephrectomy; split-liver transplants; and multivisceral transplants. All of these represent new, innovative procedures that are being performed on a regular basis only in the last few years. Given these recent dramatic changes in the surgical face of transplantation, we felt it was time for a surgical atlas of transplantation that highlighted these recent developments.

The aim of this book is to provide the reader with a comprehensive, pictorial step-by-step account of abdominal organ transplant procedures performed by contemporary transplant surgeons. Emphasis has been placed on newer procedures or procedures that have undergone significant modifications. It is recognized that there are many well-accepted techniques for the same procedure, with each having potential merit. While it is impossible to present all of these variations, an attempt has been made to describe the common variations in surgical technique.

Innovations in imaging have allowed us to organize this atlas in a format that provides the reader with the most clear and realistic view of the operative procedures. Schematic diagrams are included to complement high-quality intraoperative photographs, allowing readers to clearly visualize the course of the operative procedure. A unique feature of this atlas is a digital video file of the major operative procedures, which provides the reader with the closest possible experience to being present in the operating suite. It is hoped that this format will provide the reader with a clear visual and written description of all major abdominal transplant procedures performed by the modern transplant surgeon.

Acknowledgments

The editors gratefully acknowledge the contributing authors for their hard work in the preparation of individual chapters or sections of chapters. The help of Dr. Khalid Khwaja was greatly appreciated in the design of the illustrations used in this atlas. The videos that accompany this atlas would not have been made possible without the expertise and hard work of Dr. Bradley Linden, Eric Carolan, and Jake Gotler.

Contents

3 Nephrectomy from a Living Donor   59
Raja Kandaswamy and Abhinav Humar

4 Kidney Transplantation   91
Abhinav Humar and Arthur J. Matas

5 Pancreas Transplantation   133
Abhinav Humar, Khalid O. Khwaja, and David E.R. Sutherland

A. Osama Gaber and Hosein Shokouh-Amiri

Operative Videos

Deceased Donor

1. Multiorgan Procurement

Kidney

2. Brachiocephalic Arteriovenous Fistula
3. Hand-Assisted Laparoscopic Donor Nephrectomy
4. Benching Kidney from Deceased Donor
5. Adult Kidney Transplant (Two Arteries)
6. Pediatric Kidney Transplant

Pancreas Transplant

7. Benching Pancreas from Deceased Donor
8. Pancreas Transplant Alone: Systemic/Bladder Drainage
9. Simultaneous Pancreas Kidney (SPK) – Portal/Enteric Drainage
   Contribution by: Osoma Gaber, Hosein Shokouh-Amiri
10. Laparoscopic Distal Pancreatectomy for Living-Donor Pancreas Transplant
    Contribution by: Miguel Tan, Raja Kandaswamy, Rainer W.G. Gruessner

Liver Transplant

11. Benching Liver from Deceased Donor
12. Deceased Donor Liver Transplant – Adult Recipient
13. In-Situ Split of the Deceased Donor Liver for Adult/Pediatric Recipients
    Contribution by: Hasan Yersiz, John Renz, Ronald Busutil
14. In-Situ Split of the Deceased Donor Liver for Two Adult Recipients
15. Adult to Adult Living-Donor Liver Transplant Using the Right Lobe – Donor Procedure
16. Adult to Adult Living-Donor Liver Transplant Using the Right Lobe – Recipient Procedure

Intestinal Transplant

17. Living-Donor Intestinal Transplant

Contributors

A. Osama Gaber, MD, FACS
Methodist Transplant Institute
University of Tennessee
Memphis, TN, USA

Thomas M. Fishbein, MD
Transplant Institute
Georgetown University Hospital
Washington, DC, USA

Rainer W.G. Gruessner, MD, PhD
Department of Surgery
Division of Transplantation
University of Minnesota
Minneapolis, MN, USA

Abhinav Humar, MD, FRCS
Department of Surgery
Division of Transplantation
University of Minnesota
Minneapolis, MN, USA

Raja Kandaswamy, MBBS
Department of Surgery
Division of Transplantation
University of Minnesota
Minneapolis, MN, USA

Khalid O. Khwaja, MD
Transplant Center
Beth Israel Deaconess Medical Center
Boston, MA, USA

Arthur J. Matas, MD, FACS
Department of Surgery
Division of Transplantation
University of Minnesota
Minneapolis, MN, USA

Cal S. Matsumoto, MD
Georgetown University Hospital
Washington, DC, USA

William D. Payne, MD, FACS
Department of Surgery
Division of Transplantation
University of Minnesota
Minneapolis, MN, USA

David J. Reich, MD, FACS
Liver Transplant Program
Department of Surgery
Albert Einstein Medical Center
Philadelphia, PA, USA

John F. Renz, MD, PhD
Center for Liver Disease
New York Presbyterian Hospital
New York, NY, USA

Hosein Shokouh-Amiri, MD, FACS
Live Donor and Pediatric Liver
    Transplantation
Methodist Transplant Institute
University of Tennessee
Memphis, TN, USA

Mark L. Sturdevant, MD
Department of Surgery
Division of Transplantation
University of Minnesota
Minneapolis, MN, USA

David E.R. Sutherland, MD, PhD
Department of Surgery
Division of Transplantation
University of Minnesota
Minneapolis, MN, USA

Miquel Tan, MD
Division of Transplantation
Department of Surgery
Johns Hopkins Hospital
Baltimore, MD, USA

Hasan Yersiz, MD
Department of Hepatobiliary and Liver
    Transplant Surgery
Dumont-UCLA Transplant Center
David Geffen School of Medicine at
    UCLA
University of California, Los Angeles
Los Angeles, CA, USA

1

Multiorgan Procurement from the Deceased Donor

Standard Multiorgan Procurement

Mark L. Sturdevant and Abhinav Humar

Introduction

Organ procurement for transplantation was first accomplished by the Soviet surgeon Yu Yu Voronoy, who performed the first human kidney transplant on April 3, 1933. The donor was a 60-year-old man who died on admission to the hospital from a traumatic brain injury; the kidney was removed 6 hours postmortem and transplanted into the thigh of a 26-year-old woman with acute renal failure from mercury poisoning. The allograft did produce several milliliters of urine before the patient died 2 days after transplantation. The first attempt at liver transplantation, on March 1, 1963, by Thomas Starzl, was possible only after successful liver procurement from a child who had died after cardiac surgery, but was left on the heart-lung machine to allow for procurement.

Kidney transplantation in the 1950s and 1960s was primarily from live donors. However, in 1966 the concept of *brain death* was established in France by Guy Alexandre, who described the removal of kidneys from "heart-beating" cadavers with subsequent transplantation. In the United States, public support for this concept was overwhelming and led to the Harvard Ad Hoc Committee report in 1968 that outlined the criteria for brain death determination. The donor pool increased markedly after these policies entered clinical practice.

Advancement to the modern-day status of deceased-donor organ procurement was aided in large part by work done in organ preservation. The combined efforts of Dr. John Najarian and Dr. Folkert Belzer at the University of California–San Francisco (UCSF), starting in 1966, aimed at decreasing ischemia times and adding organ preservatives to increase organ viability. Prior to the acceptance of brain death, Belzer procured kidneys from non–heart-beating donors in the greater San Francisco area and emergently transported the organs to Najarian at Moffitt Hospital, who would have simultaneously started the recipient operation. Advances in organ preservation along with the acceptance of donation after brain death resulted in a more systematic, semielective kidney procurement, which resulted in organ delivery to recipients almost anywhere. Within 5 years a portable perfusion machine had been developed, and on December 24, 1971, a deceased-donor kidney procured in San Francisco was hand delivered by Belzer to transplant surgeon Hans Dicke in the Netherlands with a cold ischemia time of 37 hours. The transplanted kidney had excellent function 17 years later when the recipient died of a ruptured cerebral aneurysm.

The technique of multiple-organ procurement (kidney, liver, pancreas, small bowel) was first described by Starzl and his colleagues in 1984. Nakazato and his colleagues in 1992 described the technique of total abdominal evisceration with ex vivo dissection. Most centers have now added their own modifications to these pioneering techniques and differ primarily in their degree of in vivo dissection. Some centers perform extensive dissection of the organs to be recovered prior to flushing the organs with preservative solution. Other centers prefer to flush the organs early, remove the abdominal contents "en bloc", and perform the separation and dissection of the individual organs on the back table. Each technique has its potential advantages and disadvantages. Regardless of personal technique and preference, it is paramount that the transplant surgeon develops a systematic approach to safely procure the liver, pancreas, and kidneys, even in the unstable donor.

Surgical Technique

1. *Incision and exposure*: An incision extending from the sternal notch to the pubis, which is cruciated at the level of the umbilicus (Figure 1.1), provides maximal exposure for multiorgan procurements. The abdominal flaps can be folded back and held in place with sharp towel clips (Figure 1.2). This provides excellent exposure of the abdominal organs, without the need for a retractor. Only a sternal retractor is needed if the thoracic organs are to be procured. Sternotomy and division of the pericardium allows for examination of the heart while division of the ligamentous attachments to the liver allows for complete examination of the liver. A thorough abdominal exploration is then quickly performed to rule out contraindications to procurement such as malignancy or intraabdominal sepsis.

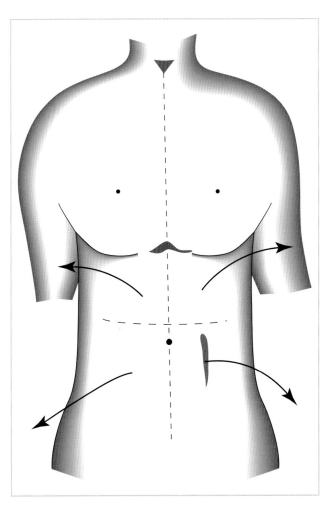

Figure 1.1

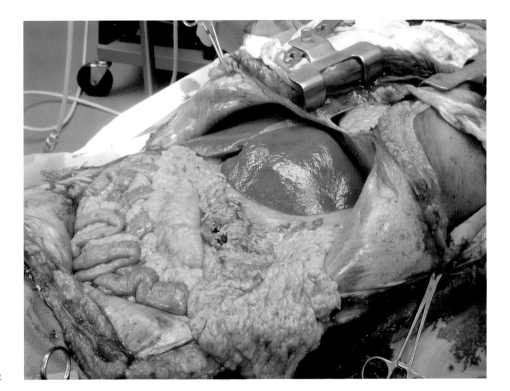

Figure 1.2

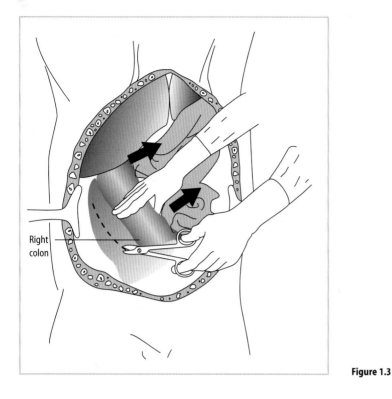

Figure 1.3

2. A Cattel-Braasch maneuver extending across the midline, with complete mobilization of the distal small bowel, right colon, and duodenum (Figure 1.3), allows for identification of the distal aorta, iliac bifurcation, and the distal inferior vena cava (IVC) (Figure 1.4).

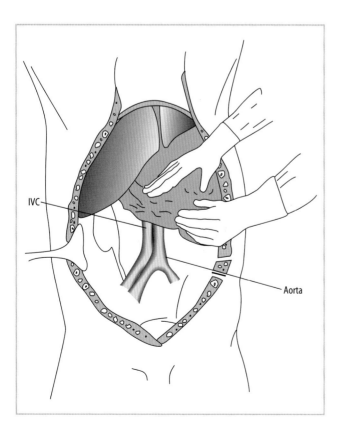

Figure 1.4

3. Division of the inferior mesenteric artery (black arrow) aids in the dissection of the distal aorta (yellow arrow and lines), which is then encircled with two umbilical tapes (Figure 1.5). This will be the site for later aortic cannulation for flushing (broken black line). The inferior vena cava sits just to the right (blue arrow).

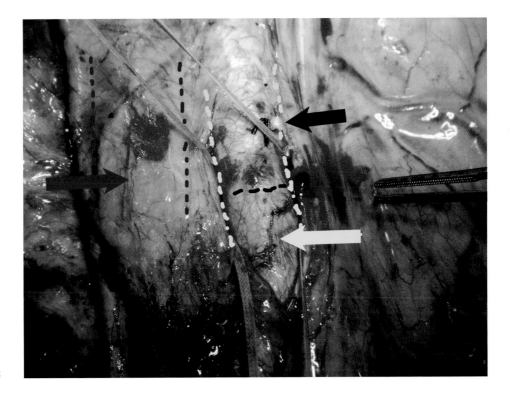

Figure 1.5

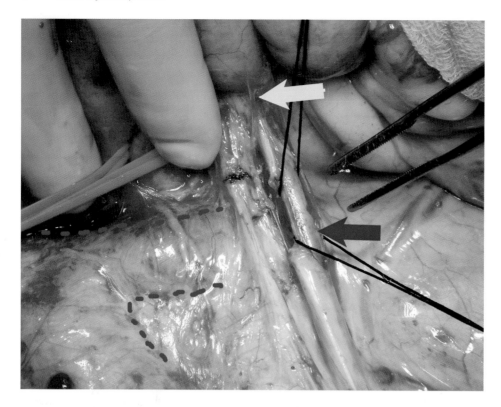

Figure 1.6

4. The inferior mesenteric vein (IMV) (blue arrow) is identified lateral to the ligament of Treitz (yellow arrow) and encircled with two silk ties in preparation for future cannulation into the portal venous circulation (Figures 1.6 and 1.7). The outline of the left renal vein (broken blue line) and its junction with the inferior vena cava is seen posterior to the IMV.

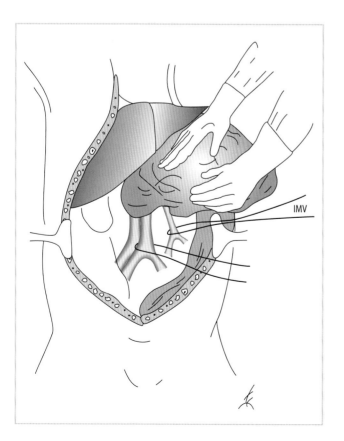

Figure 1.7

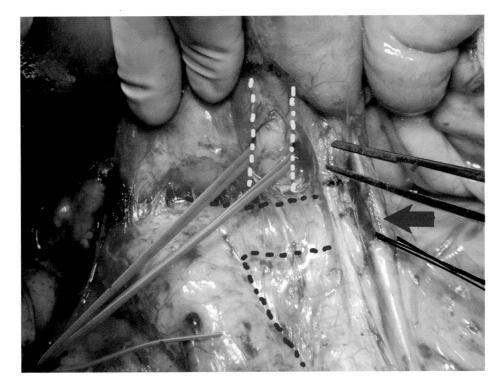

Figure 1.8

5. The third portion of the duodenum is retracted cephalad, and the superior mesenteric artery (SMA, yellow broken line) is identified, dissected free, and encircled with a vessel loop (Figures 1.8 and 1.9). This allows for occlusion of the SMA later, at the time of flushing. This limits the incidence of overperfusion injury to the pancreas. The left renal vein (broken blue line) is seen just inferior to the SMA, and the inferior mesenteric vein (blue arrow) is just lateral.

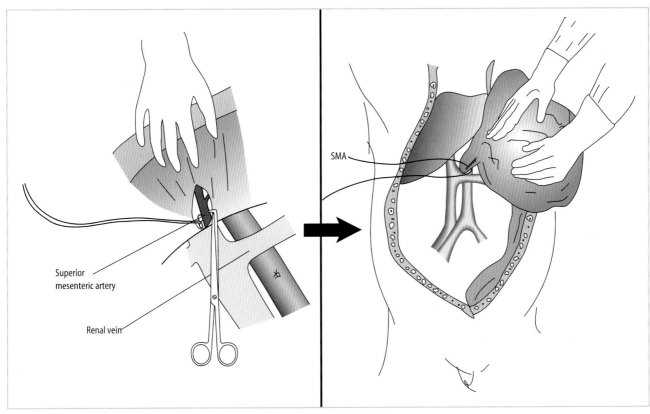

Superior
mesenteric artery

Renal vein

SMA

Figure 1.9

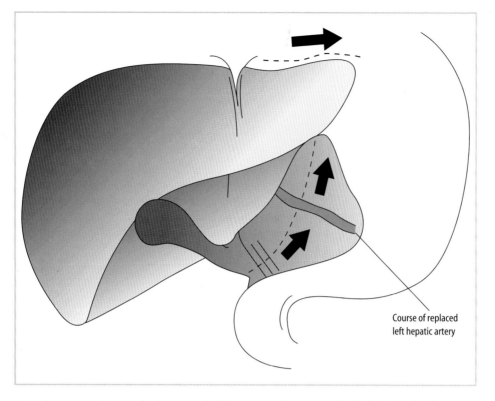

Course of replaced
left hepatic artery

Figure 1.10

6. In preparation to obtain control of the supraceliac aorta, the left triangular ligament of the liver is divided and the gastrohepatic ligament is examined and divided if no aberrant left hepatic artery is noted (Figure 1.10). If one is noted it will need to be preserved. The right diaphragmatic crus is divided, and the supraceliac aorta is identified and mobilized.

7. The supraceliac aorta is encircled with an umbilical tape (Figure 1.11). In the unstable donor, cold perfusion may be done at this point.

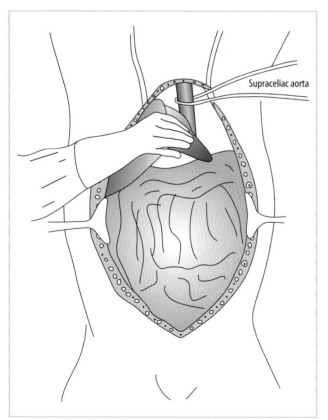

Supraceliac aorta

Figure 1.11

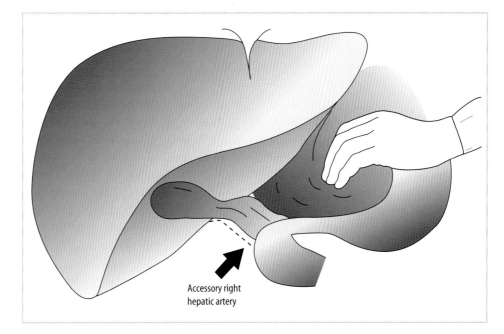

Figure 1.12

Accessory right
hepatic artery

8. The portal triad is now examined, and if present, an aberrant right hepatic artery will be palpated on the right edge of the porta hepatis, posterior to the bile duct and lateral to the portal vein. The course of an accessory or replaced right (black arrow) is shown in broken lines (Figure 1.12).

9. The common hepatic artery is identified and traced to the celiac axis, allowing for visualization and limited dissection of the splenic artery and gastroduodenal artery. The hepatic artery does not need to be completely dissected out at this time – rather, just the origin of the above branches need to be identified (Figure 1.13).

10. Limited dissection of the common bile duct (CBD, yellow arrow), which lies just to the right and anterior to the main portal vein (broken blue lines) is performed followed by ligation of the distal CBD just proximal to the pancreas. The CBD is then

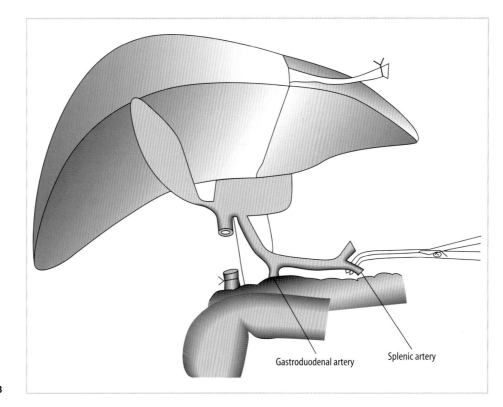

Gastroduodenal artery   Splenic artery

Figure 1.13

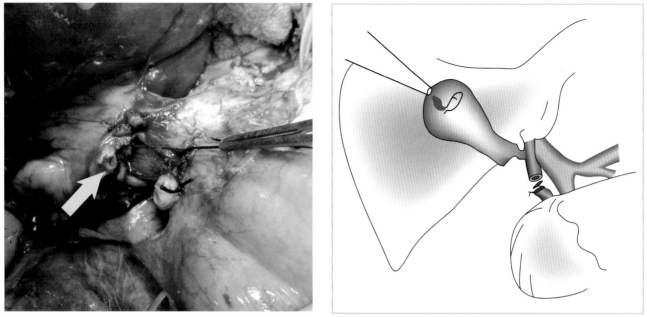

Figure 1.14

Figure 1.15

transected with a scalpel and the proximal end is left open (Figure 1.14). The gallbladder is incised and flushed with saline to clear the CBD of retained bile (Figure 1.15).

11. Systemic heparinization (300 units/kg) is performed. The distal aorta is ligated and a 24-French (F) aortic cannula (red arrow) is placed at this site. The IMV is ligated and a 14-F perfusion cannula (blue arrow) is placed (Figures 1.16 and 1.17). Alternatively, the portal vein can be cannulated directly for portal flushing.

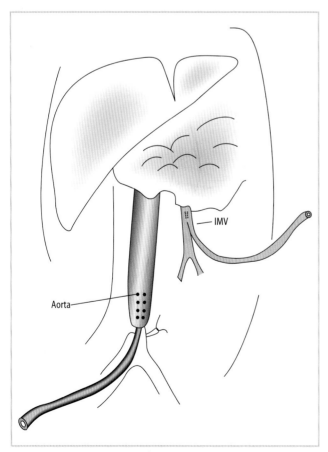

Figure 1.16

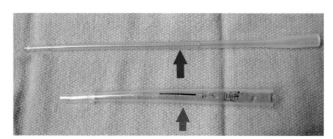

Figure 1.17

12. The supraceliac aorta is ligated or clamped and cold preservation fluid is infused via the two cannulas. The suprahepatic IVC is transected at its entrance to the right atrium in order to vent the perfusate (Figure 1.18). If heart procurement is also performed, the thoracic surgeon will incise the IVC just cephalad to the diaphragm. In adults, 5 L of preservation fluid is flushed via the aortic and inferior mesenteric vein cannulas (3 L and 2 L, respectively). The superior mesenteric artery is occluded after 1 L to avoid overperfusion of the pancreas. Slushed ice is placed into the peritoneal and pericardial cavities to complete the cooling process (Figure 1.19). Thoracic organ procurement occurs once flushing has been initiated.

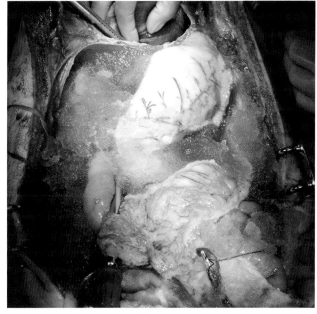

Figure 1.19

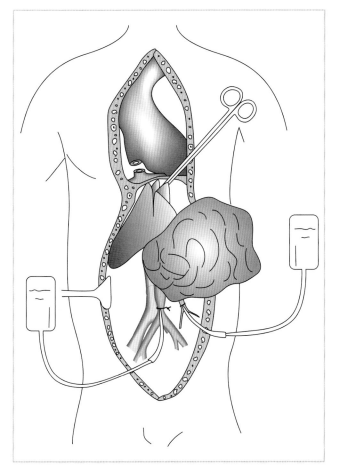

Figure 1.18

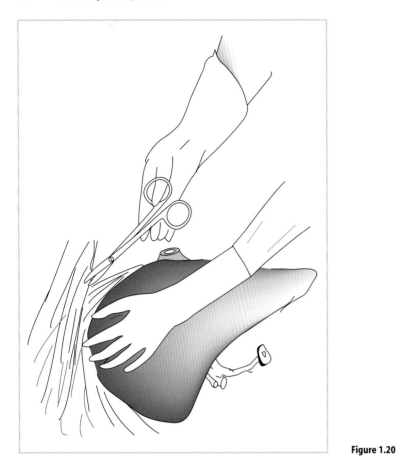

Figure 1.20

13. After the organs have been adequately flushed and the thoracic organs removed, attention is turned to the intraabdominal organs, starting first with the liver. Donor hepatectomy is started by dividing the diaphragm and ligamentous attachments to mobilize the liver (Figure 1.20).

14. The common hepatic artery is fully dissected and traced to the celiac axis where an aortic cuff is fashioned after the left gastric and splenic arteries are divided (Figure 1.21). A fine suture is placed on the distal splenic artery to aid in its identification near

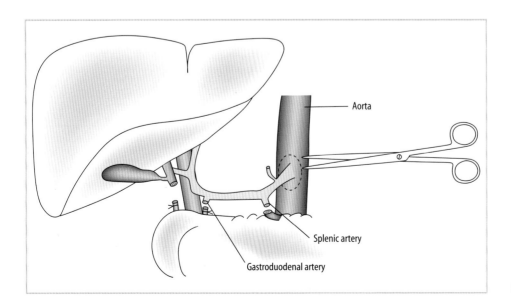

Figure 1.21

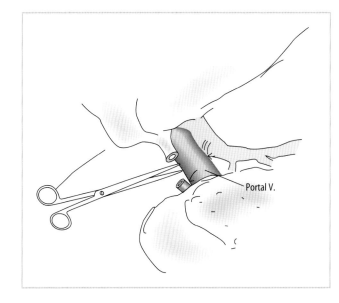

Figure 1.22

the pancreas. The gastroduodenal artery (GDA) is ligated distally near the pancreas and transected, leaving the proximal end open and available for possible reconstruction purposes.

15. Portal vein transection (blue arrow) completes division of the porta hepatis (Figures 1.22 and 1.23). If the pancreas is being procured, at least 1.5 cm of portal vein should be left with the pancreas graft.

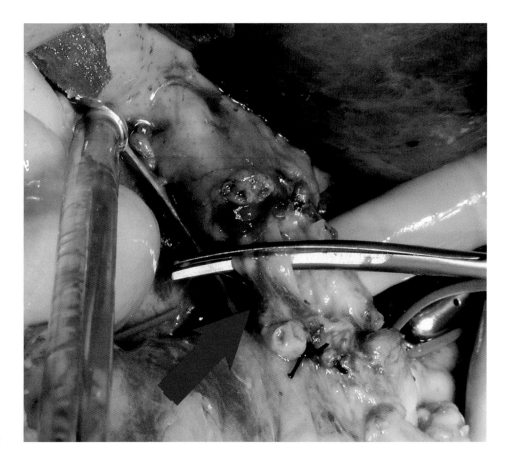

Figure 1.23

16. Transection of the infrahepatic IVC is performed cephalad to the confluences of the renal veins. The liver, along with a rim of diaphragm, is now removed (Figure 1.24).

17. The pancreas is removed next. At any juncture prior to cold perfusion, the nasogastric tube is advanced into the duodenum and 500 mL of amphotericin solution

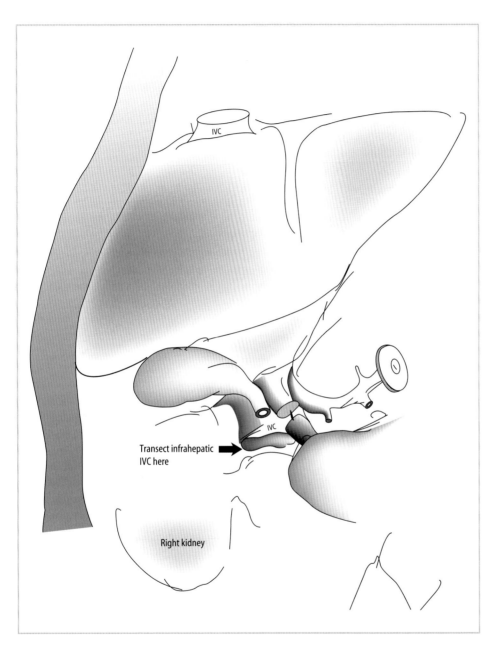

Figure 1.24

(50 mg/L) is delivered into the second portion of the duodenum. After the donor hepatectomy, the gastrocolic ligament is divided along the edge of the greater curvature of the stomach extending laterally to the spleen (Figure 1.25). This maneuver brings the entire pancreas into view for examination.

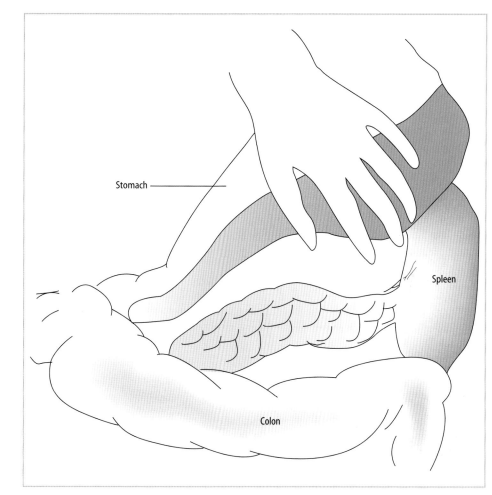

Figure 1.25

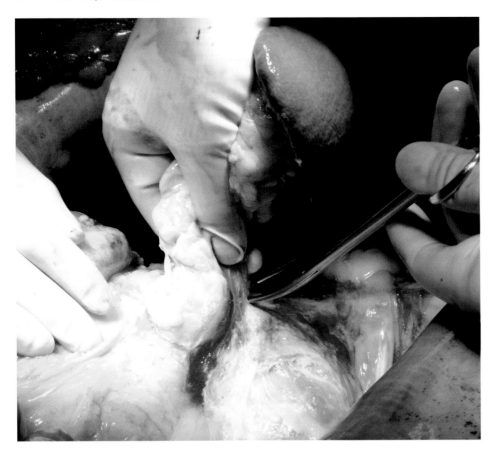

Figure 1.26

18. The ligamentous attachments to the spleen are divided next. The spleen along with the pancreatic body and tail can now be carefully mobilized from the retroperitoneum (Figures 1.26 and 1.27).

19. The first portion of the duodenum is circumferentially dissected and a mechanical stapler is used to divide the duodenum from the stomach (broken blue line) just distal

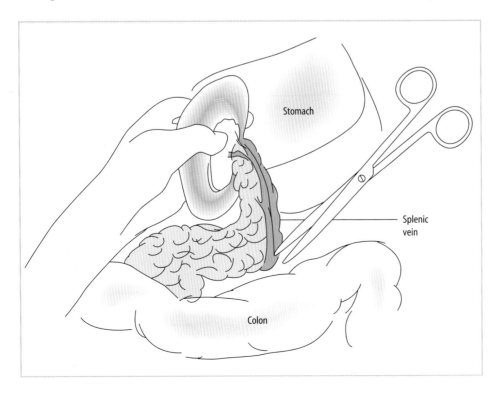

Figure 1.27

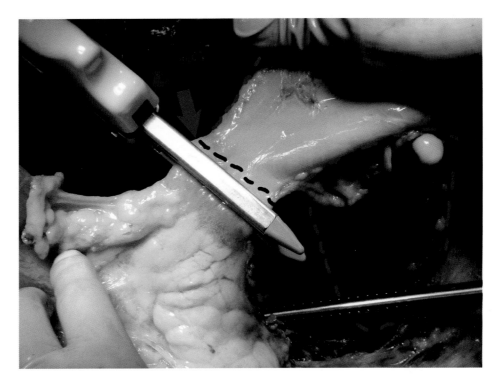

Figure 1.28

to the pylorus (blue arrow) (Figure 1.28). The stapler is also used to divide the duodenum just distal to the ligament of Treitz (Figure 1.29). The root of the transverse mesocolon, which runs along the anterior aspect of the pancreas is then divided using serial ligatures.

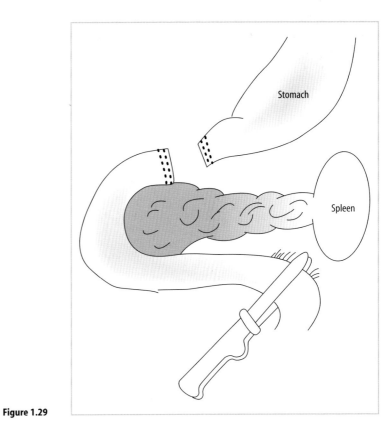

Figure 1.29

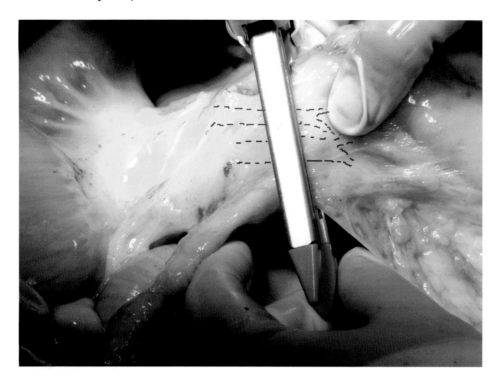

Figure 1.30

20. The IMV is ligated after the cannula is removed. The small bowel mesentery, which includes the superior mesenteric artery (SMA, broken red lines) and superior mesenteric vein (SMV, broken blue lines), is transected with a mechanical stapler (Figure 1.30).

21. The proximal superior mesenteric artery (broken red lines), which was previously encircled with a vessel loop, is now easily identified and transected flush with the aorta (Figure 1.31).

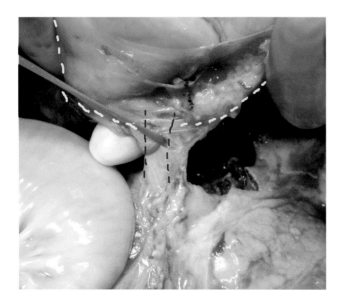

Figure 1.31

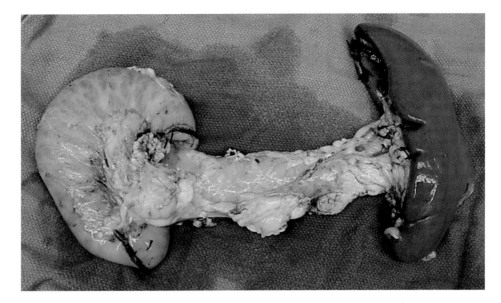

Figure 1.32

22. The pancreas is then removed en bloc with the duodenum and spleen (Figure 1.32).

23. The two kidneys are removed next en bloc with the cava and aorta. The lateral attachments to the kidney are divided and the ureters are traced caudally, and transected distally near their entrance into the bladder (Figure 1.33).

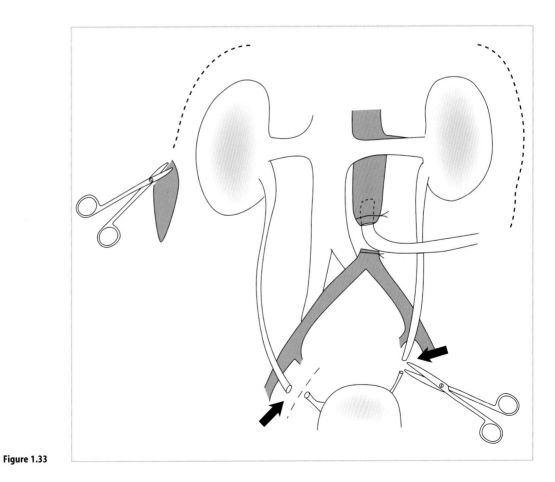

Figure 1.33

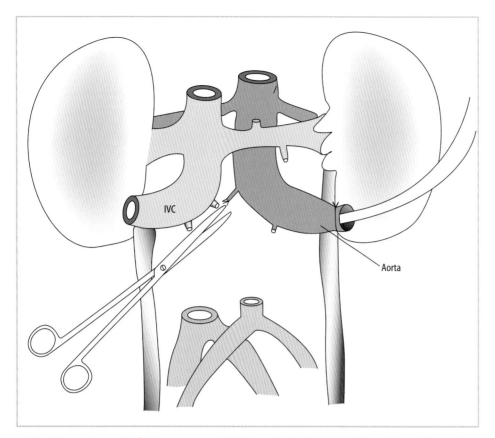

Figure 1.34

24. The aorta and inferior vena cava (IVC) are divided at their bifurcations. The ureters and these vessels are retracted cephalad and anteriorly, along with the two kidneys (solid blue lines), and dissection proceeds along their posterior aspects, anterior to the surface of the vertebral bodies and psoas muscle (broken black lines) (Figures 1.34 and 1.35).

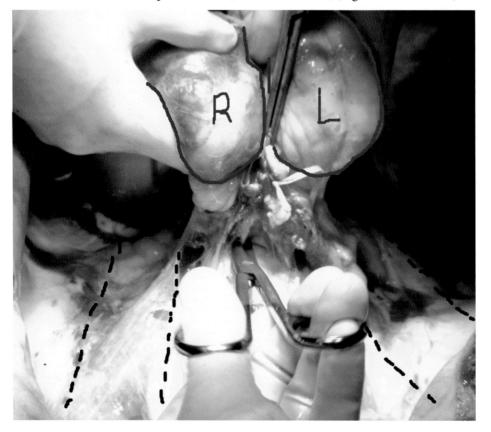

Figure 1.35

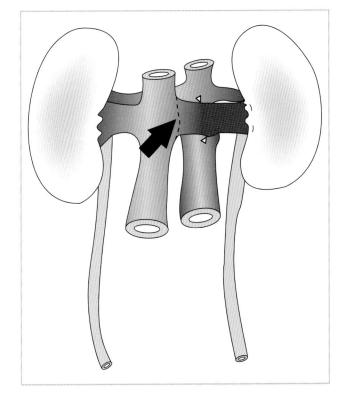

Figure 1.36

25. The kidneys are removed en bloc by transecting the aorta just proximal to the superior mesenteric artery takeoff. The IVC had been previously transected just above the renal veins during the donor hepatectomy. The kidneys are placed en bloc in cold preservation solution and are separated on the back table. Via an anterior approach, the left renal vein is identified and divided at its junction with the inferior vena cava (black arrow) (Figures 1.36 and 1.37).

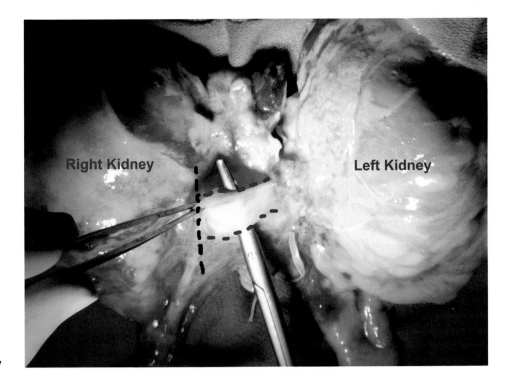

Figure 1.37

26. The aortic wall is then divided longitudinally down its center aspect, which allows for inspection of the renal artery orifices (red arrows) from within the aortic lumen (Figure 1.38).

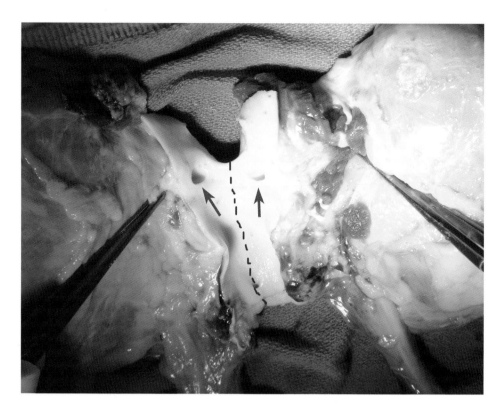

Figure 1.38

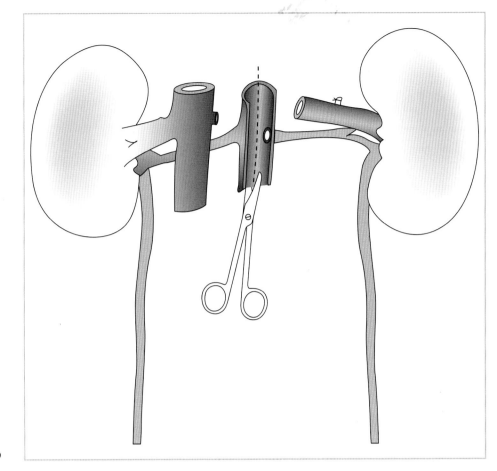

Figure 1.39

27. The posterior aortic wall is then divided between the renal artery orifices. This completes division of the right and left kidneys (Figure 1.39).

28. Finally, the iliac artery and veins are removed, to be used for possible vascular reconstructions in the pancreas and liver transplant procedures. Vessels are taken from the left and right side, starting at the common iliac vessel and extending to the distal external iliac vessels. These conduits are packaged with the pancreas and liver grafts. The deceased donor is then closed with a large suture.

Non–Heart-Beating Donor Organ Procurement

David J. Reich

Background

a) Definitions

The non–heart-beating donor (NHBD), also referred to as the donation after cardiac death (DCD) donor, is one type of expanded criteria donor that is increasingly being utilized by organ procurement organizations (OPOs) and transplant centers across the United States, Europe, and Asia to successfully boost the number of deceased donors and decrease the dire shortage of transplantable organs.[1] An NHBD death is characterized by irreversible absence of circulation, in contrast to heart-beating donor death, defined by irreversible cessation of all brain functions. Organ ischemia is minimized in the brain-dead donor because circulatory arrest typically occurs concurrently with perfusion of preservation solution and rapid core cooling. The NHBDs are less than ideal because the organs suffer ischemia during the prolonged periods between circulatory dysfunction, circulatory arrest, and subsequent perfusion and cooling. Furthermore, the surgical procedure for NHBD organ recovery, the main focus of this section, is demanding and rushed.

It is important to differentiate controlled from uncontrolled NHBDs. Uncontrolled NHBDs sustain circulatory arrest and either fail to respond to cardiopulmonary resuscitation or are declared dead on arrival at the hospital. Uncontrolled NHBD death is unplanned, so the organs suffer protracted ischemia prior to recovery. Although kidneys tolerate a short period of the resultant warm ischemia, transplantation of extrarenal organs from uncontrolled NHBDs carries a much greater risk. In contrast, controlled NHBDs undergo circulatory arrest following planned withdrawal of life support, most often in the operating room, with a donor surgical team readily available. Controlled NHBDs suffer terminal illness, usually a severe neurologic injury without the possibility of meaningful recovery or survival. Controlled NHBDs provide organs that are exposed to significantly less ischemic damage than those of uncontrolled NHBDs and in general, offer superior posttransplant function when compared with uncontrolled NHBDs.

b) History

The first human kidney, liver, and heart transplants, in 1958, 1963, and 1967, respectively, were performed using organs recovered from uncontrolled NHBDs. During the earliest years of transplantation through the 1960s, determination of death required heartbeat cessation. However, modern critical care, respirators and cardiopulmonary resuscitation made it possible to reestablish or maintain cardiopulmonary function even in the face of irreversible coma, leading to the 1968 landmark criteria for determination of brain death (Harvard neurologic definition and criteria for death).[2] These were endorsed by the major medical and legal professional associations in the United States and Europe, and for the following 25 years virtually all organ donation was from brain dead or living donors. Such donors are more desirable than NHBDs because the organs are protected from warm ischemic injury and are less prone to poor graft function. Non–heart-beating donor organ transplantation was reintroduced by the University of Pittsburgh transplant program in 1992.[3] The Pittsburgh program and the program in Madison, Wisconsin, were pivotal in initiating controlled NHBD organ transplantation and were the first to describe results of controlled NHBD kidney and liver transplantation (LTX), both in 1995.[4,5]

c) Impact of Non–Heart-Beating Donors

Over the past decade there has been increasing interest in pursuing controlled NHBD organ transplantation because results have improved and NHBDs have the potential to become a significant source of solid organs. Currently, only approximately 4% of deceased donors in the United States are NHBDs.[6] However, it has been estimated that NHBDs could increase the deceased donor pool in the United States by approximately 1000 donors per year, a 25% increase.[7] Among pediatric cadaver donors, increases of over 40% have been estimated.[8] In the United States, the number of NHBDs has steadily increased from only 42 in 1993, providing 81 organ transplants, to 270 in 2003, providing 549 transplants.[6] Some of the reasons that controlled NHBD is gaining acceptance and becoming more widespread involve increasing reluctance to prolong futile treatment and artificial life support of terminally injured and ill patients, increasing use of advance directives and health care proxies, and encouraging data on survival following NHBD organ transplantation. Families more frequently request this option in their discussions about removal of life support from patients who suffer devastating trauma or critical, irreversible illness. Certain OPOs have developed highly successful NHBD programs; in 2003, 15% of the deceased donors made possible by the Gift of Life Donor Program were NHBDs (51/344).[9] Strong OPO initiatives are crucial for increasing NHBDs. The OPOs must develop NHBD protocols; educate physicians, nurses, and other health care providers; engender enthusiasm among the OPO and transplant teams; recruit support from regional hospitals; and concentrate on public relations.[7,10]

Results Following Transplantation of Non–Heart-Beating Donor Organs

a) Kidneys

Non–heart-beating donors have provided for transplantation of kidneys, livers, some pancreata, and some lungs.[6] The majority of experience with NHBD organs is with kidney transplantation. One-year graft survival rates after uncontrolled NHBD kidney transplantation have been reported at 79% to 86%, similar to results of controlled NHBD kidney transplantation, which provides 1-year graft survival rates of 82% to 86%.[11] Comparison of 708 NHBD and 97,990 heart-beating deceased-donor renal transplants in the United States reveals that NHBD organ recipients had nearly twice the incidence of delayed graft function (DGF) (42% vs. 23%), but 1- and 5-year allograft survival rates were comparable between groups (83% vs. 87% and 61% vs. 65%, respectively).[12] Thus, in spite of temporary problems early on, renal grafts from NHBDs ultimately function as well as grafts from heart-beating donors.[12,13]

b) Livers

Several single-center experiences with NHBD LTX have been published.[14–19] Currently, uncontrolled NHBD LTX provides 1-year graft survival rates of only 17% to 55%.[4,11,19] In marked contrast, the reports on controlled NHBD LTX indicate patient and graft survival rates (76% to 90% and 72% to 90% at 1 year, respectively) that are comparable to those following heartbeating cadaver donor LTX.[1,16–18] At one institution, long-term NHBD graft loss was higher (54% vs. 81%), but half the graft losses were due to patient death with normal liver function.[16] Non–heart-beating donor LTX has not resulted in an increased incidence of primary nonfunction (0% to 11%) or hepatic artery thrombosis (0% to 5%).[1,16,18] The University of Pennsylvania group was the first to report a higher risk of major biliary complications in NHBD liver recipients (33% vs. 10%), mostly ischemic type biliary strictures and/or bile cast syndrome.[17] The group cautioned that biliary epithelium is particularly prone to ischemia-reperfusion injury, and it advocates using younger NHBDs and minimizing ischemia times. Although other groups have not experienced as high an incidence of biliary complications, it has become increasingly clear that NHBD livers are prone to ischemic-type biliary strictures, particularly those exposed to longer ischemia times. The Miami and the author's groups have shown that LTX can be safely performed using older, controlled NHBDs,[1,18] although others advise against this.[16,17] Controlled NHBD LTX may be safely performed in the face of true warm ischemia time – the interval between significant (variably defined) hypotension or hypoxemia, and initiation of perfusion – up to and perhaps somewhat beyond 20 to 30 minutes. Total warm ischemia time – the interval between stopping of mechanical ventilation and initiation of perfusion – may extend up to and perhaps somewhat beyond 30 to 45 minutes.[1]

Results of controlled NHBD LTX reported by single centers experienced in this field are superior to the results provided by one group's analysis of the United Network of Organ Sharing (UNOS) database, grouping together controlled and uncontrolled NHBD LTXs in the United States.[20] Comparison of 144 NHBD and 26,856 heart-beating donor LTXs reveals 1-year patient and graft survival rates that are lower for the NHBD cohort (80% vs. 85% and 70% vs. 80%, respectively), although the difference is not significant when comparing controlled NHBD grafts to heart-beating donor grafts. The NHBD LTX recipients required retransplantation more frequently (14% vs. 8%) and had more primary nonfunction (12% vs. 6%). Early retransplantation after NHBD LTX was more likely with donors over age 60, cold ischemia times longer than 8 hours, and recipients on life support prior to transplantation.

c) Author's Experience

At the Albert Einstein Medical Center in Philadelphia, we recently provided long-term outcomes for 22 controlled NHBD LTXs performed at our institution through 2002.[1] To date, we have performed 30 controlled NHBD LTXs using grafts procured by our team. Controlled NHBDs have provided for 7% of all LTXs (30/442) that we performed over the past 9 years. Causes of neurologic injury were trauma ($n = 14$), cerebral vascular accident ($n = 8$), and anoxia ($n = 8$). One third of the donors (10/30) were more than 50 years old; donor age ranged from 11 to 66 years. The interval between development of significant hypotension, defined as a drop in mean arterial pressure below 50 mm Hg, and the initiation of perfusion, was less than 26 minutes in all cases. The longest interval between stopping of mechanical ventilation and initiation of perfusion was 35 minutes. All donors arrested within 27 minutes of discontinuing ventilation. Perfusion was always initiated within 2 to 6 minutes of incision. Mean follow-up for the group is 39 months. Patient and graft survival rates for the 30 NHBD LTXs are the same, and comparison with the survival curves for heart-beating deceased donor LTXs that we performed during the same time period reveals no significant differences. Both patient and graft survival rates at 1 and 2 years post–NHBD LTX are 90% and 85%, respectively.

Of the nine deaths thus far, one or perhaps two are primarily related to the allografts coming from NHBDs; one patient succumbed to severe primary nonfunction and another patient to ischemic type biliary strictures. The latter patient also had severe median arcuate ligament syndrome, which very likely caused profound biliary ischemia.[15] In addition to the one primary nonfunction mentioned above (3%), there was one instance of reperfusion syndrome and another instance of poor early graft function that resolved within days. There was no case of early hepatic artery thrombosis. Ischemic type biliary strictures developed in four patients (13%); one resolved with percutaneous drainage, one succumbed as mentioned above, and two will likely require retransplantation. Notably, a significant number of the recipients developed transaminitis [mean peak alanine aminotransferase (ALT) was 1119 IU] and/or cholestasis (mean peak total bilirubin was 8 mg/dL), but in all cases the ALT quickly normalized and hyperbilirubinemia peaked within 3 weeks post-LTX and then completely resolved. Although we do not generally use T-tubes, it is our practice to place them in NHBD liver recipients to facilitate evaluation of cholestasis, should it occur.

Preoperative Maneuvers and Operative Strategy for Non–Heart-Beating Donor Organ Procurement

a) Uncontrolled Non–Heart-Beating Donors

Various postmortem measures have been used to increase the yield of transplantable organs from uncontrolled NHBDs, including cardiopulmonary resuscitation (CPR), perfusion of preservation solution using femoral vessel cannulation, and core cooling via peritoneal catheterization prior to organ retrieval.[11,19] Some protocols involve nonconsensual measures, such as CPR and cardiopulmonary bypass, and are therefore potentially ethically problematic, even though organ procurement is aborted if consent for donation is not obtained. Madrid, Spain, has an established uncontrolled NHBD organ procurement program that is based on such nonconsensual initial measures.[19]

b) Controlled Non–Heart-Beating Donors

Potential controlled NHBDs are identified by referral of dying patients to the OPO. Non–heart-beating donor management should be consistent with ethically sound protocols. In our OPO, heparin (but not phentolamine) is administered to the donor,[21] as is done by the Pittsburgh group[4]; the Madison group administers both agents.[5] Communication between the NHBD surgeon and the operating room nursing staff about conduct of the operation prior to withdrawal of support facilitates cooperation and speediness of the recovery. Upon withdrawal of support a preprinted flow sheet (see example in Figure 1.40) should be filled out by a coordinator in the operating room, documenting hemodynamic measurements every minute and the times of discontinuation of mechanical ventilation, declaration, waiting period, incision, and perfusion. After the procurement, careful assessment of the information on the flow sheet is critical for appraising the ischemic injury.

When deciding on whether to transplant a procured liver, there needs to be great emphasis on assessing the various ischemia time intervals. We particularly care about the interval between development of significant hypotension and perfusion. With all livers that we have decided to use thus far, this interval has been less than 26 minutes and no other group has routinely used NHBD livers exposed to longer true warm ischemia times; the safe limit remains unknown. If the patient remains alive 60 minutes after withdrawal of support, then organ procurement is aborted and the patient is returned to a ward for continued comfort care; in the rare instances that this occurred in our OPO, the patient always expired within the next few hours.

c) Surgical Technique

1. Most surgeons who procure NHBD organs use some modification of the super-rapid technique described by the Pittsburgh group.[4,14,17,18,22] The donor surgery should be performed by a surgeon who is experienced in rapid procurement from controlled

Patient Name _____								UNOS# _____										
OPERATING ROOM NON-HEARTBEATING ORGAN DONOR FLOW SHEET																			
INTRAOPERATIVE MANAGEMENT																			

Blood Drawn   Date _____/_____/_____   Time _____:_____   (EST)
Heparin Administered   Date _____/_____/_____   Time _____:_____   (EST)
Entered OR   Date _____/_____/_____   Time _____:_____   (EST)
Withdrawal of Support   Date _____/_____/_____   Time _____:_____   (EST)
Pronouncement   Date _____/_____/_____   Time _____:_____   (EST)
Incision   Date _____/_____/_____   Time _____:_____   (EST)
Cross-Clamp   Date _____/_____/_____   Time _____:_____   (EST)

Time From Withdrawal to Pronouncement _____ minutes
Time From Pronouncement to Cross-Clamp _____ minutes
Total Warm Ischemic Time (withdrawal to cross-clamp) _____ minutes
Flush Solution _____   1st Liter in @ ____:____   Total Flush _____ cc
Family Present for Withdrawal   ☐ Yes ☐ No   Location of Withdrawal   ☐ OR ☐ ICU ☐ PACU ☐ Other _____
Care and Comfort Administered   ☐ Yes ☐ No   Was Patient Extubated   ☐ Yes ☐ No

START TIME _____ : _____							**HEMODYNAMIC MEASUREMENTS**												
	Min 1	Min 2	Min 3	Min 4	Min 5	Min 6	Min 7	Min 8	Min 9	Min 10	Min 11	Min 12	Min 13	Min 14	Min 15	Min 16	Min 17	Min 18	Min 19	Min 20
HR																				
BP																				
RR																				
SPO2																				
	Min 21	Min 22	Min 23	Min 24	Min 25	Min 26	Min 27	Min 28	Min 29	Min 30	Min 31	Min 32	Min 33	Min 34	Min 35	Min 36	Min 37	Min 38	Min 39	Min 40
HR																				
BP																				
RR																				
SPO2																				

Figure 1.40

NHBDs. Ideally, patients undergo withdrawal of support in the operating room. Otherwise, transporting the NHBD to the operating room after declaration of death may exclude subsequent LTX because of excessive hepatic ischemia. To minimize operating and ischemic times, the potential donor should be prepared and draped prior to withdrawal of support. Instruments required for rapid entry and aortic cannulation should be chosen, including a scalpel, a pair of Kocher clamps, a moist towel, Metzenbaum scissors, a right-angle clamp, a moist umbilical tape, two Kelly clamps, a sternal saw, and abdominal and sternal retractors (Figure 1.41). As well, the cannula and tubing should be flushed and placed on the field, maintaining the containers of preservation solution in an ice bucket to prevent warming.

2. Following the above preparatory maneuvers the surgical team should exit the operating room and wait until potential procurement, to avoid conflict of interest during withdrawal of support and declaration of death. Postmortem, a midline laparotomy is performed. Upward traction on two Kocher clamps placed on each side of the umbilicus expedites rapid entry without injury to the viscera. A large scalpel is used to incise all layers of the abdominal wall.

3. A moist towel is used to retract the small intestine to the right while the sigmoid colon is retracted to the left. Although not pulsatile, the aorta is easily palpated just above its bifurcation on the left side of the vertebral column. Metzenbaum scissors are used to clear the retroperitoneum over a small segment of distal aorta in preparation for cannulation. There is no need to dissect out the inferior mesenteric artery. A right-angle clamp is used to pass a moist umbilical tape around the distal aorta, which will be used to secure the cannula. Distally, the aorta is clamped with a Kelly clamp. Next, the cannula

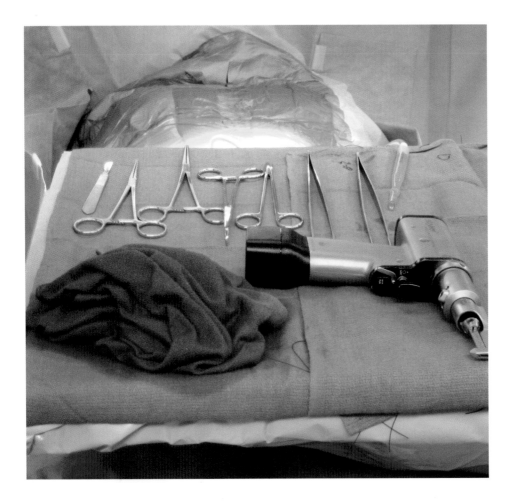

Figure 1.41

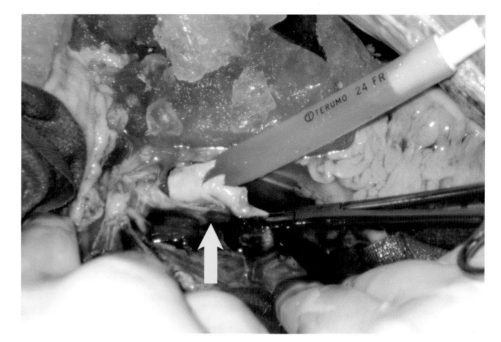

Figure 1.42

is passed cephalad through an aortotomy (Figure 1.42, yellow arrow) and secured with the umbilical tape. The flush should be started immediately at this point, without waiting to cross-clamp the proximal aorta or vent the vena cava. Using this approach, flush is typically initiated within 2 to 3 minutes of declaration of death.

4. The surgeon should not be disturbed to see a dark, purple, and somewhat engorged liver at initial inspection, as this is the typical appearance of a NHBD liver. Assessment of liver quality is best left until after perfusion, at which point the liver should appear normal. There should be a low threshold for obtaining a NHBD liver biopsy to exclude extensive centrilobular necrosis and other confounding risk factors for poor graft function, such as steatosis. Next, the round and falciform ligaments are divided sharply. The knife is used to open from the suprasternal notch to the abdomen. Median sternotomy is performed with a pneumatic saw and a Finochietto sternal retractor is placed. It is this author's preference to clamp the thoracic rather than supraceliac aorta during super-rapid procurement. The descending thoracic aorta can be easily accessed through the left thoracic cavity just above the diaphragm. The vena cava is vented above the diaphragm. A Balfour retractor is placed across the upper abdomen. Ice slush should be placed on the abdominal organs simultaneously with the sternotomy. The author infuses approximately 5 L of cold University of Wisconsin (UW) solution, containing dexamethasone 16 mg/L and insulin 40 U/L; through the adult NHBD aorta to provide a clear effluent, typically 1 L before sternotomy, cross-clamping, and venting, and then 4 L afterward. Approximately twice this volume is necessary when using HTK solution.

Liver Procurement

5. Since all the visceral dissection is performed in the cold, without blood flow and without having had opportunity to assess pulses, particular care must be taken not to damage vital structures. The hepatoduodenal ligament is divided from right to left as close to the duodenum as possible, taking care to preserve the hepatic artery. First, the common bile duct is divided and the biliary tree flushed with chilled preservation solution through an opening in the gallbladder and through the common duct directly. This maneuver is important, given concern about ischemic-type biliary strictures following NHBD LTX. The portal vein is divided at the confluence of the superior mesenteric and splenic veins. The gastroduodenal and right gastric arteries need not be clearly delineated.

6. The left lateral segment of the liver is elevated by dividing the left triangular ligament. It is safest to assume that there is a replaced or accessory left hepatic artery arising from the left gastric artery. Therefore, the lesser omentum and left gastric artery should be separated from the lesser curvature at the level of the stomach. The splenic artery is divided to the left of the midline, far from the celiac axis, and then dissected toward the aorta, so that it can be rotated to the right for exposure of the superior mesenteric artery, which lies deep to it. Unless the plan is to procure the NHBD pancreas, discussed below, the head of the pancreas should be taken with the liver to avoid transecting an aberrant right hepatic artery and to expedite organ extraction time. After a Kocher's maneuver, the duodenum and pancreatic head are elevated and retracted caudally to expose the superior mesenteric artery which is then dissected down to the aorta. Care is taken not to transect an accessory or replaced right hepatic artery by avoiding dissection on the right side of the superior mesenteric artery. Rather than taking extra time to search for a right branch, it is safest to assume that one exists and to take a common patch of superior mesenteric and celiac arteries with the liver. An aortotomy is performed between the superior mesenteric and right renal arteries and extended to provide the arterial patch.

7. The left diaphragm is then divided down toward the Carrel patch. The suprahepatic inferior vena cava is divided. The right diaphragm is then divided down to the upper pole of the right kidney. The infrahepatic inferior vena cava is then transected just above the renal veins. The liver is extricated and immediate back-table portal flush with 1 L of chilled UW solution is performed. The liver is then packaged for transport to the transplant center.

Kidney Procurement

8. Bilateral nephrectomies are then performed. The kidneys may be kept en bloc for machine perfusion, or separated and sent directly to the recipient centers. Even though NHBD organ procurement is a rushed procedure, it is still crucial to perform complete donor exploration in an effort to discern the possibility of unrecognized malignancy. It is also particularly important with NHBD grafts to perform back-table graft inspection and trimming well in advance of the recipient surgery, to ensure that it is safe to transplant the organ(s) and to allow adequate time for arterial reconstruction, if necessary.

Pancreas Procurement

9. Adding whole-organ pancreatectomy to hepatectomy during a super-rapid recovery carries risk for transecting an aberrant right hepatic artery because there is no opportunity to palpate arterial pulsations in the NHBD. Meticulous in situ dissection in search of a right branch can significantly increase extraction time. Therefore, the NHBD liver is typically removed with the pancreatic head to avoid injuring an aberrant right hepatic artery. We do not routinely procure NHBD whole pancreata when procuring NHBD livers unless there is favorable donor body habitus and other issues are optimal, such as warm ischemia time.[23] Alternatively, the liver and pancreas may be removed en bloc.

d) Premortem Cannulation Technique

The group at Madison, Wisconsin, performs consensual, preextubation (premortem) femoral vessel cannulation.[5] The NHBDs are typically taken to the operating room before withdrawal of life support. Right femoral artery and right femoral vein cannulae are inserted under local anesthesia. After cessation of respiration, lack of a monitored arterial pulse, declaration of death, and an additional wait time of 5 minutes, cold UW solution is infused into the femoral artery cannula. The femoral vein cannula is opened to gravity to decompress the venous system. Median sternotomy and midline abdominal incisions are made and the intraabdominal organs are removed en bloc or separately. Portal flush and organ separation are performed on the back table.

Ethical Issues and Professionalism

Certainly, NHBD organ procurement honors the donor's wishes, brings some comfort to the family, and benefits the recipient. It is appropriate to provide a brief overview of the ethics of NHBD organ procurement and transplantation because surgeons must be familiar with the following basic principles before working with NHBDs: individuals may not be killed for their organs or killed as a result of the removal of their organs (the "dead donor" rule), patients must not be jeopardized in order to facilitate organ procurement, euthanasia is prohibited, informed consent and respect for family wishes must not be violated, and the autonomous right of patients to refuse treatment must be upheld.[3,11,24-29] It is imperative to ensure that there is no conflict of interest between the duty to provide optimal patient care and the desire to recover organs for transplantation.[26,27,29] Specifically, the rationale for withdrawal of life support and the determination of death must be extricable from the decision to recover organs. Therefore, the patient care and organ donor teams need to be completely separate.

Several issues related to the ethics of NHBD organ procurement remain sources of debate. Interventions that improve the chance of successful donation rather than directly benefiting the donor are permitted, as long as they are consensual and do not hasten death or harm the donor, and medications routinely provided for patient comfort are permitted even if they might hasten death.[28] However, there are differing views regarding use of anticoagulants, vasodilators, narcotics, and intravascular cannulae placed premortem.[27] Another issue that is debated is whether determination of NHBD death requires loss of cardiac electrical activity or if absence of heart sounds, pulse, and blood pressure are sufficient criteria, just as they are for patients who are not organ donors.[3,11] Ultimately, the donor hospital and care team have the responsibility for defining and declaring patient death. Another important ethical question that impacts upon the warm ischemic time endured by NHBD organs relates to the duration of the waiting period used to assure irreversible death. Autoresuscitation after 1 minute of pulselessness has not been reported in the literature.[26] However, different wait times from the determination of death to organ procurement have been prescribed by various groups, ranging from 2 to 10 minutes[11,25-28]; most groups wait 5 minutes.

Conclusion

Ideally, patients who are brain dead, or will likely soon become so, should donate organs according to brain death protocols because the yield of transplantable organs from NHBDs and outcomes of NHBD organ transplantation are generally not as favorable as with heart-beating donors. Nonetheless, NHBD organ transplantation has become highly successful, bringing full circle the history of organ donation. The surge in enthusiasm about NHBDs has been fueled by several important organizations, including the Department of Health and Human Services of the United States federal government, the Institute of Medicine (IOM) of the National Academy of Science, UNOS, and various professional societies such as the Society of Critical Care Medicine.[6,11,24,28] These groups have endorsed NHBD organ procurement as an ethically effective solution for the organ shortage, have recommended standardized NHBD protocols, and have arranged significant funding for education and research about NHBD organ transplantation. Discovery of effective cytoprotective agents that could be administered to NHBDs and/or NHBD organ recipients to protect against ischemic organ injury would further expand the ability to transplant NHBD organs. Surgeons who recover organs from NHBDs must be familiar with rapid procurement techniques, as described above.

Standard Multiorgan Procurement: Selected Readings

Abu-Elmagd K, Fung J, Bueno J, et al. Logistics and technique for procurement of intestinal, pancreatic, and hepatic grafts from the same donor. Ann Surg 2000;232(5):680–687.

Boggi U, Vistoli F, Del Chiaro M, et al. A simplified technique for the en bloc procurement of abdominal organs that is suitable for pancreas and small-bowel transplantation. Surgery 2004;135(6):629–641.

D'Alessandro AM, Southard JH, Love RB, Belzer FO. Organ preservation. Surg Clin North Am 1994;74(5): 1083–1095.

Delgado DH, Rao V, Ross HJ. Donor management in cardiac transplantation. Can J Cardiol 2002;18(11): 1217–1223.

Dunn DL, Morel P, Schlumpf R, et al. Evidence that combined procurement of pancreas and liver grafts does not affect transplant outcome. Transplantation 1991;51(1):150–157.

Kootstra G, Kievit J, Nederstigt A. Organ donors: heartbeating and non-heartbeating. World J Surg 2002;26(2): 181–184.

Ojo AO, Heinrichs D, Emond JC, et al. Organ donation and utilization in the USA. Am J Transplant 2004;4(suppl 9):27–37.

St. Peter SD, Imber CJ, Friend PJ. Liver and kidney preservation by perfusion. Lancet 2002;16;359(9306): 604–613.

Starzl TE, Miller C, Broznick B, Makowka L. An improved technique for multiple organ harvesting. Surg Gynecol Obstet 1987;165(4):343–348.

Van Buren CT, Barakat O. Organ donation and retrieval. Surg Clin North Am 1994;74(5):1055–1081.

Van der Werf WJ, D'Alessandro AM, Hoffmann RM, Knechtle SJ. Procurement, preservation, and transport of cadaver kidneys. Surg Clin North Am 1998;78(1):41–54.

Non–Heart-Beating Donor: References

1. Reich DJ, Manzarbeitia CY. Non-heart-beating donor liver transplantation. In: Busuttil RW, Klintmalm GB, eds. Transplantation of the Liver. Philadelphia: WB Saunders, 2005:529–543.

2. A definition of irreversible coma: report of the Ad Hoc Committee of the Harvard Medical School to Examine the Definition of Brain Death. JAMA 1968;205:337–340.

3. DeVita MA, Vukmir R, Snyder JV, et al. Procuring organs from a non-heart-beating cadaver: a case report. Kennedy Institute of Ethics Journal 1993;3:371–385.

4. Casavilla A, Ramirez C, Shapiro R, et al. Experience with liver and kidney allografts from non-heart-beating donors. Transplantation 1995;59:197–203.

5. D'Alessandro AM, Hoffmann RM, Knechtle SJ, et al. Successful extrarenal transplantation from non-heart-beating donors. Transplantation 1995;59:977–982.

6. United Network of Organ Sharing. Donation After Cardiac Death: A Reference Guide. Richmond, VA: UNOS, 2004.

7. Edwards JM, Hasz RD, Robertson VM. Non-heart-beating organ donation: process and review. AACN Clinical Issues 1999;10:293–300.

8. Koogler T, Costarino AT Jr. The potential benefits of the pediatric nonheartbeating organ donor. Pediatrics 1998;101:1049–1052.

9. Gift of Life Donor Program. 2003 Annual Report. Philadelphia: Gift of Life Donor Program, Inc., 2004.

10. Reiner M, Cornell D, Howard RJ. Development of a successful non-heart-beating organ donation program. Prog Transplant 2003;13:225–231.

11. Institute of Medicine, National Academy of Sciences. Non-Heart-Beating Organ Transplantation: Practice and Protocols. Washington, DC: National Academy Press, 2000.

12. Rudich SM, Kaplan B, Magee JC, et al. Renal transplantations performed using non-heart-beating organ donors: going back to the future. Transplantation 2002;74:1715–1720.

13. Cho YW, Terasaki PI, Cecka M, et al. Transplantation of kidneys from donors whose hearts have stopped beating. N Engl J Med 1998;338:221–225.

14. Reich DJ, Munoz SJ, Rothstein KD, et al. Controlled non-heart-beating donor liver transplantation: a successful single center experience, with topic update. Transplantation 2000;70:1159–1166.

15. Manzarbeitia CY, Ortiz JA, Jeon H, et al. Long-term outcome of controlled non-heartbeating donor liver transplantation. Transplantation 2004;78:211–215.

16. D'Alessandro AM, Hoffmann RM, Knechtle SJ, et al. Liver transplantation from controlled non-heart-beating donors. Surgery 2000;128:579–588.

17. Abt PL, Crawford MD, Desai NM, et al. Liver transplantation from controlled and uncontrolled non-heart-beating donors: an increased incidence of biliary complications. Transplantation 2003;75:1659–1663.

18. Fukumori T, Kato T, Levi D, et al. Use of older controlled non-heart-beating donors for liver transplantation. Transplantation 2003;75:1171–1174.

19. Otero A, Gomez-Gutierrez M, Suarez F, et al. Liver transplantation from Maastricht category 2 non-heart-beating donors. Transplantation 2003;76:1068–1073.

20. Abt PL, Desai NM, Crawford MD, et al. Survival following liver transplantation from non-heart-beating donors. Ann Surg 2004;239:87–92.

21. Gift of Life Donor Program. Asystolic Cadaveric Organ Recovery Procedures Following Patient and/or Family Directed Withdrawal of Life Support. Philadelphia: Gift of Life Donor Program, Inc., 1998.

22. Olson L, Davi R, Barnhart J, et al. Non-heart-beating cadaver donor hepatectomy "the operative procedure". Clin Transplantation 1999;13:98–103.

23. Jeon H, Ortiz JA, Manzarbeitia CY, et al. Combined liver and pancreas procurement from a controlled non-heart-beating donor with aberrant hepatic arterial anatomy. Transplantation 2002;74:1636–1639.

24. Institute of Medicine, National Academy of Sciences. Non-Heart-Beating Organ Transplantation: Medical and Ethical Issues in Procurement. Washington, DC: National Academy Press, 1997.

25. Koostra G. The asystolic, or non-heartbeating, donor. Transplantation 1997;63:917–921.

26. Whetstine L, Bowman K, Hawryluck L. Pro/con ethics debate: is nonheart-beating organ donation ethically acceptable? Critical Care 2000;6:192–195.

27. Bell MD. Non-heart beating organ donation: old procurement strategy – new ethical problems. J Med Ethics 2003;29:176–181.

28. Recommendations for nonheartbeating organ donation. A position paper by the Ethics Committee, American College of Critical Care Medicine, Society of Critical Care Medicine. Crit Care Med 2002; 29:1826–1831.

29. Arnold RM, Younger SJ. Time is of the essence: the pressing need for comprehensive non-heart-beating cadaveric donation policies. Transplant Proc 1995;27:2913–2921.

Dialysis Access Procedures

Khalid O. Khwaja

Hemodialysis

Introduction

Hemodialysis is one of the main modalities for renal replacement therapy in patients with end-stage renal disease. Successful hemodialysis is contingent upon the creation of proper vascular access. Chronic vascular access was first established in 1960 by Scribner and colleagues when they created a shunt between the radial artery and the cephalic vein using an external Silastic device. However, this device was fraught with problems such as bleeding, clotting, and infection. In 1966, Breschia and Cimino described a surgical fistula between the radial artery and the cephalic vein just proximal to the wrist, thereby eliminating the external shunt and enabling a high flow system for hemodialysis. To this day, it remains the procedure of choice for patients with end-stage renal disease in need of chronic hemodialysis.

Several principles should be followed when planning vascular access surgery. In general, primary fistulas are better than prosthetic grafts due to better long-term patency and lower risk of infection and thrombosis. The upper extremity is preferable to the lower extremity and the nondominant arm should be employed first. If possible, a distal site should be selected first, preserving the upper arm for subsequent use. Careful preoperative vascular assessment is performed with palpation of the radial, ulnar, and brachial pulses; an Allen's test is performed on both sides. The superficial veins of the arm should be carefully assessed with application of a proximal tourniquet. In some cases, the cephalic vein is readily evident at the wrist, antecubital fossa area, or in the lateral aspect of the upper arm. Once a decision has been made to perform access surgery, no venipunctures or blood pressure monitoring should be performed in that arm. If no superficial veins are apparent, the venous system may be assessed by ultrasound examination of the arm. Both the cephalic and basilic systems are interrogated, as well as the deep venous system and the central veins. Patients with suspected central venous stenosis or prior catheters inserted on the ipsilateral side, or with abnormal findings on ultrasound, may be assessed by conventional venography. If central stenoses are found, they should be corrected by endovascular techniques preoperatively, or an alternate site for access should be sought.

Vascular access should be established prior to the actual need for hemodialysis, thereby avoiding temporary external catheters, which have a higher risk of infection and are also associated with central venous stenosis. This chapter discusses the technique for some common permanent access procedures.

Surgical Procedures

a) Radiocephalic Fistula

The radiocephalic fistula, as described by Breschia and Cimino, is the procedure of choice. A suitable cephalic vein just proximal to the wrist is identified preoperatively and a negative Allen's test confirmed. Although up to a third of these fistulas fail to mature, the long-term patency is excellent with as many as half of them still functioning 5 to 10 years after creation.

1. The whole arm, including the axilla, is prepped and draped. As no prosthetic device is being employed, antibiotics are not a requisite. A vertical incision is fashioned just proximal to the flexion crease of the wrist between the radial artery and the cephalic vein (black arrow). Some surgeons prefer to make an incision over the anatomic snuff box more distally and use the deep branch of the radial artery to create the fistula (grey arrow) (Figure 2.1).

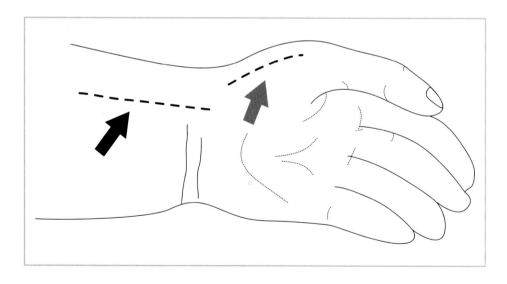

Figure 2.1

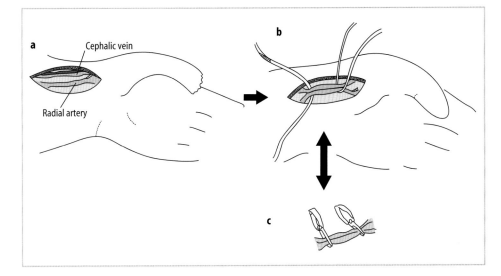

Figure 2.2

2. The incision is carried through the subcutaneous tissue, and then medial and lateral flaps are raised. Both the cephalic vein and radial artery are very superficially located and can readily be exposed (Figure 2.2a). The cephalic vein is mobilized as far proximally and distally as possible and any large branches ligated. The radial artery is also mobilized for a short distance. Once mobilization is complete, both the cephalic vein and radial artery are placed adjacent to each other in a side-by-side fashion. This can be accomplished by placing a vessel loop proximally and distally, with each loop incorporating the artery and vein. By tightening up on the loop, the two vessels are brought together (Figure 2.2b). If necessary, systemic heparin can now be administered. Control of the vessels can be achieved by tightening up on the vessel loops or by using small vascular clamps (Figure 2.2c).

3. A corresponding venotomy and arteriotomy are made in the cephalic vein and radial artery (Figure 2.3a). The arteriotomy should be limited to 6 or 7 mm to prevent a

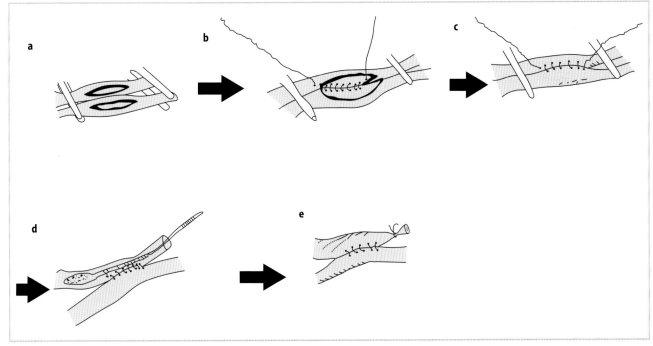

Figure 2.3

steal syndrome. A side-to-side anastomosis is then constructed using fine, nonabsorbable monofilament suture (Figures 2.3b and 2.3c). One technique is to sew the posterior wall from within the lumen, then running the suture anteriorly to complete the anastomosis. Prior to reperfusion, the anastomosis can be probed through an opening created in the distal cephalic vein (Figure 2.3d). The probe is passed sequentially up the cephalic vein and the radial artery. The distal cephalic vein is then ligated and the arterial clamps released to perfuse the fistula (Figure 2.3e).

4. Alternatively, an end-to-side or end-to-end anastomoses between the radial artery and cephalic vein can be created by dividing the vein initially (Figure 2.4a) and then anastomosing it to the artery (Figure 2.4b).

A radiocephalic fistula usually requires 8 to 12 weeks to mature. Sometimes a second procedure is required to ligate a side branch or angioplasty an area of proximal stenosis.

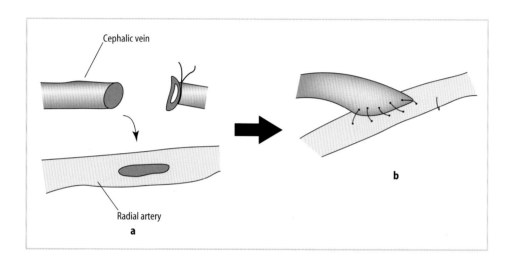

Figure 2.4

b) Brachiocephalic Fistula

If a suitable cephalic vein at the wrist is not present, then a more proximal brachiocephalic fistula may be created. In some instances, the cephalic vein might be deep in the upper arm and not clinically visible. If it is seen on ultrasound examination and has a diameter of 3 mm or more, then it may be suitable for fistula creation. Brachiocephalic fistulas have a primary failure rate of close to 10% and good long-term patency.

1. A preoperative evaluation is performed as described for the radiocephalic fistula. The whole arm is prepped from the wrist to the axilla. This procedure can be performed under local anesthetic with sedation. The elbow is examined to mark the course of the cephalic vein (red arrow) and palpated to locate the position of the brachial artery (broken red line), which lies adjacent to the basilic vein (yellow arrow) (Figure 2.5).

2. Both the brachial artery and cephalic vein can be isolated through a transverse incision either above (Figure 2.6a) or below (Figure 2.6b) the antecubital crease. The cephalic vein may require some mobilization to reach the brachial artery and may need to be dissected distally to the upper part of the forearm to gain adequate length for it to reach the artery. Frequently, an antecubital or median cubital vein (blue arrow) can be found that communicates with the cephalic vein, and this vein can be used for the

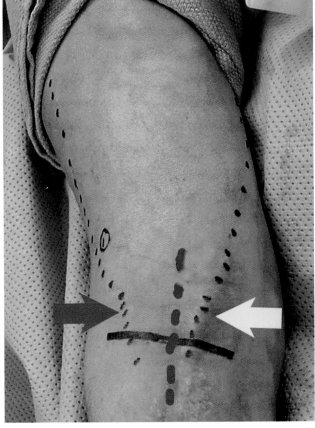

Figure 2.5

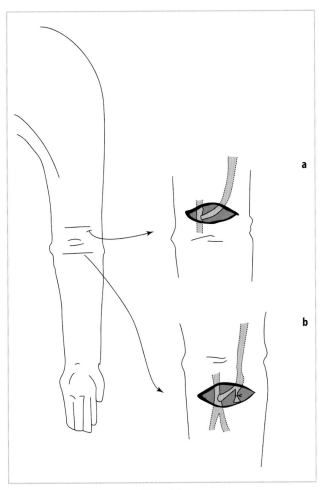

Figure 2.6

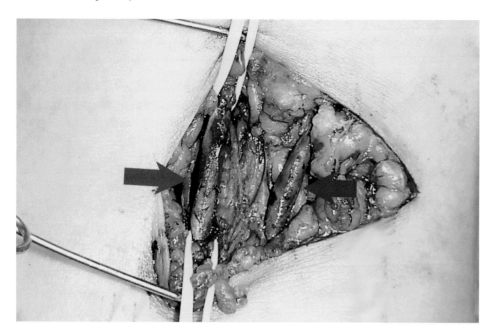

Figure 2.7

anastomosis with the distal cephalic vein being ligated (Figure 2.6b). It usually easily reaches the brachial artery (red arrow) (Figure 2.7)

3. Once an adequate length of vein is dissected free, it is divided. An end-to-side anastomosis is then constructed using fine, nonabsorbable monofilament suture (Figure 2.8). If the cephalic vein is found to be unsuitable, then the basilic vein can be used through the same approach and transposed so it runs in a more superficial course (described next). If none of these veins is suitable, a loop forearm graft can be created through the same incision. A primary brachiocephalic fistula matures in 8 to 12 weeks.

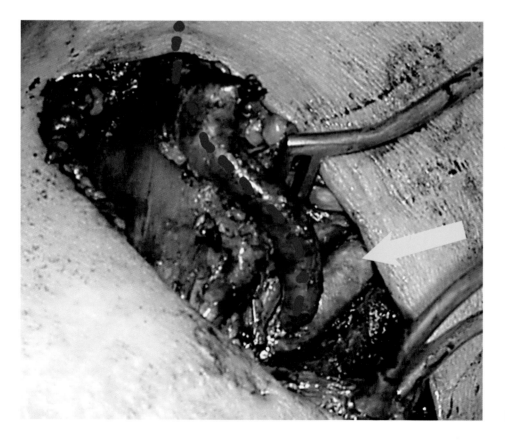

Figure 2.8

4. Sometimes the cephalic vein at the level of the elbow and above is of adequate size, but too deep to simply anastomose directly to the brachial artery. If the vein is deep, it may be difficult to cannulate for subsequent dialysis. In this case the vein can be dissected for some length above the elbow, and then brought through a tunnel created just below the skin to transpose the vein to a more superficial location. This is done by first isolating the vein either just above or below the antecubital fossa and then dissecting it further proximally as much as possible through the transverse incision. The vein is divided as far distally as possible. A longitudinal counterincision is then made higher in the arm and the same vein is isolated and mobilized into this incision (Figure 2.9). At this point it is helpful to gently dilate the vein (large blue arrow) with saline solution to ensure that there is no twisting. The vein can be marked with a pen to maintain this orientation. One is now ready to create the superficial tunnel for the vein (small blue arrows).

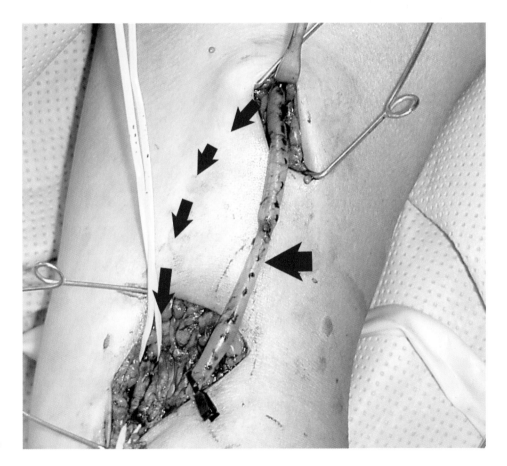

Figure 2.9

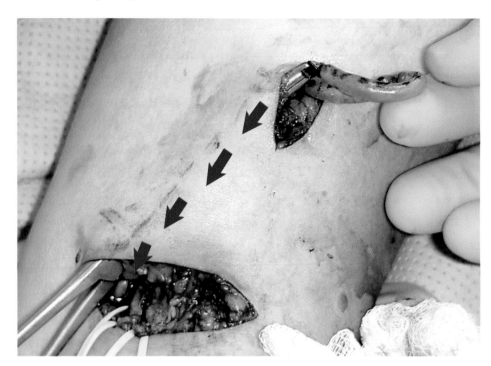

Figure 2.10

5. A subcutaneous tunnel is created for the vein using a tunneler or other blunt instrument (Figure 2.10). The tunnel should start just above the brachial artery and end at the proximal extent of the upper arm incision.

6. The cephalic vein is brought through the tunnel, making sure that the vein does not twist as it is being pulled through. The end of the vein (blue arrow) is positioned just above the brachial artery (yellow arrow), in preparation for the anastomosis (Figure 2.11).

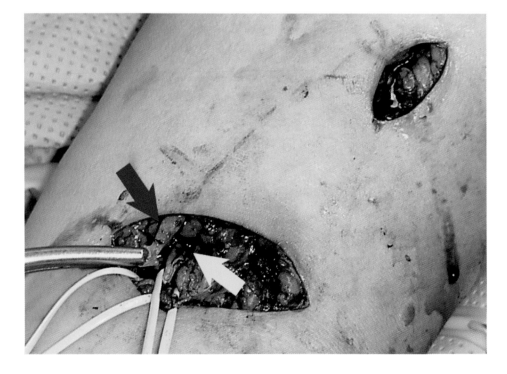

Figure 2.11

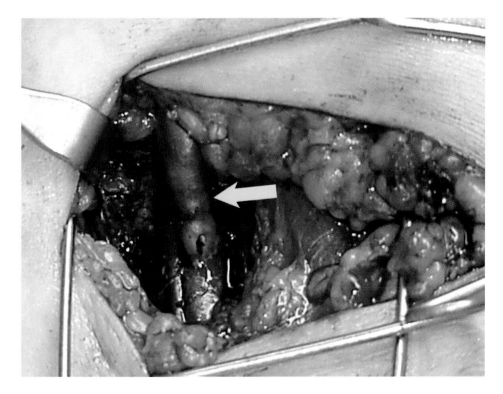

Figure 2.12

7. An end-to-side anastomosis (yellow arrow) is created between the cephalic vein and the brachial artery (Figure 2.12).

8. The arterialized vein is then inspected carefully through both incisions (blue and yellow arrows) to ensure that there is no twisting of the vein and to document that there is good flow (Figure 2.13).

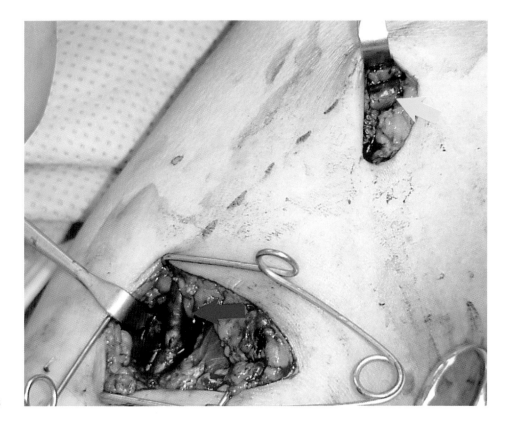

Figure 2.13

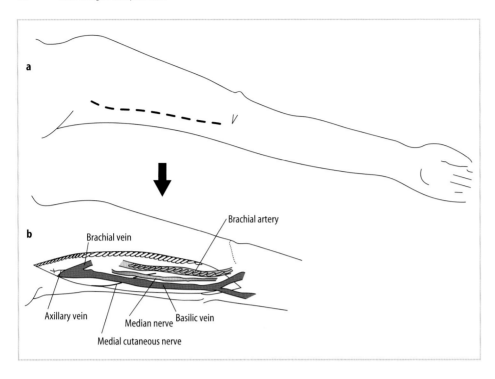

Figure 2.14

c) Basilic Vein Transposition

As the basilic vein in the upper arm runs deep to the fascia, it is protected from trauma related to venepuncture. It may be transposed to a more superficial location for dialysis access. This is a suitable option when the cephalic vein is inadequate for fistula creation. The primary patency for this fistula is about 60% to 70% and the long-term patency is similar to that of a graft.

1. The procedure can be performed with a general anesthetic or local anesthetic with sedation, though the former is preferred due to the extensive dissection involved. The whole arm is prepped, including the axilla. The incision is begun at the antecubital crease in a vertical fashion just medial to the brachial artery pulse (Figure 2.14a). The incision is carried through the subcutaneous tissue; the fascia is incised and the brachial artery exposed. The median nerve (Figure 2.15, green arrow) lies medial to the brachial artery (yellow arrow) at this location and should be identified and preserved (Figure 2.14b). Proceeding slightly more medial and still deep to the fascia, the basilic vein (blue arrow) is visualized and traced proximally, all the way to its junction with the axillary vein (Figure 2.15). At some point, usually in the proximal third of the arm, the medial

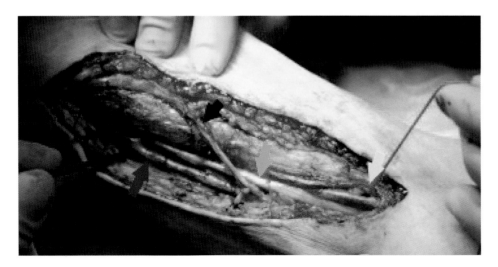

Figure 2.15

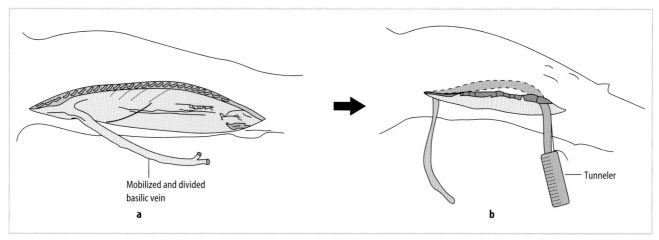

Mobilized and divided basilic vein

a

Tunneler

b

Figure 2.16

cutaneous nerve (black arrow) is encountered. This nerve usually crosses superficial to the basilic vein and, if injured, can result in numbness over the medial aspect of the arm.

2. Once the basilic vein is fully mobilized and all its branches ligated, it is divided as far distal in the arm as possible and brought superficial to the medial cutaneous nerve (Figure 2.16a). If there is adequate length, the vein can be tunneled in a more lateral, subcutaneous location (Figure 2.16b). Alternatively, a lateral flap can be created subcutaneously as a "pocket" for the vein.

3. Proximal and distal control of the brachial artery is obtained and the patient is given heparin. A 6- to 7-mm arteriotomy is then made and an end-to-side anastomosis between the basilic vein and the brachial artery is constructed using fine, nonabsorbable monofilament suture (Figure 2.17a). Clamps are then released and flow estab-

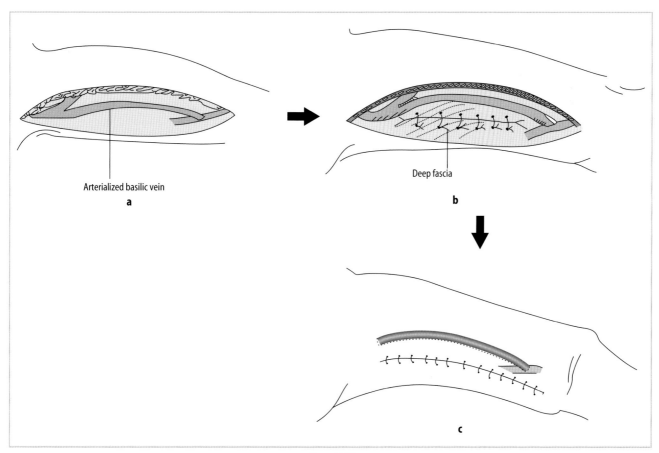

Arterialized basilic vein

a

Deep fascia

b

c

Figure 2.17

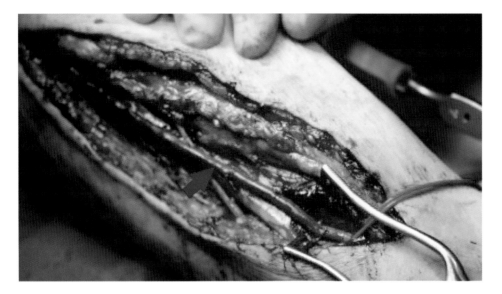

Figure 2.18

lished in the arterialized basilic vein (Figure 2.18). The deep fascia is then closed with interrupted, absorbable sutures, keeping the basilic vein superficial to the fascia (Figures 2.17b and 2.19). The basilic vein is positioned in the subcutaneous pocket, thereby relocating it in a more lateral and more superficial position (Figure 2.17c).

It generally takes about 12 weeks before the arterialized basilic vein is ready for cannulation. Some surgeons prefer a two-stage procedure for basilic vein transposition. At the first stage, the distal vein is anastomosed to the brachial artery without mobilization. The vein is then brought to a more superficial position several weeks later. The proponents of this approach feel that delayed mobilization results in less damage to the vessel wall and a better chance of maturation.

d) Forearm Loop Arteriovenous Graft

Arteriovenous (AV) grafts are reserved for patients who do not have a suitable vein for primary fistula creation. Most commonly employed grafts are made out of polytetrafluoroethylene (PTFE). The preoperative assessment is essentially the same as for fistulas. The primary patency of PTFE grafts is in the 70% to 80% range.

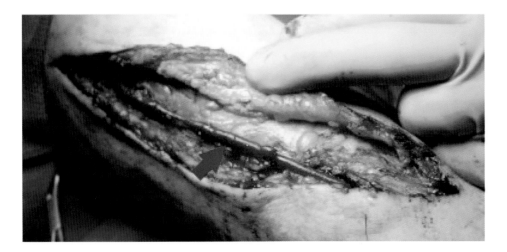

Figure 2.19

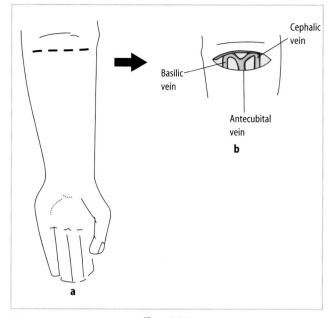

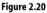

Figure 2.20

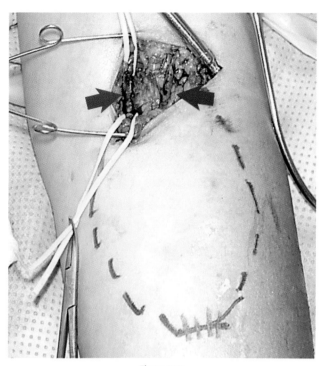

Figure 2.22

1. The procedure is usually performed under a local anesthetic with sedation. Pre-operative antibiotics are utilized. A transverse incision is fashioned below the antecubital crease (Figure 2.20a). The antecubital, cephalic, or basilic veins may be exposed in the subcutaneous layer (Figure 2.20b). Any one of these veins can be used for outflow. If these are not suitable, the graft can be drained into the deep brachial vein.

2. If a suitable superficial vein is identified, it is gently looped and preserved. The bicipital aponeurosis is then opened (Figure 2.21a). The brachial artery (red arrow), with its concomitant veins can be exposed deep to the aponeurosis (Figures 2.21b and 2.22). Care must be taken to avoid injury to the median nerve, which courses slightly deeper and medial to the artery.

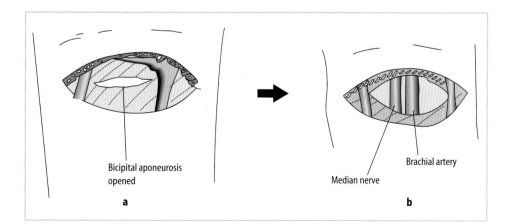

Figure 2.21

3. A tunnel in a loop configuration is then created. A counterincision is made in the middle of the arm, and a tunneling device is used to pass a PTFE graft, usually 6 mm in diameter, in a loop configuration (Figure 2.23).

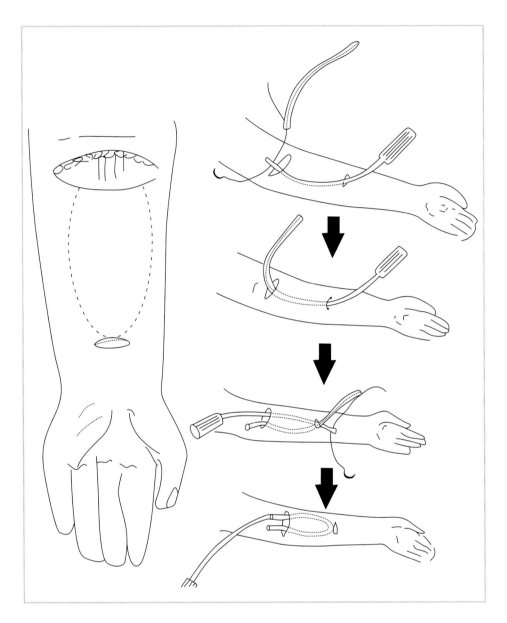

Figure 2.23

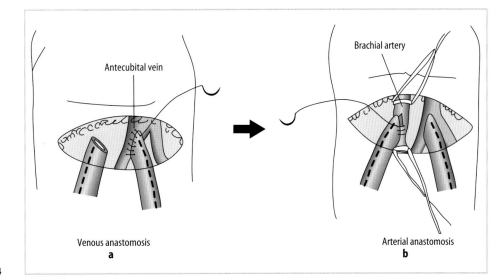

Antecubital vein

Brachial artery

Venous anastomosis
a

Arterial anastomosis
b

Figure 2.24

4. Once the graft has been tunneled, the patient can be heparinized. The arterial and venous anastomosis are performed, both in an end-to-side fashion. For the venous end, the graft can be cut at a bias to increase the diameter of the anastomosis and decrease the chances of venous stenosis (Figure 2.24a). For the arterial end, large anastomoses are avoided to decrease the chance of developing steal syndrome (Figure 2.24b).

5. The skin is closed over the completed anastomosis (Figure 2.25). It is unnecessary to close the deep fascia. The radial artery pulse is checked prior to completing the operation. Another option for a forearm graft is to place a straight graft with inflow from the radial artery at the wrist and outflow to one of the veins in the antecubital fossa.

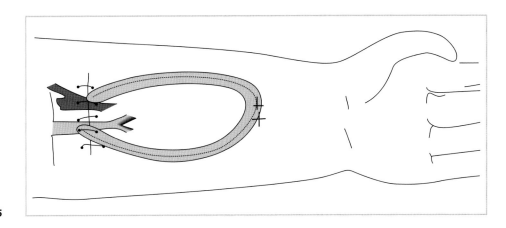

Figure 2.25

e) Upper Arm Arteriovenous Graft

An upper arm or brachial artery to axillary vein graft is possible in most patients, provided there is no central stenosis and no arterial disease. The early patency is excellent with a failure rate of only 0% to 3%. However, complications associated with the use of prosthetic material are inherent in this procedure, such as thrombosis and infection.

1. The preoperative assessment is as already described. The procedure is performed under local or general anesthesia. The whole arm including the axilla is prepped. The brachial artery can be exposed above the antecubital crease through a transverse incision. The axillary vein is usually exposed through a vertical or transverse incision made in the axilla (Figure 2.26a, c). The axillary incision is continued through the subcutaneous tissue and the fascia is opened. The axillary vein can be readily exposed or, alternatively, the brachial vein or basilic vein can be exposed more distally (Figure 2.26b). These two vessels coalesce to form the axillary vein. Any of these veins, depending on their caliber, may be used for outflow.

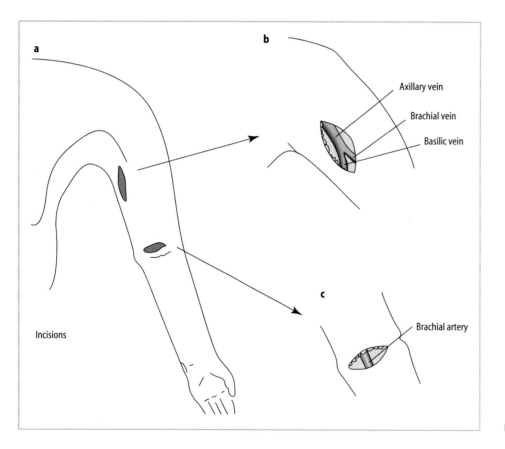

Figure 2.26

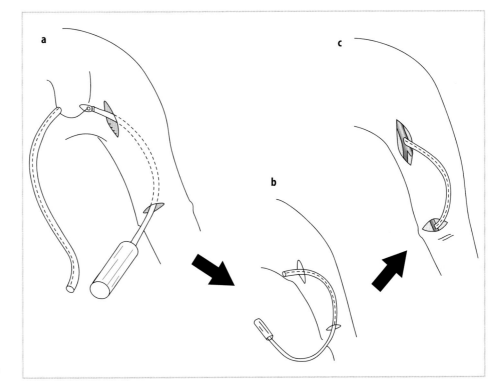

Figure 2.27

2. Using a tunneling device, a 6-mm PTFE graft is placed subcutaneously between the two incisions (Figure 2.27a, b). The graft should be directed lateral, as this is more comfortable for the patient during dialysis. Once the graft has been tunneled in its location, the patient may be heparinized. The venous end of the graft is cut at a bias to increase the diameter. An end-to-side anastomosis is then performed using a fine, monofilament, nonabsorbable suture. The arterial anastomosis is then made in a similar fashion, limiting the arteriotomy to 6 or 7 mm to avoid steal syndrome. The venous clamps are first released followed by the arterial clamps and flow in the graft established (Figure 2.27c).

f) Lower Extremity Access Procedure

Use of the lower extremity for permanent dialysis access should be limited to those situations in which all options involving the upper extremity have been exhausted or are not possible. These procedures unfortunately have a high risk of failure, poor long-term patency rates, high risk of infection, and poor tolerance by patients. Options include a primary arteriovenous fistula utilizing the saphenous vein as the conduit and the superficial femoral artery as the source of inflow. Alternatively, a prosthetic graft can be used with anastomosis to the femoral artery and saphenous vein.

1. For a primary arteriovenous fistula, the saphenous vein is completely dissected out from its junction with the main femoral vein to a level in the mid to distal thigh (Figure 2.28a). All branches are divided and the distal few centimeters of the vein is completely freed so that it can be brought close to the superficial femoral artery for anastomosis. The vein is ligated and divided distally. The superficial femoral artery is isolated at this level for an adequate length to allow for easy anastomosis. The vein is then brought to lie close to the artery. An end-to-side anastomosis is fashioned (Figure 2.28b).

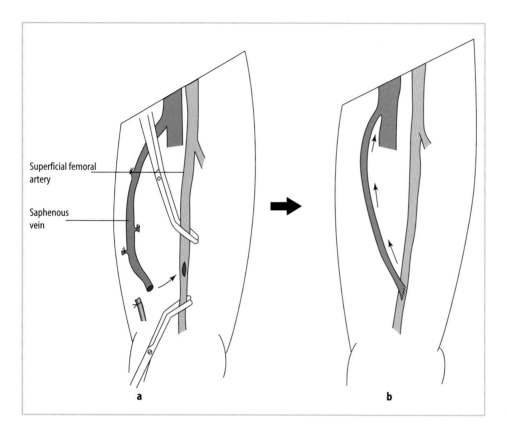

Superficial femoral artery

Saphenous vein

a   b

Figure 2.28

2. If the saphenous vein is not of useable quality for an adequate length, then a prosthetic graft can be used. A horizontal or vertical incision is made in the femoral region, directly over where the saphenous vein likely enters the main femoral vein. The artery, which lies just lateral to the femoral vein, is similarly dissected out. The graft is brought through a tunnel, similar to as with a looped graft procedure in the forearm. The ends of the graft are anastomosed to the corresponding artery and vein (Figures 2.29 and 2.30).

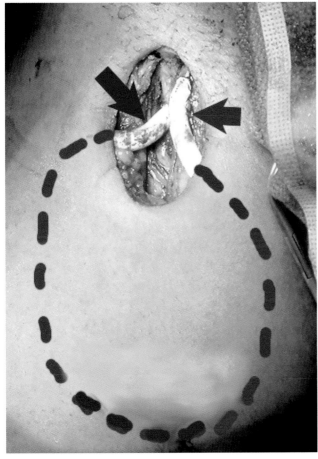

Figure 2.29

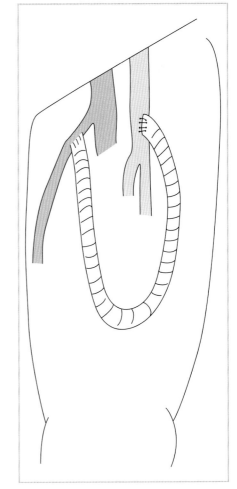

Figure 2.30

Peritoneal Dialysis

Peritoneal dialysis has been in wide usage since the 1960s. For some patients it is an effective means of renal replacement therapy. Several modalities of peritoneal dialysis are now available, but the principle remains the same – fluid and solutes are exchanged via the peritoneum.

As with hemodialysis, careful preoperative planning is required. Peritoneal dialysis may not be a viable option in patients with multiple prior abdominal surgeries as intraabdominal adhesions may preclude effective exchange of the dialysate. The patient must be competent enough to manage the machine and catheter at home. It is a useful option in patients who have difficult vascular access.

Peritoneal Dialysis Catheter Placement

a) Open Technique

In 1968, Tenckhoff developed a silicone catheter that is still used for peritoneal dialysis. Several modifications of this catheter are currently available. Most of the catheters have two Dacron cuffs, one that is implanted just above the peritoneum and the other in a subcutaneous location. Both these cuffs create an inflammatory reaction with subsequent fibrosis and adhesion, preventing bacterial ingrowth from the skin.

1. Typically, either a vertical or transverse incision is made in a paramedian location below the umbilicus (Figure 2.31). If the patient is a renal transplant candidate, the incision should be made on the left, saving the right side for the kidney.

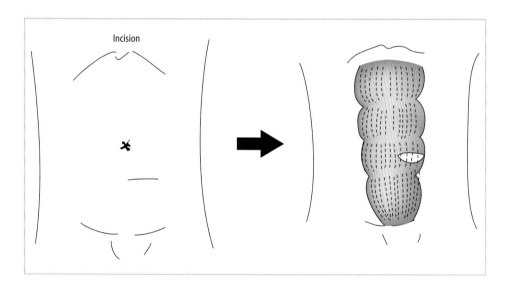

Figure 2.31

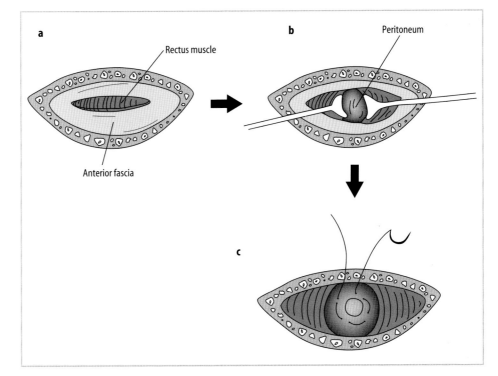

Figure 2.32

2. The incision is carried through the subcutaneous tissue and the anterior rectus sheath incised transversely (Figure 2.32a). The fibers of the rectus muscle are then split bluntly to expose the transversalis fascia and peritoneum (Figure 2.32b). An opening is made in the peritoneum and a purse-string suture placed around the opening (Figure 2.32c).

3. The catheter is then flushed and threaded over an inserting stylet. The catheter (Figure 2.33a) can then be gently fed through the peritoneal opening into the peritoneal cavity, directing it caudad (Figure 2.33b). Care must be taken to avoid injury to underlying viscera during this maneuver. The purse-string suture is tied, securing the peritoneum around the catheter.

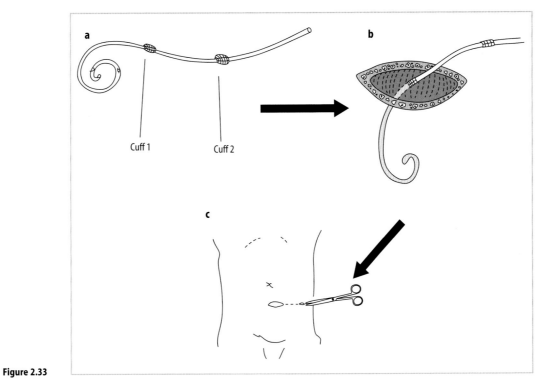

Figure 2.33

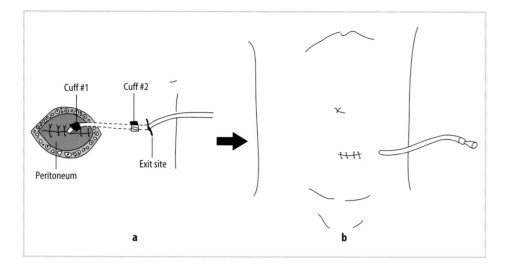

Figure 2.34

4. The first cuff is seated above the peritoneum within the body of the rectus muscle. Part of the suture may be used to directly transfix the Dacron cuff. A lateral tunnel is then created in a subcutaneous space and a small, sharp instrument passed through the tunnel into the original incision (Figure 2.33c); the free end of the catheter is grasped and pulled through. The anterior rectus sheath is then closed with nonabsorbable sutures. The second Dacron cuff is seated 1 or 2 cm away from the skin exit site to prevent erosion through the skin (Figure 2.34a). It is usually not necessary to suture the catheter to the skin. In fact, this may lead to irritation and infection of the catheter site. The skin incision is closed in standard fashion (Figure 2.34b). Prior to leaving the operating room, the catheter is tested by instilling it with saline solution and then checking for drainage by placing the catheter in a dependent position.

b) Laparoscopic Technique

The advantage of the laparoscopic method is that the catheter can be placed under direct visualization, thereby reducing the risk of visceral injury and optimizing placement. Also, with this technique, the catheter may be used right away; the open technique requires a 1 to 2-week wait. The disadvantage is that a general anesthetic is required.

1. The whole abdomen is prepped. Usually two 5-mm trocars are adequate (Figure 2.35a). Some surgeons prefer a third port as well. A 5-mm port is placed in the supraumbilical area either using the open technique or with a closed technique using a Veress needle. Pneumoperitoneum is established with CO_2 insufflation. A second 5-mm port is then placed in a paramedian position below the umbilicus. The peritoneal cavity is carefully inspected for any adhesions or other abnormalities. Adhesiolysis is performed if needed. The Silastic peritoneal dialysis catheter is then threaded over its thin inserting stylet (Figure 2.35b). The 5-mm port in the left paramedian area is then removed and the catheter with stylet is inserted through this opening under direct laparoscopic visualization (Figure 2.35c). The stylet and catheter are carefully advanced toward the suprapubic area and the catheter threaded into the peritoneal cavity (Figure 2.35d). The catheter is pushed into the abdomen until the Dacron cuff is visible. This is then seated

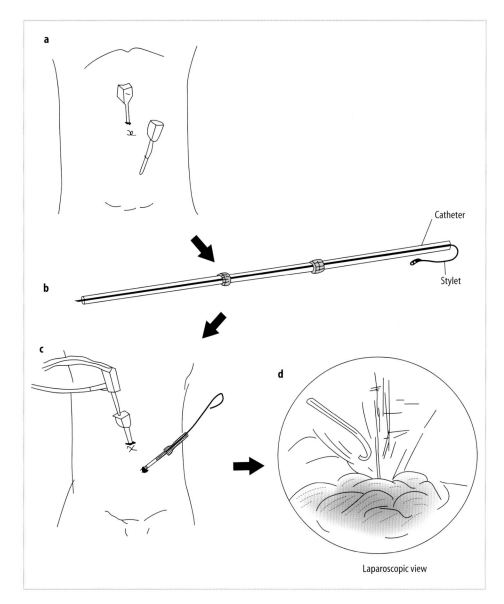

Figure 2.35

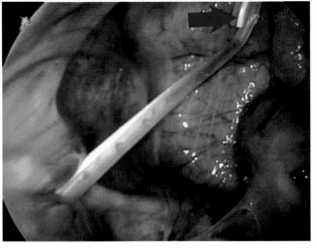

Figure 2.36

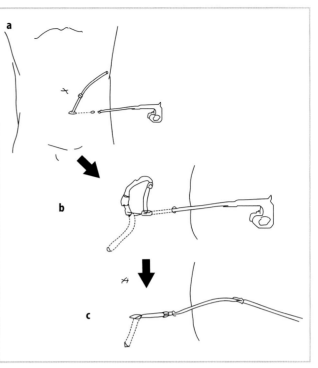

Figure 2.37

just above the peritoneum. The stylet is then completely withdrawn leaving the catheter in place, with its tip directed into the pelvis (blue arrow) (Figure 2.36).

2. A small incision is then created laterally for the catheter exit site. Using a long grasping instrument, a subcutaneous tunnel is created between this incision and the paramedian incision (Figure 2.37a). The end of the catheter is grasped and pulled out, situating the second cuff about 1 or 2 cm away from the skin exit site (Figure 2.37b). The subcutaneous tissue and skin are closed at the paramedian incision but no deeper stitches are necessary. The pneumoperitoneum is released and catheter function is tested by instilling 500 cc to 1 L of normal saline and then letting it flow out by dependent drainage. The initial port site is then closed in standard fashion (Figure 2.37c).

Selected Readings

1. Akoh JA, Sinha S, et al. A 5-year audit of hemodialysis access. Int J Clin Pract 2005;59(7):847–851.
2. Brescia MJ, et al. Chronic hemodialysis using venipuncture and a surgically created arteriovenous fistula. N Engl J Med 1966;275:1089.
3. Crabtree JH, Fishman A. A laparoscopic method for optimal peritoneal dialysis access. Am Surg 2005;71(2):135–143.
4. Diaz-Buxo JA. Access and continuous flow peritoneal dialysis. Perit Dial Int 2005;25(suppl 3):S102–104.
5. Gray RJ, Sands JJ, eds. Dialysis Access: A Multidisciplinary Approach. Philadelphia: Lippincott Williams & Wilkins, 2002.
6. Kawecka A, Debska-Slizien A, Prajs J, et al. Remarks on surgical strategy in creating vascular access for hemodialysis: 18 years of one center's experience. Ann Vasc Surg 2005;19(4):590–598.
7. Keuter XH, van der Sande FM, Kessels AG, de Haan MW, Hoeks AP, Tordoir JH. Excellent performance of one-stage brachial-basilic arteriovenous fistula. Nephrol Dial Transplant 2005;20(10):2168–2171.
8. Lin PH, Bush RL, Nguyen L, Guerrero MA, Chen C, Lumsden AB. Anastomotic strategies to improve hemodialysis access patency – a review. Vasc Endovasc Surg 2005;39(2):135–142.
9. National Kidney Foundation. Kidney Disease Outcomes Quality Initiative (NKF K/DOQI). Clinical practice guidelines for vascular access. Am J Kidney Dis 2001;37(suppl 1):s137–s181.
10. Ramage IJ, Bailie A, Tyerman KS, McColl JH, Pollard SG, Fitzpatrick MM. Vascular access survival in children and young adults receiving long-term hemodialysis. Am J Kidney Dis 2005;45(4):708–714.
11. Striker GE, Tenckhoff H. A transcutaneous prosthesis for prolonged access to the peritoneal cavity. Surgery 1971;69:70.
12. Wilson SE, ed. Vascular Access: Principles and Practice. St Louis: Mosby, 1996.

Nephrectomy from a Living Donor

Raja Kandaswamy and Abhinav Humar

Introduction

The kidney, the first organ to be used for living-donor transplants, is the most common type of organ donated by living donors today. In the Unites States, the number of living kidney donors now outnumbers the number of deceased kidney donors. Initially it was felt that only close family members could be potential donors. However, it is well recognized now that there does not need to be any direct relationship between the donor and recipient to achieve a highly successful outcome. Any healthy person is a potential kidney donor, including relatives, coworkers, friends, and acquaintances.

A living-donor kidney transplant offers significant advantage over its deceased-donor counterpart. Living-donor kidney recipients enjoy improved long-term success, avoid a prolonged wait, and are able to plan the timing of their transplant in advance. Moreover, they have a significantly decreased incidence of delayed graft function and increased potential for human leukocyte antigen (HLA) matching. As a result, living-donor transplants generally have better short- and long-term results, as compared with deceased-donor transplants. Of course, the risks to the living donor must be acceptably low. The donor must be fully aware of potential risks and must freely give informed consent. But as long as these conditions are met, the search for a living donor should not be restricted to immediate family members. Results with living, unrelated donors are comparable to those with living, related (non–HLA-identical) donors.

The preoperative evaluation of individuals who present as possible kidney donors is a crucial part of the living-donor kidney transplant process. A complete and thorough evaluation is important in minimizing the risks of the procedure for the potential donor and optimizing donor safety – the underlying principle of any living-donor procedure. The predonation evaluation of the potential donor is also critical in ensuring a successful outcome for the recipient. The evaluation process may vary slightly depending on individual center preference. But the steps of the process essentially remain the same, and can be divided into three major parts: (1) medical evaluation, (2) surgical or radiologic evaluation, and (3) psychosocial evaluation. The potential donor should satisfy each of the three parts of this evaluation process before being considered an acceptable donor. The evaluation process, at the same time as being complete, should not be overly cumbersome for the donor. It should be streamlined and efficient, invasive tests should be minimized, and it should be cost-effective. Members of a multidisciplinary team need to be involved in the evaluation process, including a nephrologist, surgeon, psychologist, social worker, and transplant coordinator.

One main goal of the preoperative medical evaluation is to ensure that the donor does not have underlying medical problems that would significantly increase the risk associated with a general anesthetic and a major operative procedure. This part of the evaluation is not too dissimilar from the evaluation for any person undergoing a major general surgical procedure. The other important part of the medical evaluation serves to identify and exclude any possibility of chronic kidney disease or kidney dysfunction in the potential donor. The medical evaluation includes the screening for viral pathogens that could potentially be significantly harmful when transmitted to the recipient. The next part of the evaluation looks at the surgical anatomy of the kidney including the blood vessels supplying the kidney. Present-day noninvasive imaging is sufficient to provide adequate preoperative information, eliminating the need for invasive tests such as angiograms. The final part of the evaluation looks at the psychosocial status of the donor, ensuring that the donor is mentally fit to donate, understands the associated risks, and is able to give informed consent without coercion.

The operative procedure for removal of a kidney for living-donor kidney transplant has changed dramatically in the last 5 years. Laparoscopic techniques have become increasingly more common, and at many centers, laparoscopic donor nephrectomy is now the preferred method for removal of the kidney. Advantages for the donor include a quicker recovery, a shorter hospital stay, and decreased postoperative pain. It is likely that laparoscopic removal of the kidney will become the standard of care at almost all centers over the next few years.

The early postoperative care of donors is very similar to that of anyone undergoing a major intraabdominal procedure. Fluid and electrolytes are monitored closely, as is the urine output. Pain and other postoperative symptoms such as nausea should be adequately controlled. Donors should be encouraged to ambulate early to minimize the risk of pulmonary complications or deep venous thrombosis. Donors should also be monitored closely for any surgical complications including postoperative bleeding, wound infections, or bowel complications.

Most donors undergoing laparoscopic nephrectomy stay in the hospital for 2 to 3 days after the procedure. The early recovery period (i.e., the first 2 weeks after surgery) involves gradual return to activities of daily living. At 2 weeks, most donors are able to tolerate mild exercise in addition to regular activities. They should wait 4 to 6 weeks before engaging in any strenuous activity or heavy lifting.

Studies have shown that laparoscopic donors experience less pain than open donors, as indicated by a decreased use of pain medicines (narcotics) after surgery. In addition, a shorter hospital stay and quicker return to full activity and work have been documented. Early to intermediate follow-up (up to 5 years) of laparoscopic donors has revealed no increase in the risk of complications, as compared with open donors. However, long-term follow-up information (i.e., 10, 20, and 30 years) is lacking. Because laparoscopic nephrectomy involves working through the abdominal cavity (in contrast to open donor nephrectomy, which is a retroperitoneal procedure), there may be a small risk of long-term intestinal obstruction due to adhesions within the abdomen. This risk remains theoretical; in fact, with other types of laparoscopic procedures in the last 20 years, no increased risk of intestinal obstruction has been consistently documented. In the short term, however, laparoscopic donors may experience bowel dysfunction (nausea, bloating, irregular bowel movements) during the first few days after surgery. Such dysfunction usually responds to a combination of bowel rest and laxatives.

Open Nephrectomy

1. The patient is positioned with the right or left flank (depending on which kidney is being removed) elevated and exposed. The incision begins posteriorly at the tip of the 12th rib and curves anteriorly in the direction of the umbilicus, stopping at the lateral border of the rectus muscle (black arrow) (Figure 3.1).

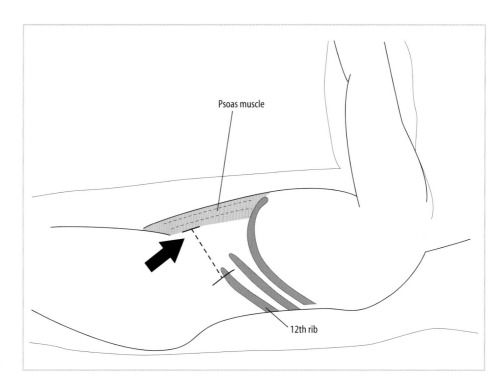

Psoas muscle

12th rib

Figure 3.1

2. The three muscular layers of the lateral abdominal wall are divided. Sometimes a small portion of the tip of the 12th rib may need to be removed. Deep to the muscular layers, the peritoneum is identified and retracted medially to visualize the retroperitoneal space. The ureter (black arrow) is identified below the lower pole of the kidney, running on the anterior surface of the psoas muscle. It is mobilized down to the pelvis, taking care not to remove the surrounding periureteral tissue. Once the ureter is mobilized, Gerota's fascia is incised and the kidney is separated from the surrounding perirenal fat (Figure 3.2).

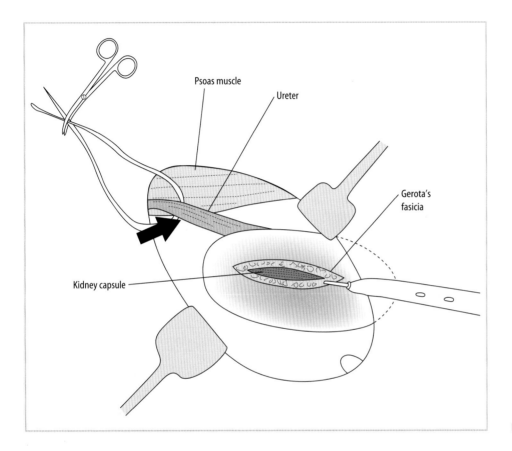

Figure 3.2

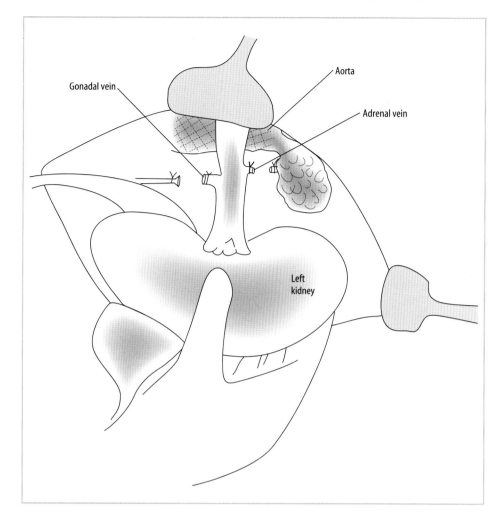

Figure 3.3

3. The renal vein is identified and mobilized proximally. For the left kidney, the vein is mobilized to the point where it lies anterior to the aorta (Figure 3.3). The gonadal vein, adrenal vein, and any lumbar veins will need to be ligated and divided. The right renal vein, however, usually has no branches draining into it. The vein on the right side is traced proximally to its junction with the inferior vena cava.

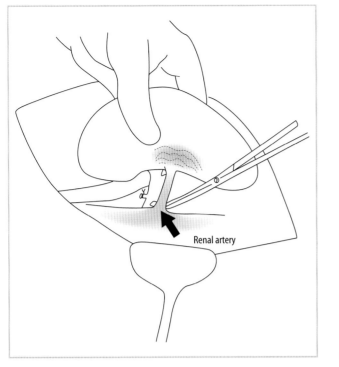

Figure 3.4

4. The renal artery is identified next, usually lying posterior and superior to the lower border of the renal vein. It is useful to retract the kidney medially and carry out the dissection along the posterior aspect of the hilum. The renal artery is mobilized to its junction with the aorta (Figure 3.4).

5. The ureter is divided distally. At this point one can easily check to ensure that the kidney is producing urine. If the function of the kidney appears adequate, the donor is given intravenous heparin. Vascular clamps are applied on the renal artery at its junction with the aorta, and on the renal vein where it runs anterior to the aorta (Figure 3.5). These structures are divided. The kidney is removed and sent to the recipient team.

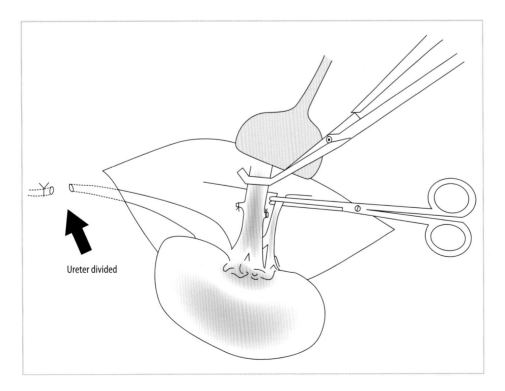

Figure 3.5

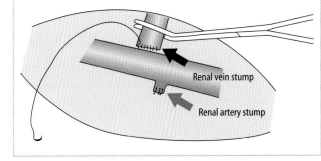

Renal vein stump

Renal artery stump

Figure 3.6

6. The vascular stumps are then oversewn with a nonabsorbable suture (Figure 3.6). After checking for hemostasis, closure is initiated. The abdominal wall is closed in layers.

Laparoscopic Donor Nephrectomy

a) Introduction

Nephrectomy from a living donor, which has been performed since the 1960s using the open technique, has been associated with a relatively long incision along the flank, often involves removal of a portion of the 12th rib, and may be associated with significant pain and significant loss of time from work and other activities. The recovery period is usually 6 weeks and sometimes longer. However, long-term results with open donor nephrectomy in terms of quality and longevity of life have been excellent.

The short-term disability caused by open donor nephrectomy was the impetus to seek an alternative – a less invasive method that would result in a smaller incision, less pain, and faster recovery. Even though laparoscopic nephrectomy for disease had been performed as early as 1991, laparoscopic donor nephrectomy was first performed in the United States in 1995. Early concerns about an increased incidence of delayed graft function and graft thrombosis were quickly dispelled as experience in the field grew. Currently, over 60% of living donors in the United States are performed using the laparoscopic technique.

Laparoscopic donor nephrectomy can be performed using a variety of techniques. These include hand-assisted, pure laparoscopic, robotic hand–assisted, and robotic pure laparoscopic. The main advantages of the hand-assisted techniques are that they are easier to adapt for a surgeon with little experience in advanced laparoscopy, they provide an added safety margin in case of emergencies, and they provide tactile feedback while operating. The disadvantages of the hand-assisted techniques include a slightly larger incision than would be required to deliver the kidney, and restricted areas where the incision can be placed to facilitate reaching to the kidney. Usually, upper midline incisions are used for a hand-assisted left nephrectomy, although some surgeons do this using a lower midline or even a Pfannenstiel incision. Pure laparoscopic technique, which is most commonly employed by advanced laparoscopic surgeons, offers the advantage of placing the incision below the belt line, where it is better concealed. Also, the size of the incision is usually smaller since the kidney is delivered using a bag. Theoretically, the pain would be expected to be lower, since upper midline incisions are more painful than lower incisions in the abdomen. In the last few years, the addition of the surgical robot to assist in donor nephrectomy led to the use of this technique by some centers. Again, as with traditional laparoscopy, this can be done either with or without hand assistance. The advantages of using a robotic system are as follows:

1. A 360-degree articulating wrist for the operating arms, providing greater flexibility and maneuverability;
2. Tremor-free operation due to a stabilization system built in;

3. Increased magnification of the robotic console;
4. Binocular vision at the console, providing a three-dimensional image.

The major disadvantages of the robotic system are as follows:

1. Lack of tactile feedback from the end of the instrument to the console;
2. Fixed port and patient positions with limited range of movement, which may sometimes limit moving from the upper pole of the kidney down to the pelvis to dissect the ureter;
3. Expense associated with the robotic system.

At our center, we have been performing laparoscopic donor nephrectomy since December 1997, and have performed over 650 such cases. We started with the hand-assisted technique, but now perform donor nephrectomy by all of the different techniques, including robotic-assisted pure laparoscopic nephrectomy. The technique chosen is based on the individual patient and surgeon's preference. Open donor nephrectomy is only performed, however, when there is a specific patient request.

b) Preoperative Preparation

The patient, after undergoing routine donor evaluation, including tests of kidney function and general health, is imaged using a computed tomography (CT) renal angiogram to look for vascular and parenchymal anomalies. This noninvasive technique provides excellent images of the vascular and parenchymal anatomy of the kidney, including its collecting system. The following CT angiogram, for example, clearly demonstrates three renal arteries supplying the right kidney and two arteries supplying the left kidney (Figure 3.7).

With bilateral single arteries and normal kidneys, we preferentially perform a left donor nephrectomy. However, if there are two left renal arteries and a single right renal artery, we would perform a right renal nephrectomy. We have generally avoided nephrectomy in donors who have more than two arteries, rather choosing a different donor if possible. The patient is given bowel preparation instructions the night before surgery and a dose of second-generation cephalosporin 30 minutes prior to incision.

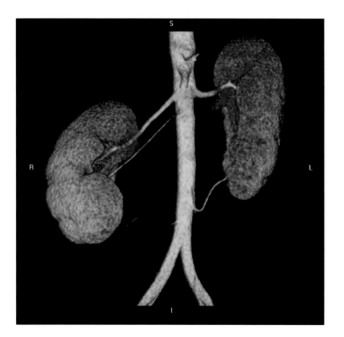

Figure 3.7

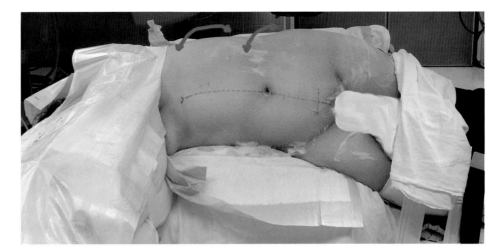

Figure 3.8

Positioning is done similarly for all the different techniques of laparoscopic nephrectomy, with the patient in a lateral position. The kidney rest is elevated; the table is retroflexed to open up the angle between the rib cage and the iliac crest. The patient is secured and placed with a bean bag and tapes as needed (Figure 3.8). The table can then be rotated from side to side to move the patient from a pure lateral to an almost supine position, as needed.

c) Hand-Assisted Laparoscopic Nephrectomy

1. A 6- to 7.5-cm incision (depending on surgeon hand size) is made in the midline [above the umbilicus for a left nephrectomy (Figure 3.9), below or around the umbilicus

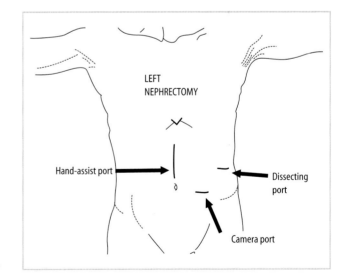

Figure 3.9

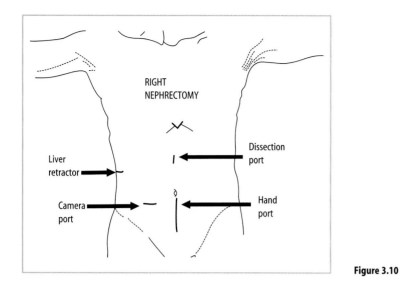

RIGHT
NEPHRECTOMY

Dissection
port

Liver
retractor

Camera
port

Hand
port

Figure 3.10

for a right nephrectomy (Figure 3.10)]. Any one of a number of different hand port devices can be used. With the hand inside the abdomen, the other ports required are inserted. For a left nephrectomy this includes one 10- to 12-mm port just slightly inferior and lateral to the umbilicus (camera port) and a second port about 8 cm lateral to the first one (dissecting port). On the right side, an additional 5-mm port is inserted for the liver retractor.

2. With the hand in the abdomen, pneumoperitoneum is achieved. The hand may be removed and inserted as necessary (Figure 3.11). It is useful to insert a small gauze sponge into the abdomen to help wipe fluid and blood. Care should be taken to keep an accurate count of sponges inserted.

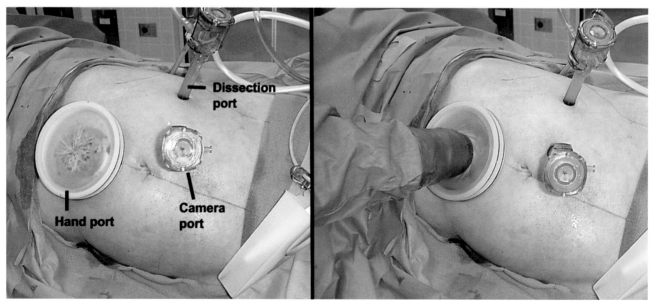

Figure 3.11

3. The left colon is mobilized extensively, starting at the splenocolic ligament and extending inferiorly to the pelvic brim. The colon is reflected medially to visualize the retroperitoneal space and the kidney enclosed in Gerota's fascia (Figure 3.12).

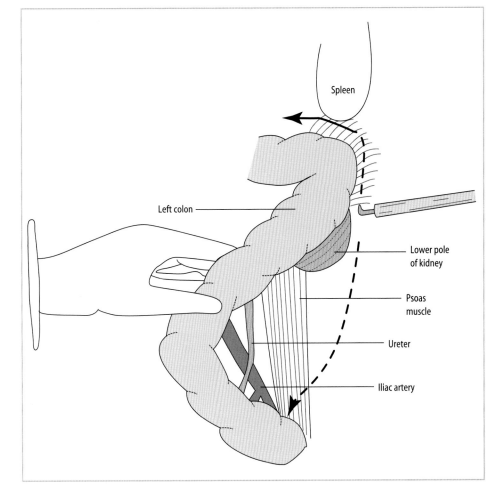

Figure 3.12

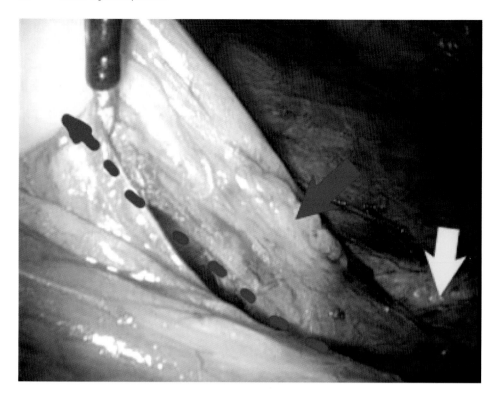

Figure 3.13

4. The ureter and gonadal vein are identified at the level of the pelvic brim just where it crosses the iliac artery (yellow arrow). Often these two structures are close together, and the two can be encircled and maintained together in one bundle (blue arrow) (Figure 3.13) to help preserve the vascular tissue adjacent to the ureter.

5. The gonadal vein (blue arrow) is divided at this location (Figure 3.14). The ureter/gonadal bundle proximal to this site is then dissected further upward (broken blue line) toward the kidney.

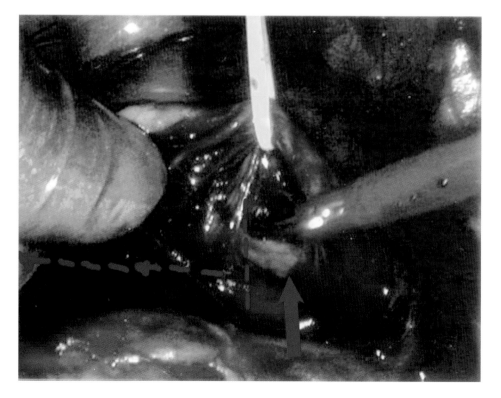

Figure 3.14

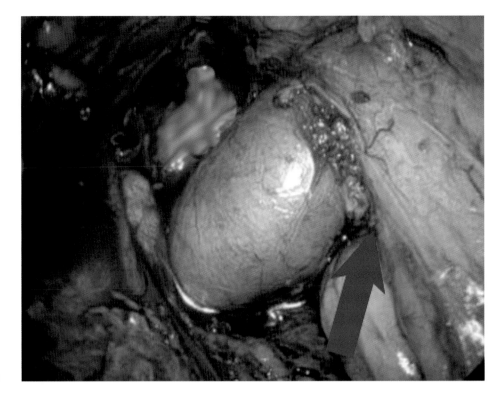

Figure 3.15

6. On the left side, the gonadal vein serves as a useful landmark to locate the renal vein. Following the gonadal vein superiorly will lead to its junction with the renal vein (yellow arrow) (Figure 3.15). On the right side, the gonadal vein drains into the inferior vena cava, not the right renal vein. However, locating the anterior surface of the cava on this side will allow one to identify its junction with the right renal vein.

7. The renal vein is then dissected and mobilized circumferentially, staying well away from the hilum (Figure 3.16). On the right there are usually no branches, but on the left the adrenal (yellow arrow), gonadal (blue arrow), and lumbar branches need to be identified and divided.

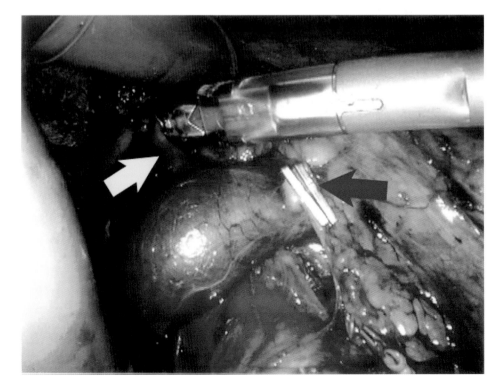

Figure 3.16

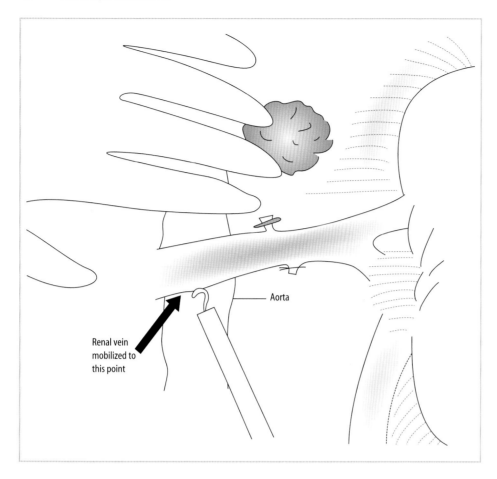

Figure 3.17

8. With the vein dissected free circumferentially, it is mobilized further proximally for adequate length. Usually freeing the left vein to the point where it passes anterior to the aorta is sufficient (Figure 3.17). On the right, the vein is mobilized to its junction with the inferior vena cava.

9. With the vein displaced in a cephalad direction (blue arrows), the location of the renal artery (red arrow) can be seen and palpated. The artery is identified by dividing the ganglion tissue anterior to it (Figure 3.18).

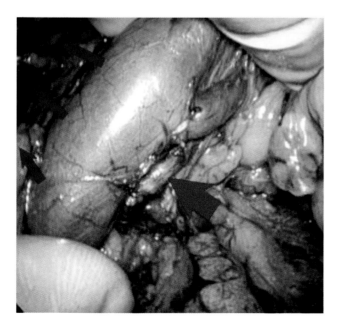

Figure 3.18

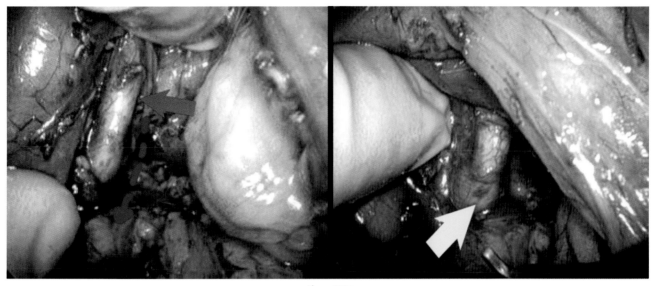

Figure 3.19

10. The renal artery is then traced proximally to its junction with the aorta (Figure 3.19).

11. With the vascular and ureteral dissection complete, mobilization of the kidney is performed (Figure 3.20). This can be done in a stepwise fashion starting with the superior and medial attachments to the adrenal gland, mobilizing the upper pole and upper lateral aspect of the kidney, proceeding from the inferior pole along the lateral aspect of the kidney, and then reflecting the kidney medially to free it along its posterior aspect.

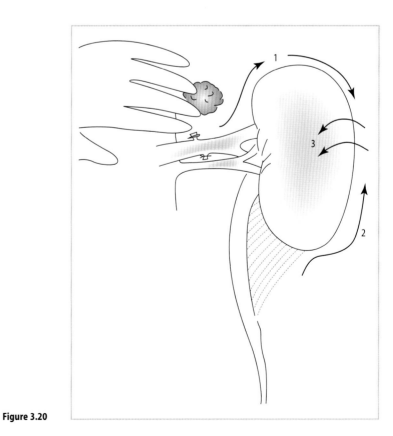

Figure 3.20

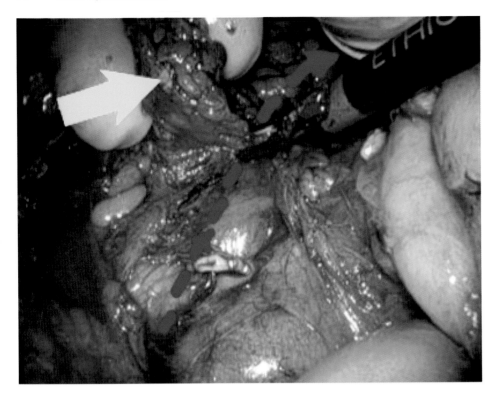

Figure 3.21

12. The adrenal gland (yellow arrow) is identified first and carefully separated from the upper medial aspect of the kidney (blue line) (Figure 3.21). This area tends to be quite vascular and this step is best accomplished with an instrument such as a harmonic scalpel.

13. The kidney is then completely mobilized from the upper pole to the lower pole along its lateral aspect. Care should be taken to preserve the triangle of tissue between the ureter and lower pole of the kidney, as extensive dissection here can disrupt the blood supply to the ureter (Figure 3.22).

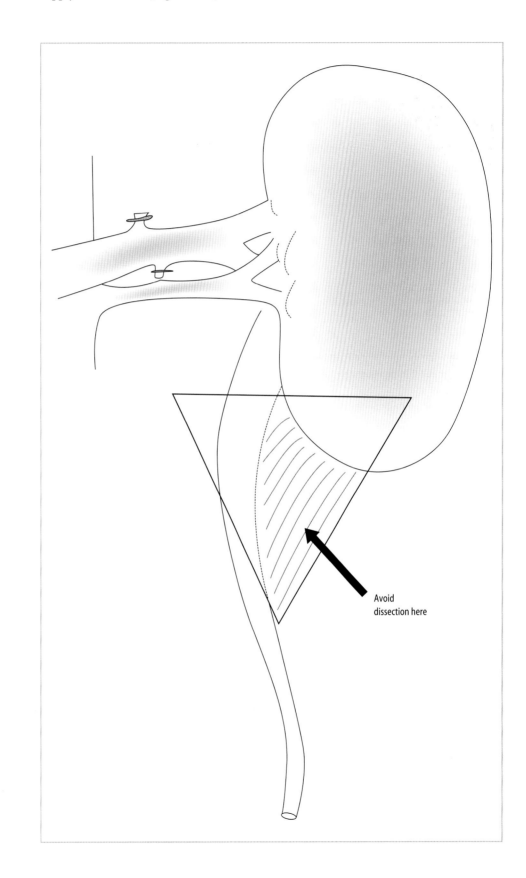

Avoid
dissection here

Figure 3.22

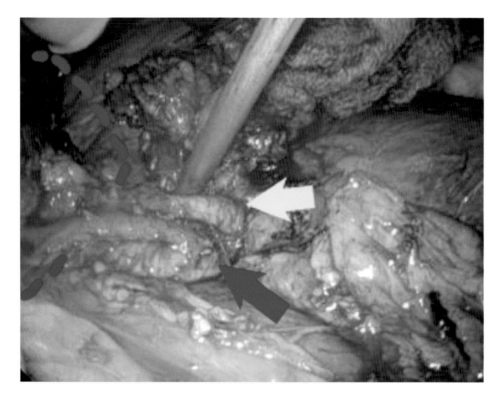

Figure 3.23

14. With the kidney rotated medially, the posterior attachments, including ganglion tissue along the posterior aspect of the renal artery (yellow arrow) and renal vein (blue arrow) can be divided (Figure 3.23). The kidney is now ready for removal.

15. The ureter (yellow arrow) is mobilized further into the pelvis as needed with regard to length. It is then divided using hemoclips or plastic locking clips. At this point one should check that there is urine production from the kidney (blue arrow) (Figure 3.24). If there is not, it is wise to release the pneumoperitoneum, give diuretics, and wait for evidence of urine.

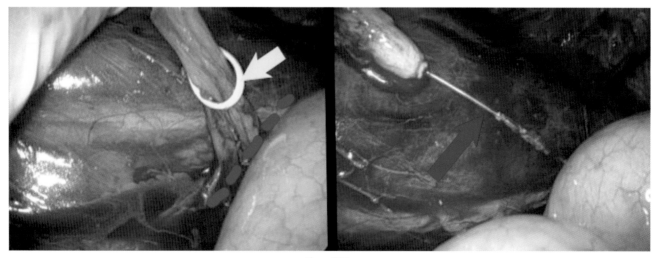

Figure 3.24

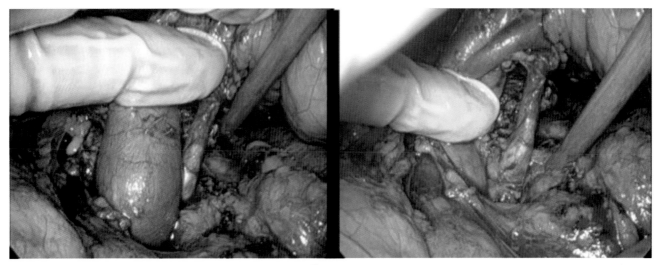

Figure 3.25

16. The donor is given heparin in preparation for removal of the kidney. The kidney is grasped with one hand and retracted out laterally to stretch out the renal artery and vein. Retracting the vein cephalad gives excellent exposure at this point to the renal artery at the point of its junction with the aorta (Figure 3.25).

17. The artery can now be divided using either locking clips or a vascular stapler (Figure 3.26). It is useful at this point to insert the stapler through the camera port and place the camera in the dissection port – this gives the straightest approach for the stapler to reach the artery. Our preference is to use a noncutting stapler to get maximal length on the artery. The staple line can be reinforced with a hemoclip, but we do not use hemoclips in isolation for fear of dislodgment.

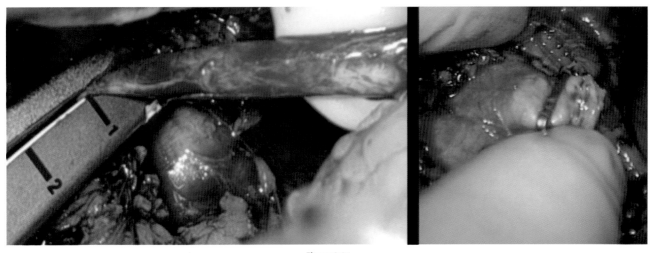

Figure 3.26

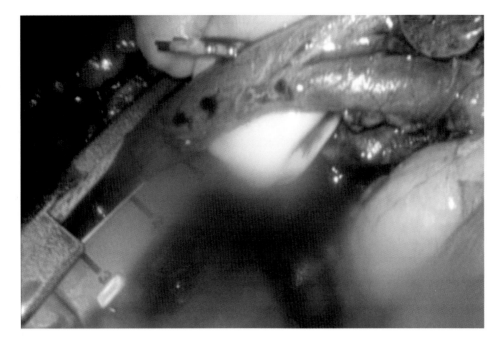

Figure 3.27

18. The vein is divided with a stapler also, and the kidney removed through the hard-port site (Figure 3.27). The kidney is then flushed.

19. A careful check is then made for hemostasis. Areas to inspect specifically include the vascular stumps (blue arrow), the adrenal bed (yellow arrow), and the distal stump of the divided ureter (Figure 3.28).

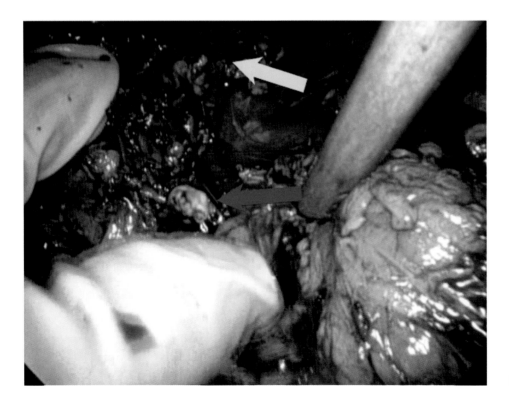

Figure 3.28

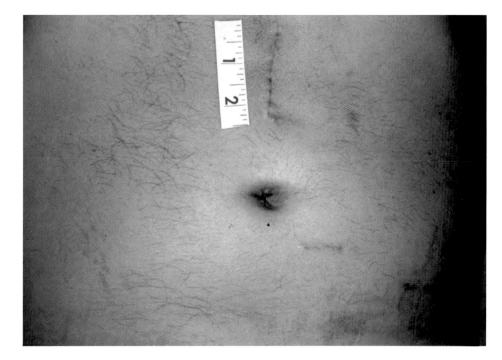

Figure 3.29

20. All incisions, including the 10- to 12-mm port sites are closed. The appearance of the incisions at 2 weeks postdonation is shown (Figure 3.29).

d) Pure Laparoscopic Technique

The pure laparoscopic technique varies in port placements as shown. Ports 1 or 2 can act as a camera port while the other two are dissecting ports (Figure 3.30). The Pfannenstiel incision is low and small. Details of the dissection are discussed in the following section.

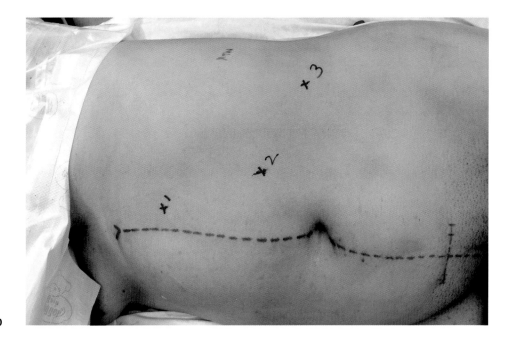

Figure 3.30

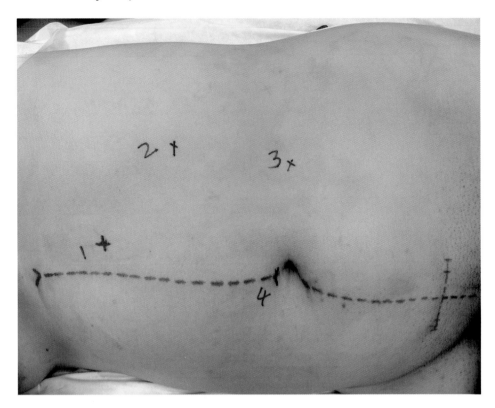

Figure 3.31

e) Robotic-Assisted Technique

1. Port placements are shown (Figure 3.31). We use the inverted triangle for the robotic ports (1, 2, and 3). Port number 4 is in the umbilicus, and is the assistant's port (for retracting, placing clips, or using the stapler).

2. A Veress needle (blue arrow) is used to insufflate the abdomen with CO_2 to 12 mm Hg (Figure 3.32). In lean patients pressures as low as 8 mm Hg could be used, whereas in others up to 15 mm Hg may be required.

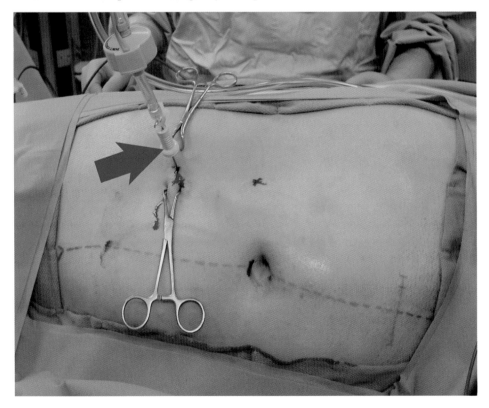

Figure 3.32

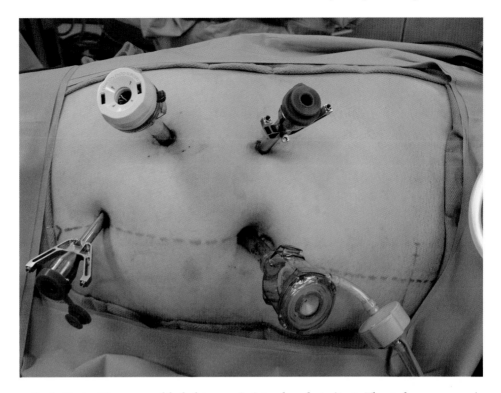

Figure 3.33

3. A 10- to 12-mm nonbladed trocar is introduced at site 2. The 0-degree scope is inserted through the trocar to provide visual assistance as the fascia and peritoneum are penetrated. This helps minimize the risk of injury to the bowel. Subsequently two 7-mm ports (DaVinci ports) are places at sites 1 and 3. These are inserted under visual guidance from the inside. Finally, a 10- to 12-mm bladed trocar is inserted through the umbilicus (Figure 3.33)

4. The robotic system is docked in position and the 0-degree camera is inserted using visual guidance. The forceps in the left port and the hook in the right port are inserted to position of function (Figure 3.34). The assistant sits next to the patient with easy access to port 4. In robotic hand–assisted cases the right hand of the assistant is inserted through a midline handport. In pure laparoscopic robotic cases the assistant helps using the umbilical port (yellow arrow). The surgeon is ready to sit at the console and begin. The surgeon should have undergone the standard training offered by the manufacturer

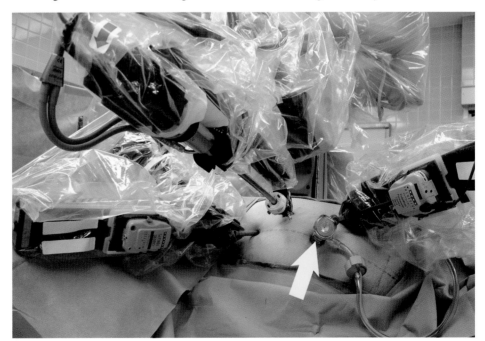

Figure 3.34

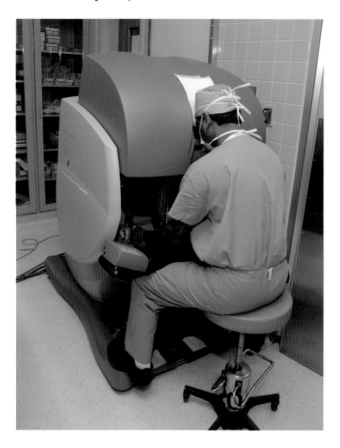

Figure 3.35

and should be certified to operate the system. The surgeon should sit at a comfortable height and operate with user-friendly ergonomics (Figure 3.35).

5. The first step in dissection of the left side is mobilization of the left colon by taking down the line of Toldt from the splenic flexure to the sigmoid colon. This is done using a Harmonic scalpel or electrocautery. Once the colon is reflected medially, Gerota's fascia is identified and traced medially to the renal vein (Figure 3.36).

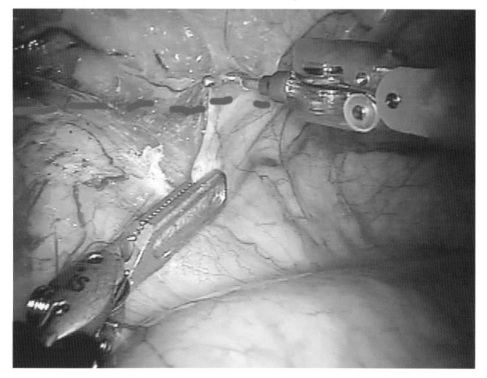

Figure 3.36

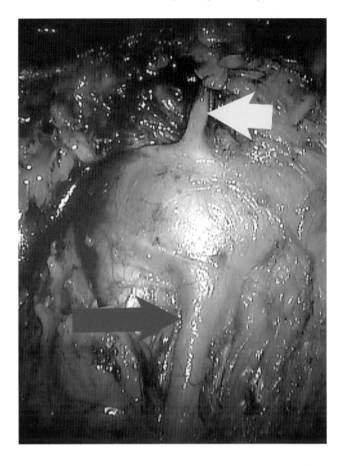

Figure 3.37

6. The renal vein is dissected well away from the hilum. This will expose the adrenal and the gonadal veins (Figure 3.37). Fine dissection around the vein is done using hook electrocautery taking care to avoid heat injury to the vasculature.

7. The venous branches of the renal vein including gonadal (yellow arrow, Figure 3.38), adrenal, and one or more lumbar veins can be divided between hemoclips, or, if less than 7 mm in diameter, can be divided with an electrocautery device.

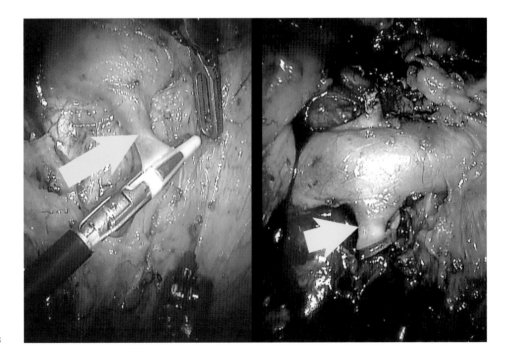

Figure 3.38

8. Cephalad displacement of the renal vein usually exposes the renal artery. Thick ganglionic tissue anterior to the artery will have to be divided to get a good view of it. The artery is dissected circumferentially to its junction with the aorta (yellow arrow, Figure 3.39).

9. Once the branches of the renal vein have been divided, circumferential dissection proximally to get adequate length is carried out.

10. Having completed the vascular dissection from the anterior side, the kidney should now be released from its superior and medial attachments. The adrenal gland is separated from the kidney. This step could be complicated by small bleeding due to venous hypertension of the adrenal gland. The Harmonic scalpel may help minimize blood loss.

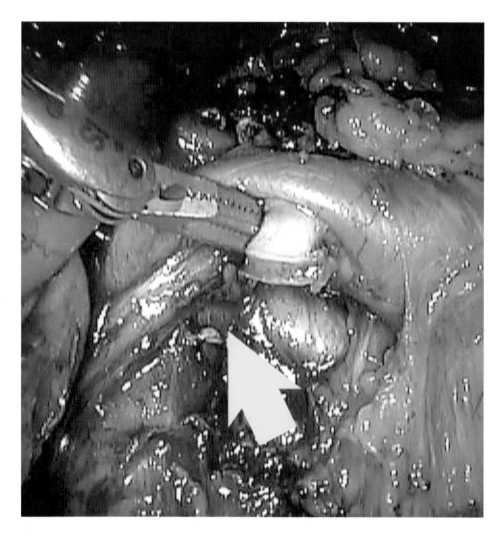

Figure 3.39

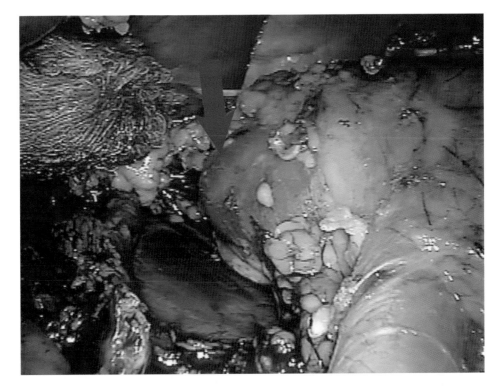

Figure 3.40

11. Dissection is then carried out around the upper pole (blue arrow). It is preferable, whenever possible, to free the upper pole first before the lower pole is dissected (Figure 3.40). This prevents the kidney from retracting upward and making the upper pole dissection more difficult.

12. Next, the inferior medial aspect of the kidney is dissected just lateral to the gonadal vein. The ureter (blue arrow) is usually identified in this position. It is then dissected down to its crossing of the iliac artery, taking care not to damage the periureteral vessels (Figure 3.41).

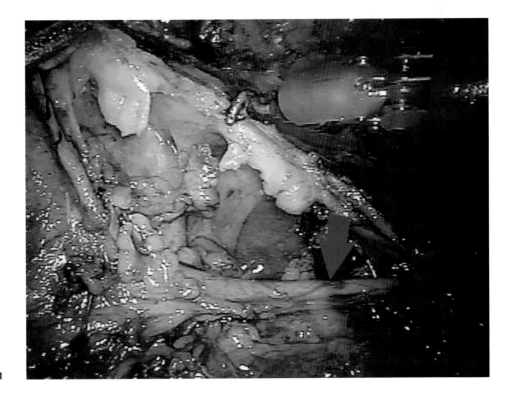

Figure 3.41

13. The inferior pole is then freed lateral to the ureter, and dissection is carried along to the lateral and posterior attachments of kidney to facilitate a posterior view. Once the posterior attachments are released, the kidney can be slipped medially to expose the vessels from the posterior side. This ensures complete release of all attachments of the kidney except the vessels (blue arrow) and the ureter (Figure 3.42). The kidney is now ready for removal.

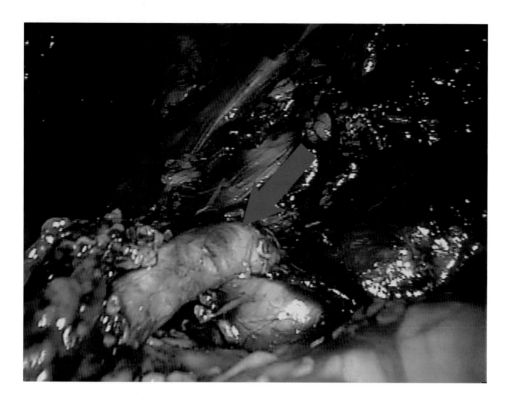

Figure 3.42

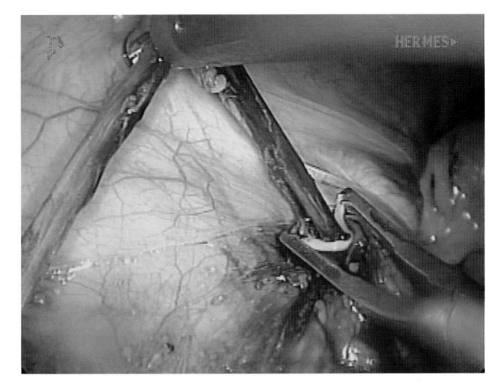

Figure 3.43

14. Next, the ureter is divided after clipping distally. A locking clip can be used for the purpose (Figure 3.43). The cut end of the ureter should be inspected for urine production. If urine output is absent or low, then letting down the pneumoperitoneum and waiting a few minutes may help. Forced diuresis is facilitated throughout the case using mannitol and furosemide.

15. At this point the pneumoperitoneum is released and a 6-cm Pfannenstiel incision is made. The fascial incision is midline. An endoscopic bag is inserted through a peritoneal purse string. The bag is deployed and the kidney and ureter placed in it (Figure 3.44).

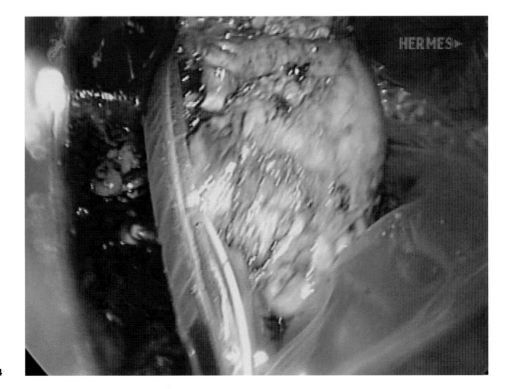

Figure 3.44

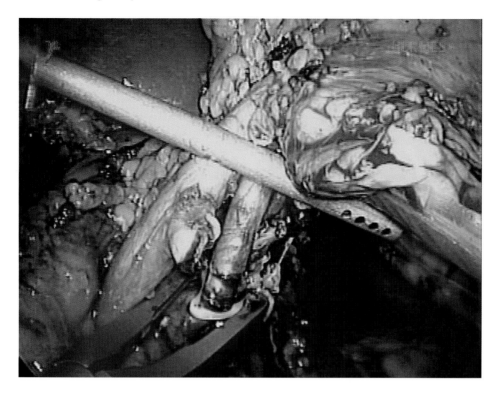

Figure 3.45

16. The only structures outside the bag are the renal artery and vein. After administration of 70 U/kg heparin, the renal artery is double clipped with locking clips and divided distally (Figure 3.45).

17. Then the vein is divided using a 35-mm articulating endovascular linear cutting stapler. Care should be taken to avoid catching any unwanted structures in the stapler (e.g., superior mesenteric artery). At the same time the stapler should be pushed far enough proximally to get maximal length on the vein. Alternatively, a noncutting stapler could be used to get slightly more length. This is our routine on the right side. Protamine is given to reverse the heparin once the vessels are ligated.

18. The kidney is now completely enclosed by turning the mouth of the bag upward. The mouth of the bag is then closed and it is withdrawn through the incision after the pneumoperitoneum is released and the peritoneotomy extended manually.

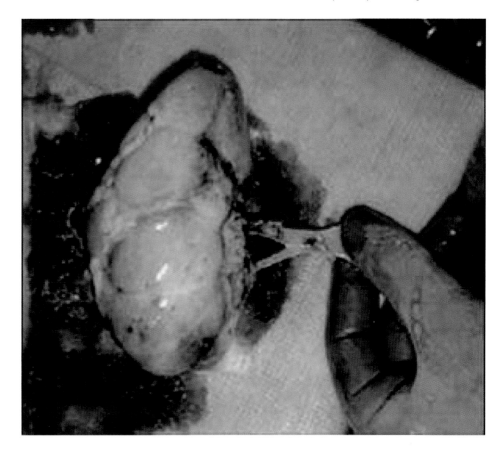

Figure 3.46

19. The kidney is flushed immediately to minimize warm ischemia time (Figure 3.46). The peritoneotomy is closed to facilitate pneumoperitoneum repair.

20. The vascular stumps are inspected for adequacy and hemostasis. The adrenal gland should also be inspected for venous oozing.

21. The ports are closed using a laparoscopic closing device.

Selected Readings

Clayman RV, Kavoussi LR, Soper NJ, et al. Laparoscopic nephrectomy. N Engl J Med 1991;324(19):1370.

Daily PP, Chavin KD. Laparoscopic live donor nephrectomy: the single surgeon technique. J Am Coll Surg 2003;197(3):519–520.

Dasgupta P, Challacombe B, Compton F, Khan S. A systematic review of hand-assisted laparoscopic live donor nephrectomy. Int J Clin Pract 2004;58(5):474–478.

Derweesh IH, Goldfarb DA, Abreu SC, et al. Laparoscopic live donor nephrectomy has equivalent early and late renal function outcomes compared with open donor nephrectomy. Urology 2005;65(5):862–866.

Flowers JL, Jacobs S, Cho E, et al. Comparison of open and laparoscopic live donor nephrectomy. Ann Surg 1997;226(4):483–489.

Horgan S, Benedetti E, Moser F. Robotically assisted donor nephrectomy for kidney transplantation. Am J Surg 2004;188(4A suppl):45S–51S.

Jacobs SC, Flowers JL, Dunkin B, Sklar GN, Cho E. Living donor nephrectomy. Curr Opin Urol 1999;9(2): 115–120.

Johnson MW, Andreoni K, McCoy L, et al. Technique of right laparoscopic donor nephrectomy: a single center experience. Am J Transplant 2001;1(3):293–295.

Kacar S, Gurkan A, Akman F, Varylsuha C, Karaca C, Karaoglan M. Multiple renal arteries in laparoscopic donor nephrectomy. Ann Transplant 2005;10(2):34–37.

Leventhal JR, Kocak B, Salvalaggio PR, et al. Laparoscopic donor nephrectomy 1997 to 2003: lessons learned with 500 cases at a single institution. Surgery 2004;136(4):881–890.

Melcher ML, Carter JT, Posselt A, et al. More than 500 consecutive laparoscopic donor nephrectomies without conversion or repeated surgery. Arch Surg 2005;140(9):835–839.

Odland MD, Ney AL, Jacobs DM, et al. Initial experience with laparoscopic live donor nephrectomy. Surgery 1999;126(4):603–606; discussion 606.

Oyen O, Andersen M, Mathisen L, et al. Laparoscopic versus open living-donor nephrectomy: experiences from a prospective, randomized, single-center study focusing on donor safety. Transplantation 2005;79(9): 1236–1240.

Pietrabissa A, Boggi U, Moretto C, Ghilli M, Mosca F. Laparoscopic and hand-assisted laparoscopic live donor nephrectomy. Semin Laparosc Surg 2001;8(2):161–167.

Rajab A, Mahoney JE, Henry ML, et al. Hand-assisted laparoscopic versus open nephrectomies in living donors. Can J Surg 2005;48(2):123–130.

Ruiz-Deya G, Cheng S, Palmer E, Thomas R, Slakey D. Open donor, laparoscopic donor and hand assisted laparoscopic donor nephrectomy: a comparison of outcomes. J Urol 2001;166(4):1270–1273.

Schostak M, Wloch H, Muller M, et al. Living donor nephrectomy in an open technique; a long-term analysis of donor outcome. Transplant Proc 2003;35(6):2096–2098.

Terasaki PI, Cecka JM, Gjertson DW, Takemoto S. High survival rates of kidney transplants from spousal and living unrelated donors. N Engl J Med 1995;333:333–336.

Tooher RL, Rao MM, Scott DF, et al. A systematic review of laparoscopic live-donor nephrectomy. Transplantation 2004;78(3):404–414.

4

Kidney Transplantation

Abhinav Humar and Arthur J. Matas

Introduction

In the last 35 years, few fields of medicine have undergone the rapid advances that have been seen with kidney transplantation. From the development of the surgical techniques necessary for transplantation at the beginning of the century, to the dawn of modern transplantation with the introduction of immunosuppressants in the late 1950s, and to its current status as the treatment of choice for end-stage renal disease (ESRD), renal transplantation has enjoyed remarkable progress. The surgical techniques for organ transplantation, including methods of vascular anastomosis, were developed in animal models by Carrel and Guthrie in the early 1900s. The first clinical deceased renal transplant was performed in 1933 by the Ukrainian surgeon Voronoy, with unsuccessful results secondary to the immunologic barrier. In the 1950s these obstacles were circumvented by performing the procedure between identical twins. The era of modern renal transplantation began with the introduction of the immunosuppressive agent azathioprine, and renal transplantation was established as a viable option for the treatment of ESRD.

For the majority of individuals with ESRD, transplantation results in superior survival, improved quality of life, and lower costs as compared with chronic dialysis. There are very few absolute contraindications and so most patients with ESRD should be considered as potential candidates. The surgery and general anesthesia, however, impose a significant cardiovascular stress. The subsequent lifelong chemical immunosuppression is also associated with considerable morbidity. Therefore, evaluation of a potential recipient must focus on identifying risk factors that could be minimized or may even contraindicate a transplant.

The preoperative evaluation can be divided into four phases: medical, surgical, immunologic, and psychosocial. The medical evaluation begins with a complete history and physical examination. Mortality after transplantation is just as likely to be due to underlying cardiovascular disease as to infectious and neoplastic complications of immunosuppression. Any history of congestive heart failure, angina, myocardial infarction, or stroke should be elicited. Patients with symptoms suggestive of cardiovascular disease or significant risk factors (e.g., diabetes, age over 50, previous cardiac events) should undergo further cardiac evaluation. Any problems identified should be treated appropriately (medically or surgically). Patients with suspected cerebrovascular disease should undergo evaluation with carotid duplex Doppler studies.

Untreated malignancy and active infection are absolute contraindications to transplantation because of the requisite lifelong immunosuppression. Following curative treatment of malignancy, an interval of 2 to 5 years is recommended prior to transplantation. This recommendation is influenced by the type of malignancy, with longer observation periods for neoplasms such as melanoma or breast cancer and shorter periods for carcinoma in situ or low-grade malignancies such as basal cell carcinoma of the skin. Chronic infections such as osteomyelitis or endocarditis must be fully treated. Other areas of the medical evaluation should concentrate on gastrointestinal problems such as peptic ulcer disease, symptomatic cholelithiasis, and hepatitis.

The surgical evaluation should concentrate on identifying vascular or urologic abnormalities that may affect transplantation. Evidence of vascular disease that is revealed by the history (e.g., claudication or rest pain) or the physical examination (e.g., diminished or absent pulse, bruit) should be evaluated further by Doppler studies or angiography. Severe aortoiliac disease may make transplantation technically impossible; one option in these patients is a revascularization procedure such as an aorto-bifemoral graft prior to the transplant. Areas of significant stenosis proximal to the planned site of implantation may need preoperative balloon angioplasty or stenting. Urologic evaluation should rule out chronic infection in the native kidney, which may require nephrectomy pretransplant. Other indications for nephrectomy include very large polycystic kidneys, significant reflux, and uncontrollable renal vascular hypertension. Children especially require a complete genitourinary tract examination to evaluate reflux and bladder outlet obstruction.

An assessment of the patient's immunologic status involves determining blood type, tissue type [human leukocyte antigens (HLAs) A, B, DR], and the presence of any cytotoxic antibodies against HLAs (because of prior transplants, blood transfusions, or pregnancies).

A psychosocial evaluation is necessary to ensure that patients understand the nature of the transplant procedure, with its attendant risk. They must be capable of following the medical regimen after the transplant. Patients who have not been compliant with their medical regimen in the past must demonstrate a willingness and capability to do so, before they undergo the transplant.

Living donors are preferred over deceased donors. Recipients of living-donor organs enjoy improved long-term success, avoid a prolonged wait, and are able to plan the timing of their transplant in advance. Moreover, they have a significantly decreased incidence of delayed graft function. All of these advantages contribute to a lower incidence of early acute rejection and to improved graft and patient survival rates. While there is significant benefit for the recipient, there is no physical benefit for the living donor, only the potential for harm. Therefore, it is paramount that the risks of donation be acceptably low, and that the donor is fully aware of the potential risks and has freely given informed consent.

The surgical technique for renal transplantation has changed very little from the original pelvic operation described in 1951. The most common approach today is the standard pelvic operation, with retroperitoneal placement of the kidney, allowing easy access for percutaneous renal biopsy. Usually, the right iliac fossa is chosen because of the more superficial location of the iliac vein on this side. The procedure involves two vascular anastomoses (renal artery and vein) and the ureter to bladder anastomosis.

The initial postoperative care is not unlike that of other surgical patients. Fluid and electrolyte status, vital signs, central venous pressure, and urine output are carefully monitored. Special issues include immunosuppression and monitoring for transplant-related surgical and medical complications unique to these patients. Potential surgical complications specific to the kidney transplant include renal artery or vein thrombosis, ureteral leak, and ureteral stricture.

Outcomes after kidney transplantation have steadily improved over the past three decades, thanks to improvement in maintenance immunosuppression, antirejection therapy, organ retrieval techniques, perioperative care, and treatment of posttransplant infectious complications. Most centers now report patient survival rates exceeding 95% during the first posttransplant year for all recipients. Transplants from living donors have a clear advantage over those from deceased donors; reported 5-year patient survival rates after living and deceased donor transplants are approximately 90% and 80%, respectively. Compared with dialysis, the survival advantage after a transplant is probably greatest for diabetics.

Benching the Kidney from a Deceased Donor

Kidneys from a deceased donor are generally procured with a significant amount of the surrounding tissue including the surrounding perineal fat, the adrenal gland, and portions of the aorta and inferior vena cava (IVC). The two kidneys may also be procured en bloc. This wide dissection minimizes the risk of damage to the renal hilum at the time of procurement. Therefore, the first step of the deceased-donor kidney transplant procedure is to adequately prepare the graft to render it suitable for transplant. The basic steps involved are inspection of the organ, dissection of the artery and vein, and removal of the surrounding perirenal fat.

a) Procedure

1. The kidney is oriented in its anatomic position to allow for careful inspection of the renal artery (red arrow), the renal vein (blue arrow), the ureter, and the parenchyma. Placing a small clamp on the distal ureter (yellow arrow) is helpful in keeping the proper orientation of the kidney (Figure 4.1). The vessels are inspected for evidence of damage or atherosclerotic disease. The parenchyma should also be inspected for evidence of lesions or traumatic injury.

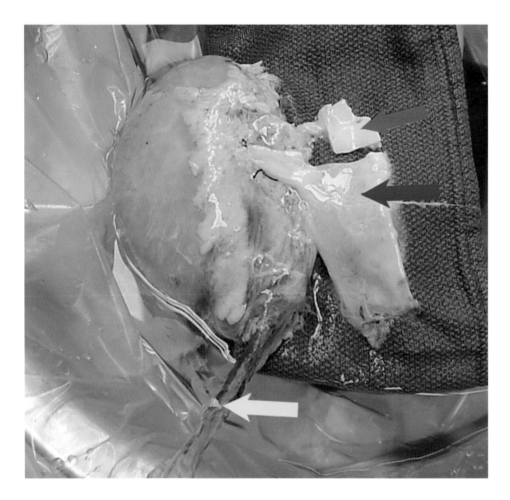

Figure 4.1

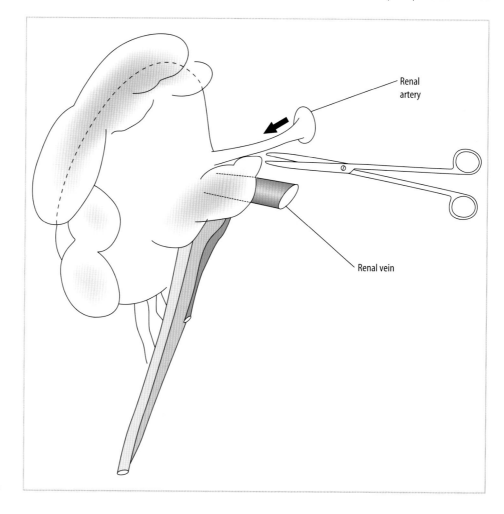

Renal
artery

Renal vein

Figure 4.2

2. The renal artery is dissected free from the surrounding hilar tissue and an appro-priate sized aortic patch is fashioned (Figure 4.2).

3. The renal vein is then similarly dissected for an adequate length. Branches including the adrenal, gonadal, and lumbar all need to be divided and ligated. These branches are usually present on the left renal vein, but the right renal vein usually has no branches. For a left kidney, there is usually adequate length so that the inferior vena cava does not need to be included (Figure 4.3).

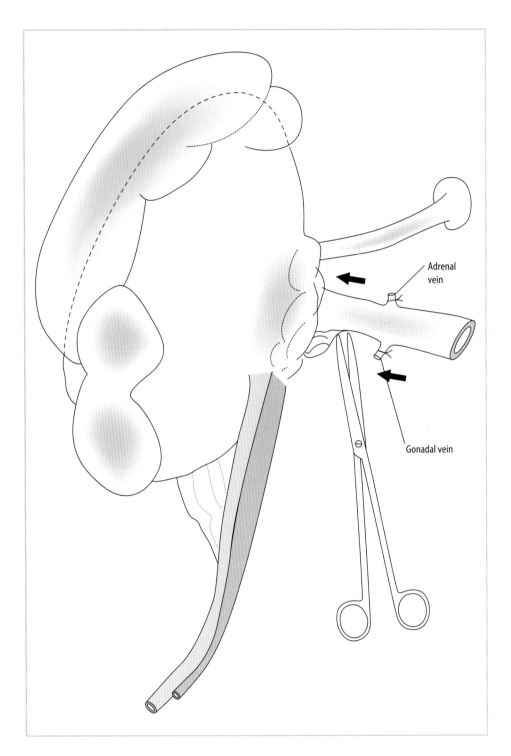

Adrenal vein

Gonadal vein

Figure 4.3

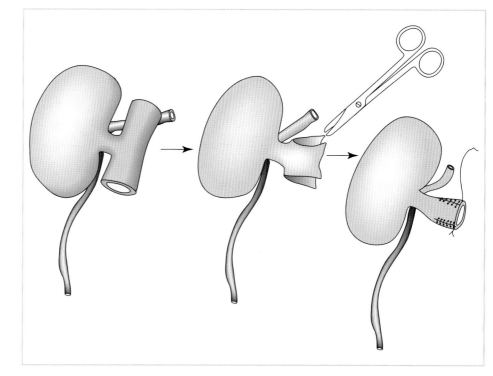

Figure 4.4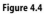

4. With a right kidney, the right renal vein may sometimes be short. If so, it can be lengthened by using a segment of the IVC, transecting it transversely superior and inferior to the renal vein, and then closing the edges of the transected IVC using a fine running vascular suture (Figures 4.4 and 4.5).

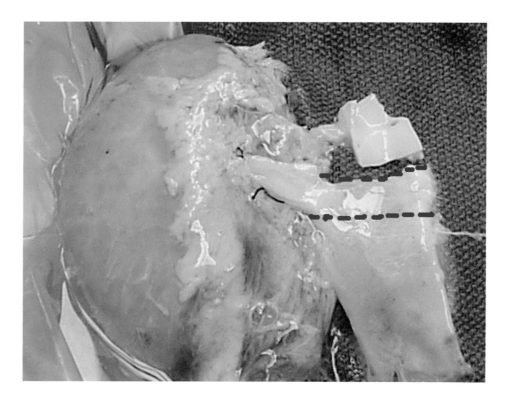

Figure 4.5

5. The surrounding perineal fat is then removed from the kidney, taking care not to injure the capsule. This is started from the medial aspect of the upper pole, where the adrenal gland is identified and removed. The dissection continues along the upper pole and then the lateral aspect of the kidney (gray arrows). Care should be taken not to carry the dissection too extensively in the lower pole, as this may devascularize the ureter. The fat (black arrow) in the triangle formed by the lower pole, the hilar vessels, and the ureter (Figure 4.6) should not be separated from the kidney, to preserve blood supply to the ureter.

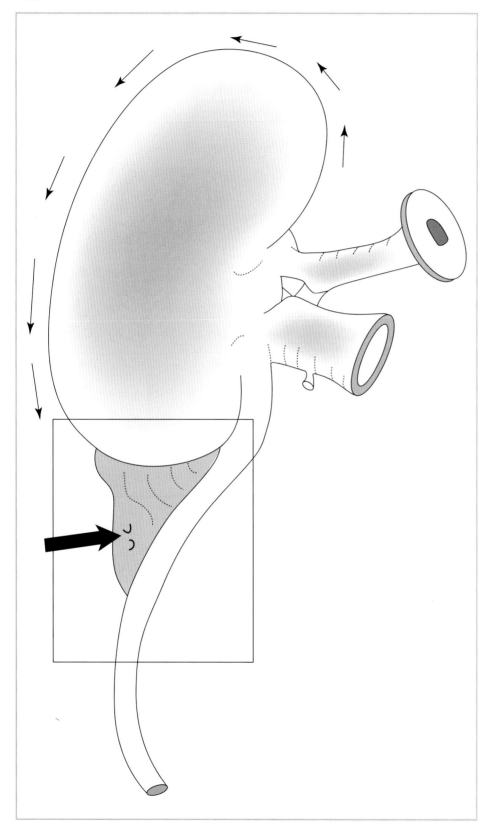

Figure 4.6

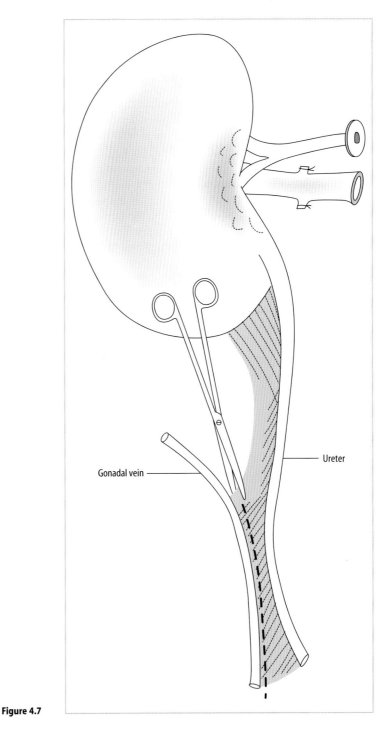

Gonadal vein

Ureter

Figure 4.7

6. Minimal dissection should be done around the ureter, but the accompanying gonadal vein may be removed (Figure 4.7). The kidney is now ready for implantation.

Adult Kidney Transplant

The standard kidney transplant for an adult recipient is usually a heterotopic procedure with the kidney placed in a retroperitoneal location, either in the right or left iliac fossa. The right iliac fossa is usually preferred, unless a future pancreas transplant is planned, or a kidney transplant was previously performed in the right fossa. In these cases, the left fossa is chosen.

In certain situations, an intraperitoneal placement of the kidney may be the better option. If the procedure is performed with a simultaneous pancreas transplant, then the kidney is best placed intraperitoneally, on the opposite side of the pancreas. In very small pediatric patients (usually <20 kg), an intraperitoneal position usually allows for more space and anastomosis to larger vessels for inflow and outflow. Lastly, in the recipient with multiple previous transplants, or with other previous procedures on both the right and left iliac vessels, an intraperitoneal location allows one to stay away from the site of previous surgery, and use the distal aorta and IVC for graft implantation if necessary.

Regardless of the location of the kidney, for adult recipients the vascular anastomoses are generally performed to the iliac vessels. For arterial inflow, the common iliac artery, internal iliac artery, or external iliac artery may be used. Generally, the external iliac artery is preferred, but if it is diseased or small in caliber, then there should be no hesitation in using the common iliac artery. Ultimately, the best option is to place the kidney in the fossa prior to selecting a site for the anastomosis, and choose the site where the renal artery will lie most naturally without significant tension, redundancy, and angulation.

The iliac vein is used for venous outflow – again most commonly the external iliac vein. However, the optimal site should be chosen based on the position of the kidney. The branches of the iliac vein are more variable than the artery. There may be one dominant internal iliac vein or several smaller ones. If the graft renal vein is short, or the recipient iliac vein deep, then the branches of the iliac vein may be divided. This allows the vein to be brought up into a more superficial position, making the anastomoses simpler.

Urinary continuity is restored by connecting the transplant ureter to the bladder. This may be done with or without a stent. Several different techniques have been described for performing this anastomosis. The key goals are to ensure that the ureter is not under tension or too redundant, and that it is well vascularized and perfused at its most distal position where the anastomosis will be performed. It is advisable to create some form of tunnel for the distal aspect of the transplant ureter to diminish urinary reflux.

a) Operative Procedure

1. With the patient in the supine position, a "hockey-stick" – shaped incision is made in the lower quadrant (purple line) (Figure 4.8). The incision starts in the midline, one or two finger widths above the pubic bone (solid black line). The incision extends laterally, gently curving upward until the lateral edge of the rectus muscle is reached (broken red line). The incision is then extended superiorly along the lateral edge of the rectus.

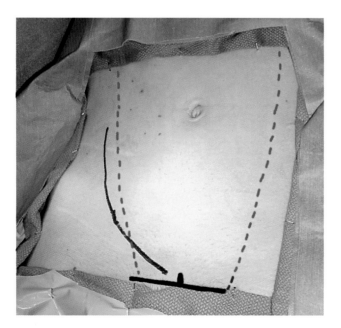

Figure 4.8

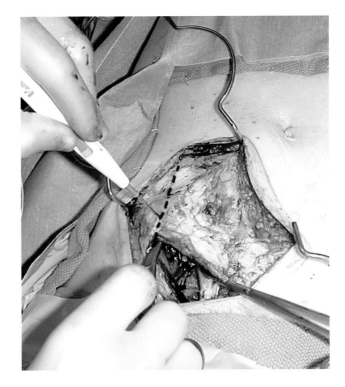

Figure 4.9

2. The incision is deepened to the fascia. Starting medially, and going laterally, the anterior sheet of the rectus muscle is incised (Figure 4.9). At the lateral edge of the rectus muscle, the fascial incision is carried superiorly just lateral to the edge of the rectus muscle (broken line) (Figure 4.10). This is where the muscular layers of the lateral abdominal wall start to form the anterior and posterior sheets of the rectus muscle. Relatively little actual muscle needs to be divided with this approach. Medially it is usually not necessary to divide the rectus muscle, but mobilizing it down to its attachment to the pubic bone helps in later exposure of the bladder.

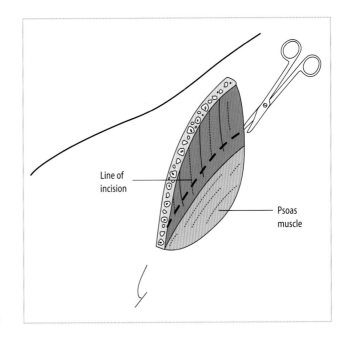

Line of
incision

Psoas
muscle

Figure 4.10

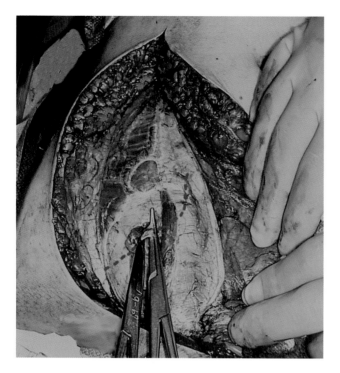

Figure 4.11

3. The inferior epigastric vessels are encountered in the middle to lower portion of the incision once the fascia is incised (broken blue line) (Figure 4.11). These vessels are divided between ligatures.

4. As the incision is deepened, the next structure to be encountered is the round ligament in females and the spermatic cord in males (broken yellow lines) (Figure 4.12). The round ligament can be divided, but the spermatic cord should be preserved and a vessel loop passed around it.

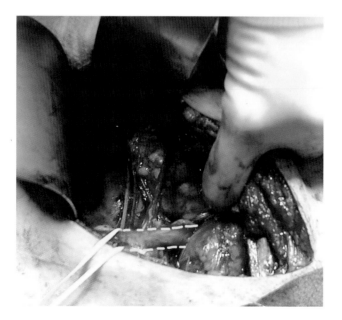

Figure 4.12

5. The peritoneum is then gently reflected medially toward the midline using one hand to retract the peritoneum (broken blue line) and the cautery to divide loose connections. This allows visualization of the retroperitoneal space, with the underlying psoas muscle (broken yellow line) (Figure 4.13).

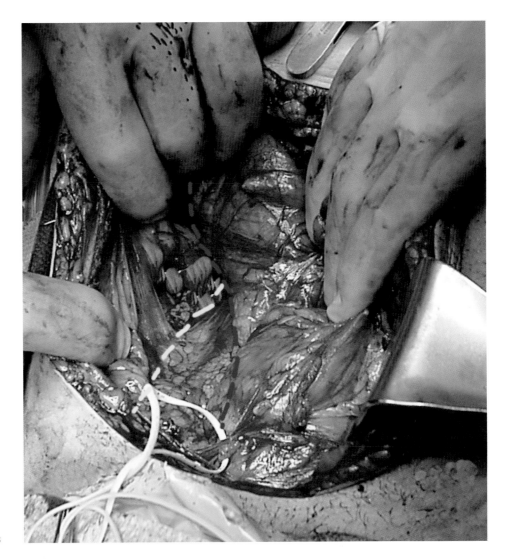

Figure 4.13

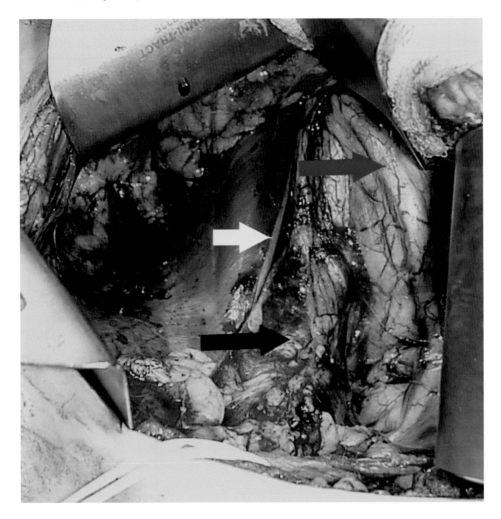

Figure 4.14

6. A self-retaining retractor is inserted at this point. An outline of the iliac vessels (black arrow) can be seen at the base of the wound with the genitofemoral nerve (yellow arrow) laterally and the native ureter (blue arrow) medially (Figure 4.14). Where the ureter enters the pelvis is a good landmark to locate the bifurcation of the common iliac artery into its internal and external branches. Care should be taken to ensure that the blades of the retractor do not impinge and occlude the iliac vessels proximally.

7. The external iliac artery is dissected free and mobilized for an adequate length to allow for subsequent clamp placement and anastomosis. Lymphatics (yellow arrow) overlying the artery should be carefully ligated to diminish the risk of lymphocele formation (Figure 4.15).

8. The external iliac vein (blue arrow), usually lying just medial to the artery (yellow arrow), is subsequently isolated. If the iliac vein is deep, or the transplant renal vein short, the internal iliac venous branches can be divided to place the vein in a more superficial

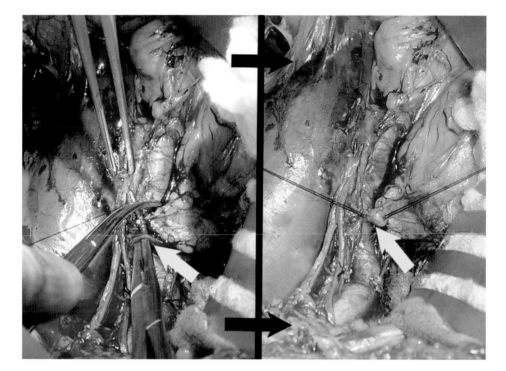

Figure 4.15

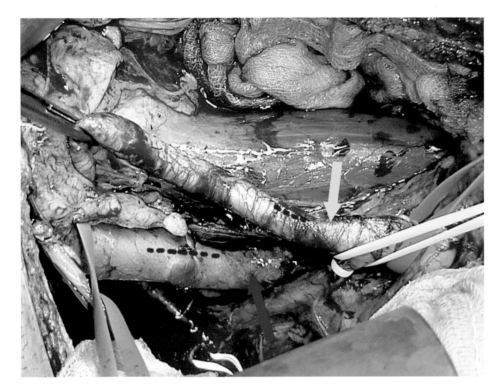

Figure 4.16

position. It is usually a good idea once the vascular dissection is finished to place the kidney in the iliac fossa to determine the best location to perform the venous and arterial anastomosis. These locations can be marked with a marking pen (broken purple line) (Figure 4.16).

9. Usually the venous anastomosis is performed first. Clamps are placed proximally and distally on the vein and an appropriate-sized venectomy is made. There are several ways to perform the actual anastomosis. One technique is to place four sutures (Figure 4.17): one at the upper end of the anastomosis, one at the lower end (solid lines), and one each on the two sides (broken lines).

10. The four sutures are tied and the superior stitch is sewn circumferentially around the anastomosis, with the primary surgeon suturing his/her side and the assistant the

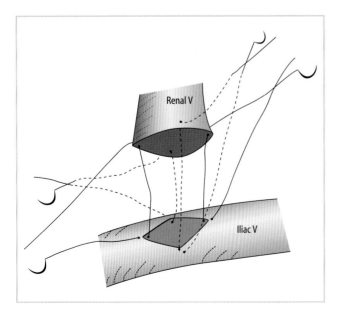

Figure 4.17

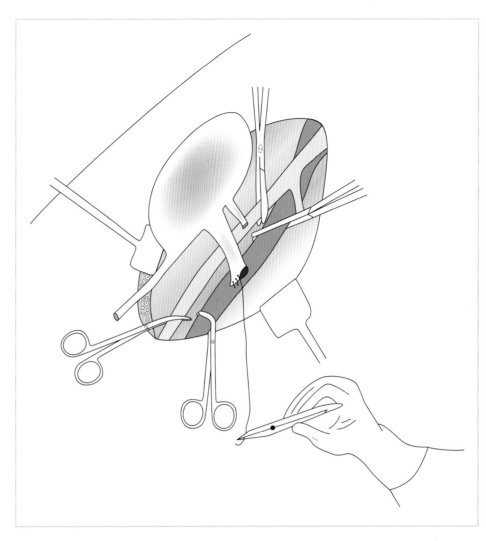

Figure 4.18

other side (Figure 4.18). In this manner the renal vein is anastomosed to the iliac vein in an end-to-side fashion (blue arrow) (Figure 4.19).

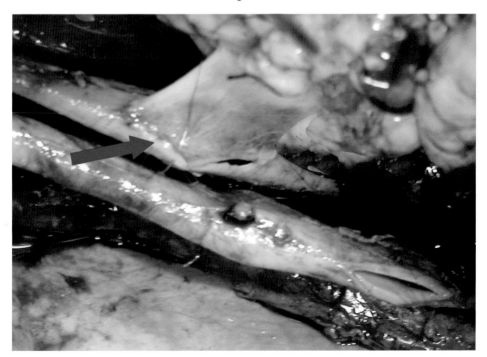

Figure 4.19

11. The arterial anastomosis can be performed in a similar fashion after clamping the artery and making an appropriate sized arteriotomy. If there is no aortic cuff present on the artery (as with a living donor transplant), then a small circular arteriotomy is made on the iliac vessel (yellow arrow) (Figure 4.20). A vascular punch device, as shown

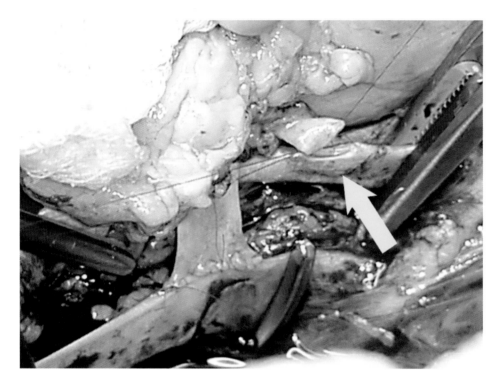

Figure 4.20

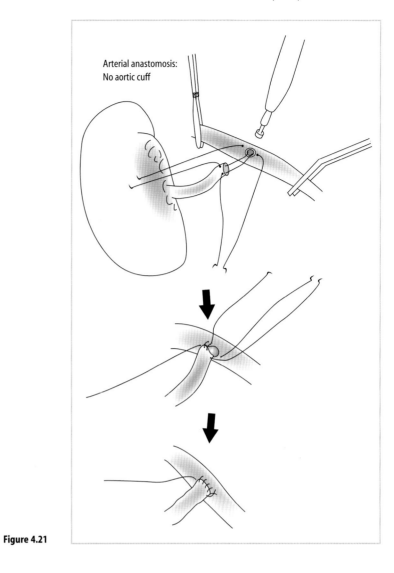

Arterial anastomosis:
No aortic cuff

Figure 4.21

(Figure 4.21), may be useful for this step. The clamps are removed after this anastomosis, and the kidney allowed to reperfuse.

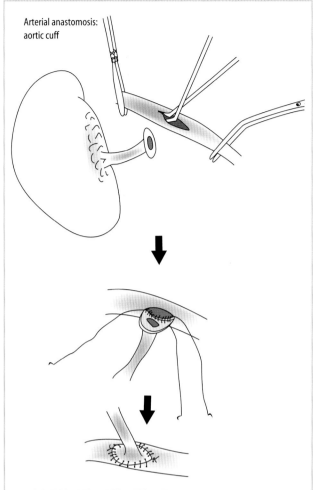

Arterial anastomosis:
aortic cuff

Figure 4.22

12. If there is a patch present around the renal artery, then a straight arteriotomy can be made on the recipient vessel, and the patch sewn to the arterial wall (Figure 4.22).

13. There are several methods to perform the ureter to bladder anastomosis including the Ledbetter-Pollitano, Litch, and anterior one-stitch techniques. The latter two techniques are subsequently described. The distal ureter is adequately prepared by trimming to an appropriate length, ligating the accompanying ureteral vessels (black arrows), and spatulating the distal end (Figure 4.23).

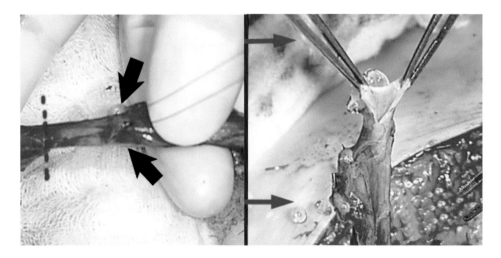

Figure 4.23

14. The retractors are repositioned to expose the bladder (Figure 4.24). It is helpful to fill the bladder and clamp the urinary catheter at this point. An incision is made

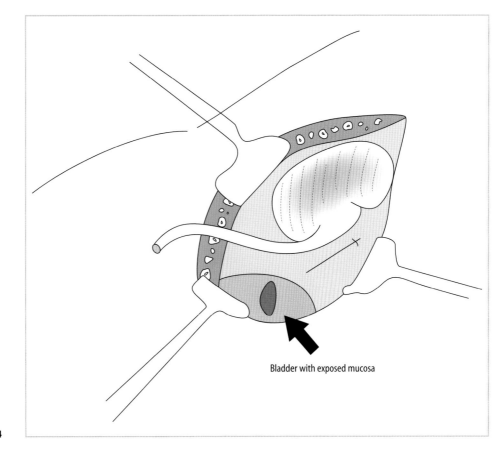

Bladder with exposed mucosa

Figure 4.24

through the detrusor muscle, exposing the underlying mucosa, but not going through it (black arrow) (Figure 4.25).

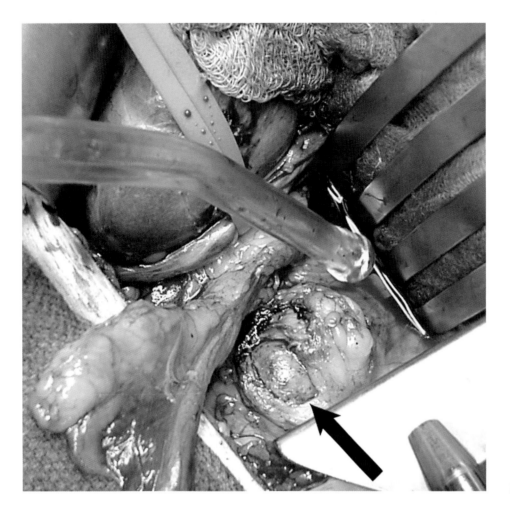

Figure 4.25

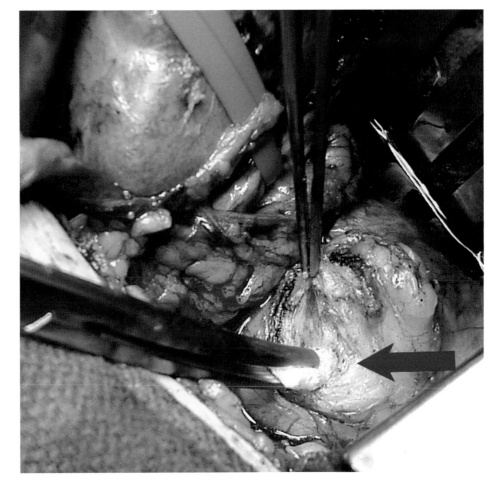

Figure 4.26

15. The detrusor muscle is then gently separated from the underlying mucosa (Figure 4.26). This can be done bluntly with gauze (blue arrow). This step is useful for creation of the subsequent tunnel, which will cover the distal part of the ureter.

16. With the Litch technique, an incision is made in the bladder mucosa and the distal spatulated end of the ureter is anastomosed for the bladder mucosa using a fine running absorbable suture (Figure 4.27). Triangulating the anastomosis is a useful technique here. One suture is placed in the heel, and one at each of the two distal corners. The heel stitch is then tied and run toward the tops.

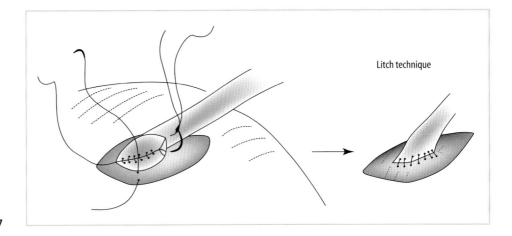

Litch technique

Figure 4.27

17. With an anterior one-stitch technique a double-ended suture is placed in the spatulated end of the ureter with the two needles on the "inside" aspect of the ureter (Figure 4.28a). These two sutures are then brought through a small opening made in the bladder mucosa with the needles exiting the bladder further distally (Figure 4.28b). These sutures are then used to pull the ureter into the bladder. The ureter is then secured to the anterior wall of the bladder by tying the anterior double-ended stitch (Figure 4.28c).

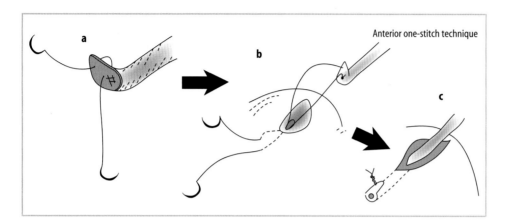

Figure 4.28

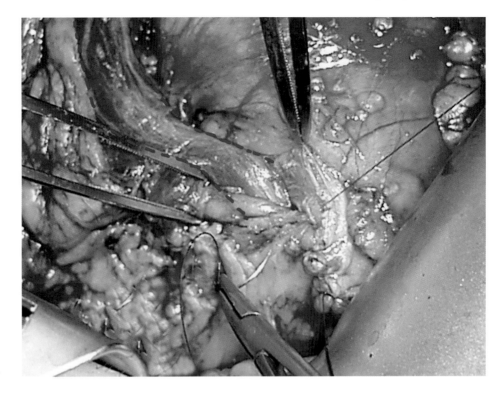

Figure 4.29

18. With either technique the detrusor muscle is then closed over the distal 5 to 6 cm of transplant ureter (broken blue line) to prevent reflux (Figures 4.29 and 4.30).

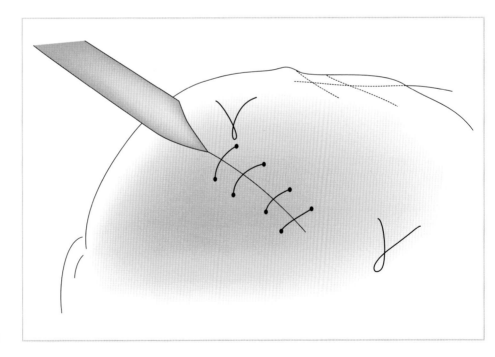

Figure 4.30

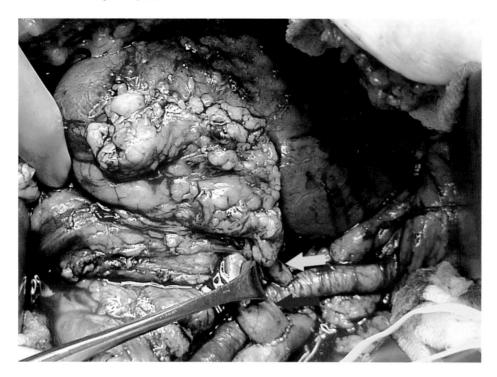

Figure 4.31

19. The kidney is then placed in a position such that there is no angulation or twisting of the renal artery (yellow arrow) or the renal vein (blue arrow) (Figure 4.31). The incision is then closed by approximating the fascia using a running or interrupted suture.

Surgical Variations

a) Pediatric Recipient Kidney Transplant

The surgical techniques for kidney transplantation in pediatric recipients, especially in the older child, are not very different from the techniques described for adult recipients.

1. For recipients ≤20 kg, we prefer an intraperitoneal approach using a kidney from an adult-sized living donor. The kidney is placed on the right side, behind the right colon (Figure 4.32). Anastomosis is generally to the distal aorta and cava.

2. The procedure is started with a long midline incision to enter the peritoneal cavity. The right colon (blue arrow) is mobilized and reflected medially to expose the right

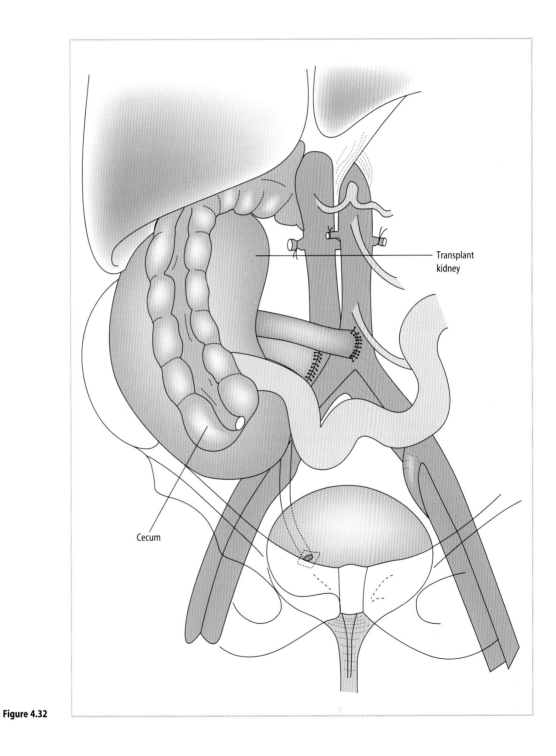

Figure 4.32

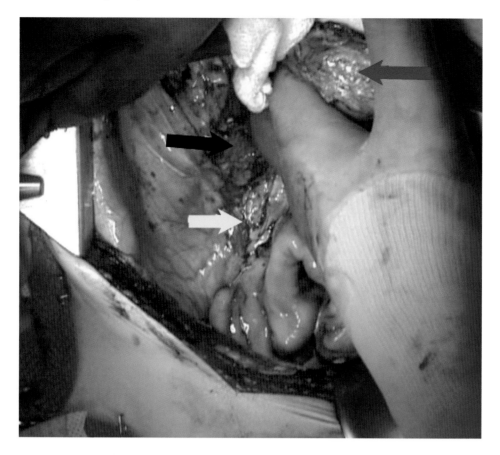

Figure 4.33

retroperitoneal area, including the psoas muscle (black arrow) and the distal aorta/
proximal iliac vessels (yellow arrow) (Figure 4.33).

3. The infrarenal cava (blue arrow), infrarenal aorta (yellow arrow), and proximal iliac
vessels are isolated and encircled (Figure 4.34).

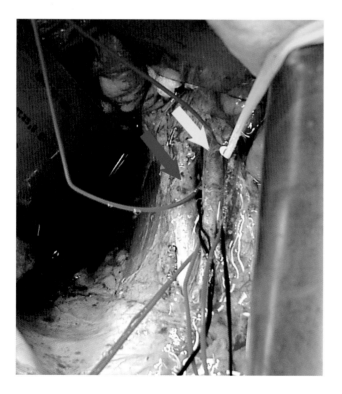

Figure 4.34

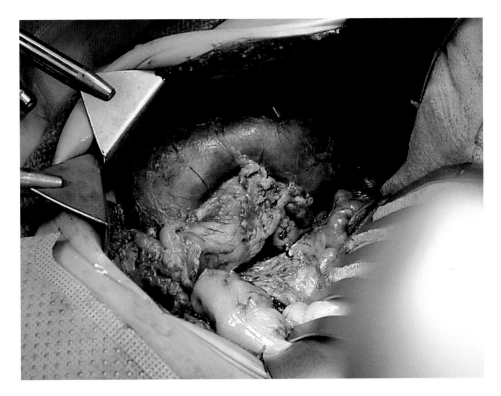

Figure 4.35

4. The renal artery is anastomosed to the distal aorta and the renal vein is anastomosed to the distal cava (Figure 4.35), in a manner similar to that described for adult recipients. The bladder anastomoses can also be performed as previously described for adults. The colon is then returned to its proper position, lying anterior to the transplanted kidney. The incision is then closed.

b) Pediatric Donor En-Bloc Kidneys

Kidney from small pediatric donors (<15 kg) can be used in adult recipients. In this situation, however, both kidneys should be transplanted en bloc into the one recipient.

1. The kidneys are prepared on the back table. The aorta and cava are left intact with the two kidneys. The proximal ends of the cava and aorta are oversewn (Figure 4.36). The distal ends can then be used to perform the anastomoses to the recipient vessels.

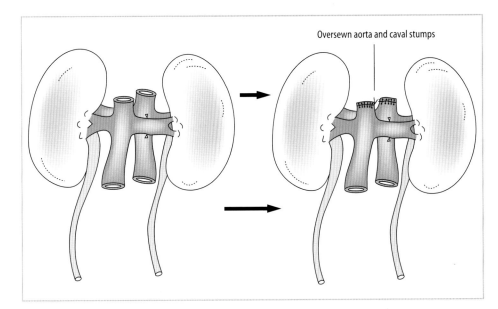

Oversewn aorta and caval stumps

Figure 4.36

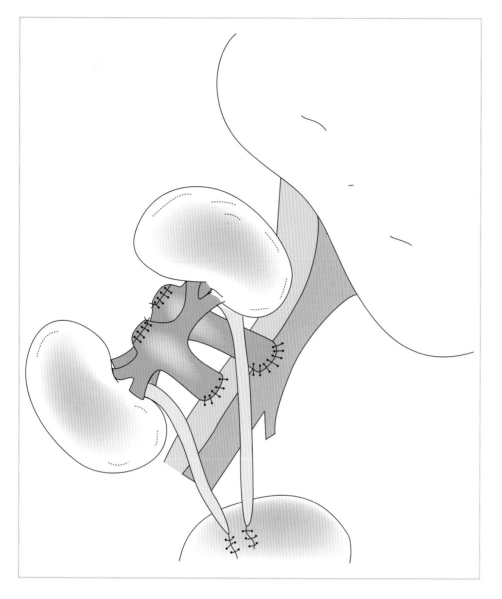

Figure 4.37

2. The anastomoses are performed to the iliac vessels of the recipient. The two ureters can be anastomosed separately into the recipient bladder (Figure 4.37).

c) Multiple Renal Arteries

Multiple renal arteries are present in 10% to 15% of cases. Many different options are possible for reconstruction, depending on size of the vessels, location of the vessels, donor source (living vs. deceased), and quality of the recipient vessels.

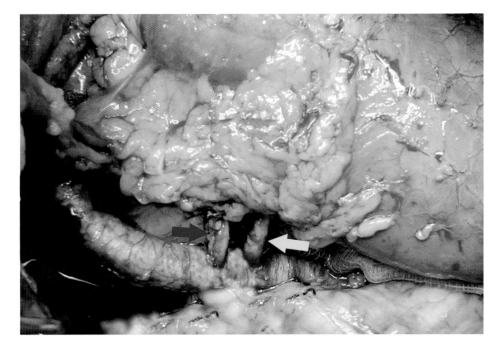

Figure 4.38

1. Often the two arteries (yellow and blue arrow) are implanted separately, either to the external or common iliac vessels (Figure 4.38) ...

2. ... or one to the external iliac and one to the internal iliac artery (Figure 4.39).

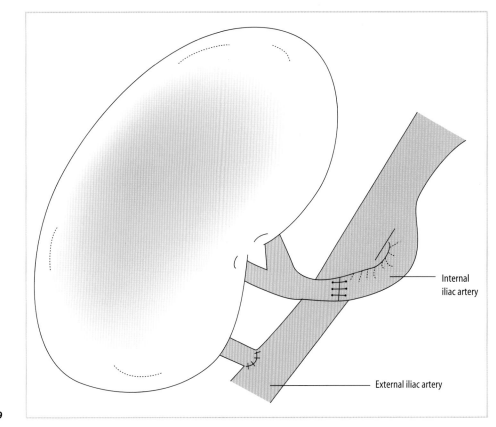

Internal iliac artery

External iliac artery

Figure 4.39

3. The two vessels can be reconstructed on the back table so that only one anastomosis is required in the recipient. If an aortic patch is present on the two vessels, the two patches can be sewn together (Figure 4.40).

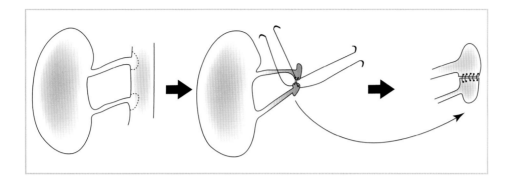

Figure 4.40

4. Another option is to connect one vessel to the other in an end-to-side fashion. As shown in this example with three renal arteries, artery 1 and 2 have been sewn together with a common patch (broken blue line), while artery 3 has been anastomosed to artery 1 in an end-to-side fashion (broken yellow line) (Figure 4.41).

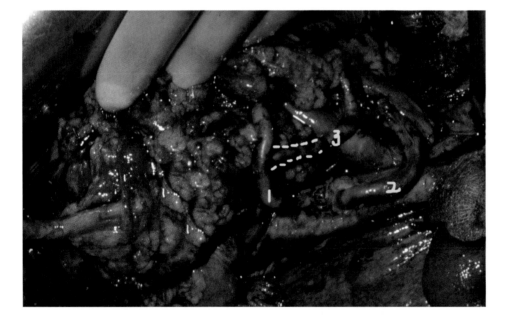

Figure 4.41

Surgical Complications and Their Management

Surgical complications remain an important potential cause of graft loss after kidney transplants. They may also result in graft dysfunction that must be differentiated from medical and immunologic causes of graft dysfunction. The initial presentation of surgical problems may be very similar to nonsurgical problems such as rejection or drug toxicity. Even if these complications do not affect graft function, they nonetheless may account for significant morbidity in the recipient, or may even result in death. For all of these reasons, it is crucial that all persons involved in the postoperative care of kidney transplant recipients be aware of the potential surgical complications that may occur, thus allowing for rapid diagnosis and initiation of treatment. Common surgical complications include the following.

a) Hemorrhage

Bleeding is uncommon after kidney transplants; it usually occurs from unligated vessels in the graft hilum or from the retroperitoneum of the recipient. Risk factors include recipient obesity, the presence of antiplatelet agents, and the need for anticoagulation. A falling hematocrit level, hypotension or tachycardia, and significant flank pain should all raise concern regarding the possibility of bleeding. Surgical exploration is seldom required, because the bleeding often stops spontaneously. However, ongoing transfusion requirements, hemodynamic instability, and compression of the kidney by hematoma are all indications for surgical reexploration.

b) Renal Artery Thrombosis

This complication usually occurs early posttransplant; it is an uncommon event, with an incidence of <1%. However, it is a devastating complication, usually resulting in graft loss. Typically, it occurs secondary to a technical problem, such as intimal dissection or kinking or torsion of the vessels. Presentation is with a sudden cessation of urine output. Diagnosis is easily made with color flow Doppler studies. Urgent thrombectomy is indicated, but the transplanted kidney has no collateral vessels, and its tolerance of warm ischemia is very poor. Therefore, most of these grafts cannot be salvaged and require removal.

c) Renal Artery Stenosis

Stenosis of the renal artery, a late complication, is generally much more common than renal artery thrombosis. Renal artery stenosis has a reported incidence of 1% to 10%. Most cases are identified within the first few years posttransplant. Recipients may present with poorly controlled hypertension, allograft dysfunction, and peripheral edema; physical examination may detect a bruit over the kidney. Doppler studies are a good screening tool with high sensitivity and specificity. A magnetic resonance angiogram or computed tomography (CT) angiogram can be performed to confirm the diagnosis.

First-line treatment for symptomatic lesions uses interventional radiologic techniques, usually angioplasty with or without a stent. Initial success rates of about 80% have been reported with angioplasty, albeit with a fairly significant recurrence rate. Some lesions are less amenable to angioplasty. For example, anastomotic strictures and long strictures are less likely to be treated successfully with angioplasty and have a higher risk of angioplasty complications. Potential complications with any angioplasty procedure include rupture or thrombosis of the vessel, which can lead to graft loss. Surgery is reserved for stenoses that do not respond to radiologic techniques. Possible options include reimplantation of the vessel, patch angioplasty, and surgical bypass. While the success rate with surgery is generally good, it may be technically very difficult because of the extensive fibrosis that often develops around the transplanted kidney. Graft loss at the time of attempted surgical correction is a potential risk.

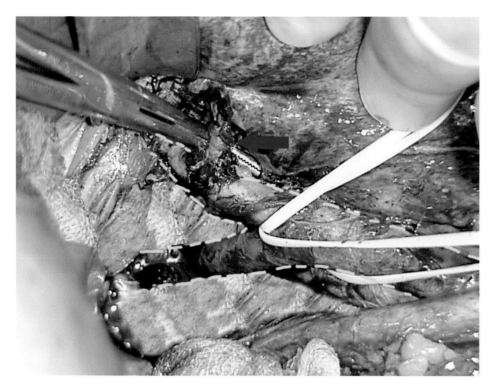

Figure 4.42

1. If surgery is indicated, one useful technique is to use the internal iliac artery to bypass a proximal stenosis. The surgery should be approached from an intraperitoneal route. The transplant renal artery distal to the stenosis is isolated (broken blue line) (Figure 4.42). The internal iliac artery (broken yellow line) is isolated and mobilized deep into the pelvis. Here it is divided (black arrow) (Figure 4.43).

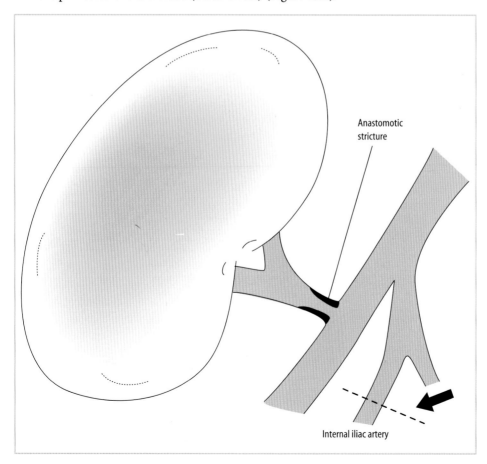

Anastomotic stricture

Internal iliac artery

Figure 4.43

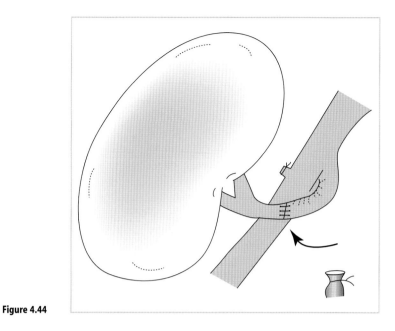

Figure 4.44

2. The transplant renal artery is then divided and anastomosed to the divided internal iliac artery (black arrow) (Figures 4.44 and 4.45).

d) Recipient Arterial Complications

Arterial complications that affect the recipient vessels (most commonly the iliac vessels) are much less common, but can be equally devastating. Early events, such as iliac artery thrombosis or intimal dissection, can be limb-threatening as well as potentially lead to

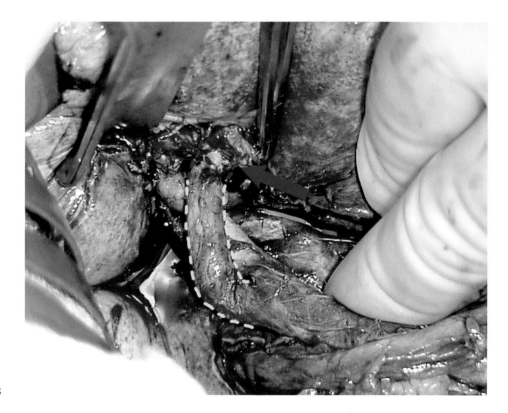

Figure 4.45

graft loss. Late complications, such as pseudoaneurysms or fistulas, can lead to significant hemorrhage. Predisposing risk factors include underlying peripheral vascular disease, deep infections, and insulin-dependent diabetes. Iliac artery thrombosis results in an ischemic extremity, which usually occurs very early postoperatively (at times, even intraoperatively). If the problem is recognized intraoperatively, it should be immediately resolved (e.g. an intimal dissection is repaired by tacking the intima to the arterial wall.) At the end of every transplant procedure, a quick vascular exam and inspection of the lower extremities should be performed. If an ischemic extremity is noted, immediate surgical exploration with balloon thrombectomy is essential to salvage the limb and prevent long-term sequelae.

Occlusive disease of the iliac artery proximal to the site of renal artery anastomoses may clinically mimic renal artery stenosis. Occlusive lesions may develop as a result of progressive peripheral vascular disease, or they may represent an injury from the vascular clamp placed on the artery at the time of the transplant. Patients may present with deteriorating renal function, hypertension, and buttock claudication. On physical examination of such patients, diminished femoral pulse should make the clinician suspicious of occlusive disease. This disease tends to be very amenable to treatment with radiologic techniques such as angioplasty and stenting.

e) Renal Vein Thrombosis

This complication, like its arterial counterpart, usually results in graft loss. Causes include angulation or kinking of the vein, compression by hematomas or lymphoceles, anastomotic stenosis, and extension of an underlying deep venous thrombosis. Most cases occur early, usually within the first 10 days posttransplant. Patients may present with a tender swollen graft and/or hematuria. Doppler studies are again the best diagnostic tool. Urgent thrombectomy is indicated, but for most patients, graft salvage is not possible; graft nephrectomy is usually required. However, graft salvage is possible if thrombectomy can be achieved soon after the event (usually within 1 hour). Even if graft salvage is not possible, urgent reexploration should be performed, because such grafts can become very swollen and edematous, with a risk for rupture and subsequent hemorrhage.

f) Venous Thromboembolism

Venous thromboembolic complications that affect the recipient vessels (deep venous thrombosis and pulmonary embolism) are not uncommon. The incidence of deep venous thrombosis is close to 5%; the incidence of pulmonary embolism is 1%. Usually two peaks in incidence are reported – one early in the postoperative period (likely related to operative factors) and a second peak at around 4 weeks (perhaps related to a rising hematocrit level). Risk factors include older recipient age, diabetes, thrombophilic disorders, and a history of deep venous thrombosis. For recipients with such risk factors, prophylaxis with low-dose heparin is recommended.

g) Aneurysms and Fistulas

Other potential vascular problems include arteriovenous fistulas and aneurysms. Most aneurysms that occur posttransplant are pseudoaneurysms, usually resulting from partial disruption of the arterial anastomosis. Some aneurysms are associated with a local infection, though this association is more common after pancreas transplants. Patients may be asymptomatic, with the abnormality being noted on a routine ultrasound exam. However, hypotension and abdominal pain due to rupture of the aneurysm may also occur. Sometimes, expansion of the aneurysm results in local pressure symptoms before rupture. Ultrasound is a good screening test, but a further definitive tool, such as angiography, is necessary – unless the patient presents with a rupture, in which case an immediate repair is indicated. The technique of repair depends on the presence or absence of infection or if the patient presents with massive bleeding. If either infection or massive bleeding is present, graft salvage is usually not possible; instead, graft nephrectomy and repair of the recipient vessels with autogenous vein usually represents the best option. In a more elective setting without infection, pseudoaneurysm repair and graft salvage may be possible.

Arteriovenous fistulas may occur in the kidney graft parenchyma after a biopsy. They are easily detected by Doppler studies. Asymptomatic fistulas can simply be observed, because most will resolve spontaneously. Fistulas that occur with significant hematuria can be managed by selective arterial catheterization and embolization.

h) Urologic Complications

Urinary tract complications, manifesting as leakage or obstruction, generally occur in 2% to 10% of kidney recipients. The underlying cause is often related to poor blood supply and to ischemia of the transplant ureter. Rarely life-threatening, urinary tract complications can result in significant morbidity for immunocompromised recipients or in significant, long-term graft damage.

Urine Leaks

Leakage most commonly occurs early. It is usually from the anastomotic site. Causes other than ischemia include undue tension created by a short ureter, and direct surgical injury to the ureter (usually at the time of procurement). Presentation is usually early (before the 5th posttransplant week); symptoms include fever, pain, swelling at the graft site, increased creatinine level, decreased urine output, and cutaneous urinary drainage. Diagnosis can be confirmed with a hippurate renal scan. Early surgical exploration with ureteral reimplantation is indicated for very early leaks, for large leaks, or for leaks that do not respond to conservative measures. Many leaks, however, may be managed by using the principles of drainage and stenting. Drain placement to evacuate a urinoma and urinary tract stenting (usually by percutaneous nephrostomy and stent placement) can successfully manage many urine leaks posttransplant.

Obstruction

Obstruction may present early or late. Early obstruction may be due to edema, blood clots, hematoma, and kinking. Late obstruction is generally due to scarring and fibrosis from chronic ischemia. Presentation is usually with an elevated serum creatinine level. An ultrasound exam, assessing for hydronephrosis, is a good initial tool. A furosemide renogram is useful in less obvious cases of obstruction; a percutaneous nephrostogram is the most specific test. Initial treatment with percutaneous transluminal dilatation (PTD), followed by internal or external stent placement, has yielded good results. If such treatment is not successful, then surgical intervention is indicated. For very distal strictures, the transplanted ureter may be reimplanted into the bladder. If the stricture

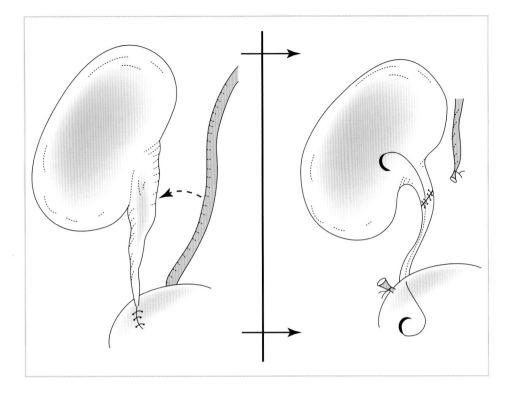

Figure 4.46

is more proximal, then the native ureter can be used to bypass the obstruction (Figure 4.46).

Hematuria

Another potential urinary complication is hematuria. Mild hematuria is not infrequent. It is usually observed in the first 12 to 24 hours posttransplant. In most patients, it resolves spontaneously. More extensive bleeding may result in retained blood clots and urinary tract obstruction, which is the most common cause of sudden cessation of urine output immediately posttransplant. Continuous bladder irrigation usually restores diuresis, but if not, cystoscopy may be necessary to evacuate the clot and cauterize the source of the bleeding.

Lymphoceles

The incidence of lymphoceles (fluid collections of lymph that generally result from cut lymphatic vessels in the recipient) is 1% to 15%. Careful ligation of all lymphatics seen at the time of iliac vessel dissection can help minimize the incidence of lymphoceles. Lymphoceles usually do not occur until at least 2 weeks posttransplant. Symptoms, if present, are generally related to the mass effect and compression of nearby structures (e.g., ureter, iliac vein). An ultrasound exam confirms a fluid collection, but percutaneous aspiration may be necessary to rule out other complications such as urinoma, hematoma, or abscess.

Many lymphoceles are clinically asymptomatic; if so, they usually are less than 3 cm, resolve spontaneously over time, and do not require any therapeutic intervention.

Symptomatic lymphoceles require drainage, which can be achieved either by surgery or by percutaneous radiologic methods. The standard surgical treatment is creation of a peritoneal window to allow for drainage of the lymphatic fluid into the peritoneal cavity, where it can be absorbed. Either a laparoscopic or an open approach can be used. Another option is percutaneous insertion of a drainage catheter, with or without scle-

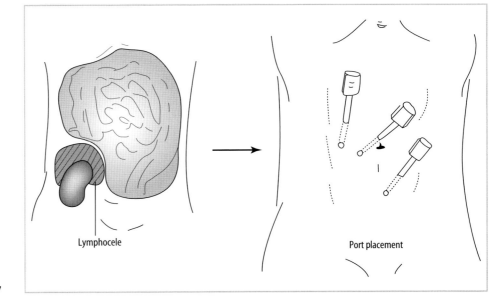

Figure 4.47

rotherapy; however, this option is associated with some risk of recurrence or infection. A variant approach is to initially drain the lymphoceles percutaneously after inserting a drainage catheter; sclerotherapy is then attempted via this catheter. If the lymphoceles continue to drain, if they recur, or if they were not amenable to percutaneous drainage initially, then a laparoscopic or open peritoneal window should be created surgically.

1. Laparoscopically the lymphocele is drained from the inside of the peritoneal cavity (Figure 4.47).

2. The lymphocele is identified from the inside of the peritoneal cavity by its bulging (solid arrows) (Figure 4.48a). Intraoperative ultrasound may be useful to identify the exact location of the lymphocele. A circular rim of peritoneum is excised (Figure 4.48b) to allow for internal drainage of the lymphocele (Figure 4.48c).

Wound Complications

Wound complications are now probably the most common types of complication posttransplant. They usually do not result in graft loss or death, but can result in

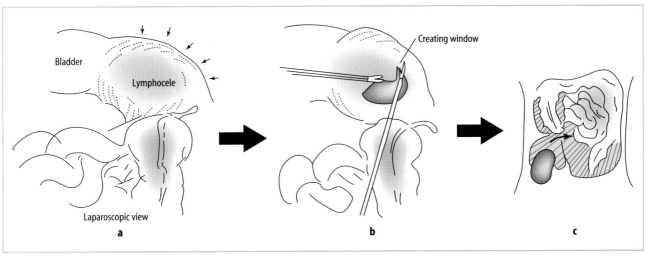

Figure 4.48

significant morbidity with prolonged hospitalization or rehospitalization. In certain situations, wound complications may also be associated with inferior graft survival rates. Wound complications can be broadly categorized into infectious and noninfectious complications.

Wound Infections

Wound infections generally occur earlier after a surgical procedure as compared with noninfectious wound complications. The incidence of wound infections after kidney transplants is about 5%, a figure consistent with that reported in the urologic literature for nontransplant procedures of similar magnitude. A kidney transplant is generally considered a clean-contaminated case: the bladder is opened, and some urine is usually spilled in the operative field. The added stress of immunosuppressive drugs, including prednisone, probably also has some impact on the risk for wound infections posttransplant.

Wound infections may be either superficial or deep (i.e., to the fascia). Deep infections are generally related to complications such as urinary leaks. Superficial infections, more common than deep infections, are related to contamination from skin organisms or from urine (during the bladder anastomosis). Obesity is probably the biggest risk factor for a wound infection posttransplant. Other risk factors include a urine leak, the need for a reoperation, and perhaps the use of the newer, more powerful immunosuppressive medications.

Treatment depends on whether the wound infection is superficial or deep. Deep infections are treated with drainage – either by surgery or by percutaneous drainage – and, usually, antibiotics. Superficial infections are usually treated by opening the surgical wound and allowing it to heal by secondary intention; antibiotics are usually not necessary, unless the recipient has significant cellulitis or systemic symptoms.

Noninfectious Wound Complications

These include early fascial dehiscence and late incisional hernias. Recipient obesity is the most significant risk factor. These will generally require surgical repair.

Selected Readings

1. Adams J, Gudemann C, Tonshoff B, Mehls O, Wiesel M. Renal transplantation in small children – a comparison between surgical procedures. Eur Urol 2001;40(5):552–556.
2. Ali-El-Dein B, Osman Y, Shokeir AA, Shehab El-Dein AB, Sheashaa H, Ghoneim MA. Multiple arteries in live donor renal transplantation: surgical aspects and outcomes. J Urol 2003;169(6):2013–2017.
3. Bay WH, Hebert LA. The living donor in kidney transplantation. Ann Intern Med 1987;106:719–727.
4. Bitker MO, Benoit G. Surgical aspects of kidney transplantation in France in 1997. Eur Urol 1998;34(1): 1–5.
5. Breza J, Navratil P. Renal transplantation in adults. BJU Int 1999;84(2):216–223.
6. Calne RY, Alexondre GP, Murray JE. A study of the effects of drugs in prolonged survival of homologous renal transplants in dogs. Ann NY Acad Sci 1962;99:743–749.
7. Carrel A. The transplantation of organs. NY Med J 1914;99:839–851.
8. Cecka JM, Terasaki PI. The UNOS scientific renal transplant registry. Clin Transplant 1992;6:1–16.
9. Doehn C, Fornara P, Fricke L, Jocham D. Laparoscopic fenestration of posttransplant lymphoceles. Surg Endosc 2002;16(4):690–695.
10. Greneir N, Douws C, Morel D, et al. Detection of vascular complications in renal allografts with color Doppler flow imaging. Radiology 1991;178:217–223.
11. Guthrie CC. Blood vessel surgery and its applications. New York: Longmans Green, 1912.
12. Hakim NS, Benedetti E, Pirenne J, et al. Complications of ureterovesical anastomosis in kidney transplant patients: the Minnesota experience. Clin Transplant 1994;8:504–507.
13. Hamilton DNH, Reid WA. Yu Yu Voronoy and the first human kidney allograft. Surg Gynecol Obstet 1984;159:289–294 .
14. Johnson EM, Remucal M, Pandian K, et al. Complications and risks of renal donation. J Am Soc Nephrol 1996;7(9):1934.

15. Jones JW, Hunter DR, Matas AJ. Successful percutaneous treatment of ureteral stenosis after renal transplantation. Transplant Proc 1993;25:1038.
16. Kinnaert P, Hall M, Janssen F, Vereerstraeten P, Toussaint C, Van Geertruyden J. Ureteral stenosis after kidney transplantation: true incidence and long-term follow-up after surgical correction. J Urol 1985;133:17–20.
17. Makowka L, Sher L. Handbook of Organ Transplantation. Georgetown, TX: R.G. Landes, 1995.
18. Matas AJ, Tellis VA, Karwa GL. Comparison of post-transplant urologic complications following extravesical ureteroneocystostomy by a "single-stitch" or "mucosal" anastomosis. Clin Transplant 1987;1:159–163.
19. Merrill JP, Murray JE, Harrison JH. Successful homotransplantation of the human kidney between identical twins. JAMA 1956;160:277–282.
20. Murray JE, Merrill JP, Harrison JH, et al. Prolonged survival of human-kidney homografts by immunosuppressive drug therapy. N Engl J Med 1963;268:1315–1323.
21. Osman Y, Shokeir A, Ali-el-Dein B, et al. Vascular complications after liver donor renal transplantation: study of risk factors and effects on graft and patient survival. J Urol 2003;169(3):859–862.
22. Plainfosse MC, Menoyo Calonge V, Beylouve-Mainard C, Glotz D, Duboust. Vascular complications in the adult kidney transplant recipient. J Clin Ultrasound 1992;20:517–527.
23. Shoskes DA, Hanbury D, Cranston D, Morris PJ. Urological complications in 1,000 consecutive renal transplant recipients. J Urol 1995;153(1):18–21.
24. Suthanthiran M, Strom TB. Renal transplantation. N Engl J Med 1994;331:36.
25. Thomalla JV, Lingeman JE, Leapman SB, Filo RS. The manifestation and management of late urological complications in renal transplant recipients: use of the urological armamentarium. J Urol 1985;134:944–948.
26. Zinke H, Woods JE, Aguila JJ. Experience with lymphoceles after renal transplantation. Surgery 1973;77:444–450.

5

Pancreas Transplantation

Abhinav Humar, Khalid O. Khwaja, and David E.R. Sutherland

Standard Procedure

The world's first clinical pancreas transplant was performed at the University of Minnesota on December 16, 1966, to treat a uremic diabetic patient. Since that time, nearly 15,000 pancreas transplants have been performed around the world, the majority in the United States.

A successful pancreas transplant can establish normoglycemia and insulin independence in diabetic recipients. It also has the potential to halt progression of some secondary complications of diabetes. No current method of exogenous insulin administration can produce a euglycemic, insulin-independent state akin to that achievable with a technically successful pancreas graft. Pancreas transplants are performed to improve the quality of life over that achieved by the alternative treatment – exogenous insulin administration. But as a treatment for type 1 diabetes, pancreas transplants have not yet achieved widespread application in all diabetics because the operative procedure is associated with complications, albeit of increasingly lower incidence, coupled with long-term side effects of immunosuppression, which together may exceed the complications due to diabetes. Thus, pancreas transplants are preferentially performed in diabetic patients with renal failure who are also candidates for a kidney transplant, and who would require immunosuppression to prevent rejection of the kidney. A pancreas transplant alone is appropriate for diabetics whose day-to-day quality of life is so poor from a management standpoint (e.g., labile serum glucose with ketoacidosis or hypoglycemic episodes, progression of severe diabetic retinopathy, nephropathy, neuropathy, or enteropathy) that chronic immunosuppression is justified to achieve insulin independence.

a) Pretransplant Evaluation

Pancreas transplant procedures may be divided into three major recipient categories: (1) simultaneous pancreas-kidney (SPK) transplant; (2) pancreas transplant after a kidney transplant (PAK); and (3) pancreas transplant alone (PTA). All uremic type 1 diabetics who are candidates for a kidney transplant should be considered potential candidates for a pancreas transplant. The benefits of the pancreas transplant (e.g., insulin independence, protection of the new kidney from recurrent disease) should be weighed, on an individual basis, against the risks of the procedure (surgical complications, increased incidence of infection, malignancy, etc.).

The pretransplant evaluation does not differ substantially from that which is undertaken for diabetic kidney transplant recipients. Examination of the cardiovascular system is most important because significant coronary artery disease may be present without symptoms. Noninvasive testing may not identify such disease, so coronary angiography is performed routinely. In PTA candidates, detailed neurologic, ophthalmologic, metabolic, and renal function testing may be needed to assess the degree of progression of secondary complications. Once patients are placed on a waiting list, their medical condition should be reassessed yearly or more frequently.

b) Surgical Technique

The initial preparation of the donor pancreas is a crucial component of a successful transplant. Examination at this time is often the best and only way to confirm suitability of the organ for transplantation. If sclerotic, calcific, or markedly discolored, the pancreas should not be used. Prior to implantation, a surgical procedure is undertaken to remove the spleen and any excess duodenum, ligate blood vessels at the root of the mesentery, and perform a vascular reconstruction to connect the donor superior mesenteric and splenic arteries, most commonly using a reversed segment of donor iliac artery as a "Y graft." The pancreas graft is then implanted via an anastomosis of the aforementioned arterial graft to the recipient common iliac artery and a venous anastomosis of the donor portal vein to the recipient iliac vein or superior mesenteric vein, using an intraperitoneal approach. Generally, the kidney is placed in the left iliac fossa and the pancreas in the right iliac fossa during SPK transplantation. Once the pancreas is revascularized, a drainage procedure must be performed to handle the pancreatic exocrine secretions. Options include anastomosing the donor duodenum to the recipient bladder or to the small bowel, the latter either in continuity or to a Roux-en-Y limb.

c) Postoperative Care

In general, pancreas transplant recipients do not require intensive care monitoring in the postoperative period. Laboratory values – serum glucose, hemoglobin, electrolytes, and amylase – are monitored daily, the former more frequently if normoglycemia is not immediately achieved. Nasogastric suction and intravenous fluids are continued for the first several days until bowel function returns. In the early postoperative period, regular insulin is infused to maintain plasma glucose levels at less than 150 mg/dL, because chronic hyperglycemia may be detrimental to beta cells. In recipients who undergo bladder drainage, a urinary catheter is left in place for 10 to 14 days. At most centers, some form of prophylaxis is instituted against bacterial, fungal, and viral infections. In addition, many centers routinely institute some form of prophylaxis against venous or arterial thrombosis of the allograft.

One crucial aspect of posttransplant care is monitoring for acute rejection and complications (both surgical and medical) or the pancreas graft. Rejection episodes may be identified by an increase in serum creatinine (in SPK recipients), a decrease in urinary amylase (in recipients with bladder drainage), an increase in serum amylase, and, in the later stages, an increase in serum glucose levels. In cases where a kidney transplant biopsy would not be helpful (PAK or PTA), a percutaneous biopsy of the pancreas can be obtained under ultrasound or computed tomography (CT) guidance or via cystoscopy in bladder-drained allografts.

d) Results

The International Pancreas Transplant Registry (IPTR) maintains data on pancreas transplants. Analyses of IPTR data have been published yearly since the mid-1980s. The results (particularly as measured by long-term insulin independence) have continually improved over time. Patient survival rates are not significantly different between the three main recipient categories and are >90% at 3 years posttransplant. Most deaths are from preexisting cardiovascular disease; the mortality risk of a pancreas transplant per se is extremely low (e.g., patient survival at 1 year for PTA recipients is >95%). Pancreas graft survival rates at 1 year remain higher in the SPK (85%) than in the PAK category and PTA (80%) categories, according to IPTR data. The differences, in part, are due to the decreased ability to monitor for rejection episodes in enteric-drained solitary pancreas transplant recipients. With improving immunosuppressive protocols and the decreasing incidence of acute rejection, the difference between the three categories has been steadily decreasing since the late 1990s.

e) Islet Cell Transplantation

Islet cell transplantation involves the extraction of islets of Langerhans from organ donors through a complex purification process. These are the cells responsible for the production of insulin. These cells are then injected into the recipient, usually into the portal vein. They then engraft into the parenchyma of the liver and secrete insulin. If successful, islet cell transplants can provide excellent moment-to-moment control of blood glucose, without the need for a major surgical procedure necessary with a whole organ transplant. The problem to date, however, has been very poor long-term results with these types of transplants. More recently, however, some centers have reported encouraging results with islet transplants, with insulin independence rates similar to those seen with pancreas transplants. Several modifications have allowed for these improved results including improvements in the isolation and preparation of the islets and immunosuppressive regimens that do not involve the use of steroids.

Benching the Pancreas from a Deceased Donor

Careful benching of the pancreas graft is a crucial part of the operative procedure, and in some ways may be the most important part of it. Preparation of the organ begins with the multiorgan procurement from the deceased donor, as has been described previously. Minimal handling of the pancreas during the procurement is important to minimize any trauma to the organ. After the organ is removed, the period of cold ischemia to the graft should be minimized, as there is good evidence to suggest that the incidence of surgical complications after transplant increases with prolonged (>20 hours) preservation time.

The basic steps involved in bench preparation of the cadaver pancreas prior to implantation are as follows:

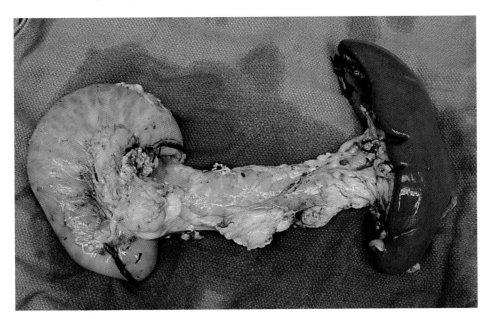

Figure 5.1

- Careful inspection of the organ for quality and evidence of trauma
- Removal of the spleen
- Removal of excess fat and surrounding tissues from the body and tail
- Isolation of the splenic and superior mesenteric arteries and the portal vein, with removal of excess ganglion tissue from the posterior aspect of the pancreas
- Removal of excess duodenum
- Ligation of vessels at the root of the mesentery
- Placement of a Y graft on the two arterial vessels

a) Surgical Procedure

1. Bench preparation of the pancreas graft begins with a careful evaluation of the appearance and feel of the pancreas. Grafts with significant fatty infiltration into the parenchyma, or areas of traumatic injury, or a hard fibrotic feel to palpation should not be used. A suitable (Figure 5.1) vs. an unsuitable pancreas (Figure 5.2) for transplant are shown.

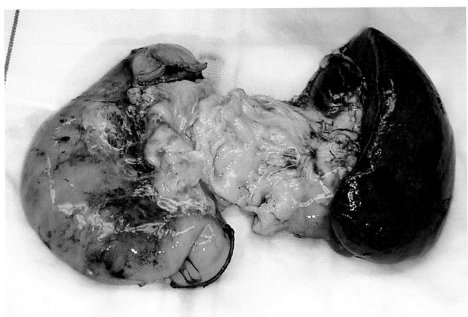

Figure 5.2

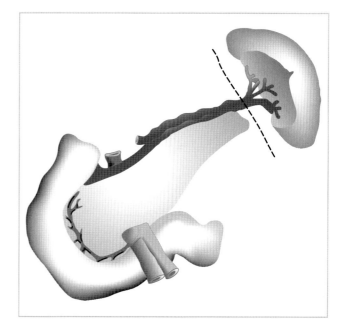

Figure 5.3

2. Splenectomy should be performed by dividing the splenic artery (red arrow) and vein close to the splenic hilum (Figures 5.3 and 5.4). The pancreatic parenchyma can sometimes extend far into the splenic hilum (broken blue line) (Figure 5.4), and care should be taken not to injure the tail of the pancreas.

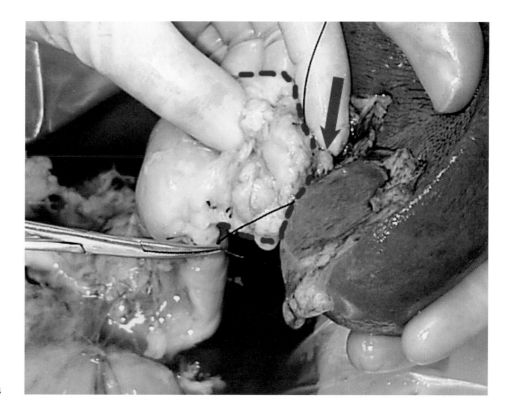

Figure 5.4

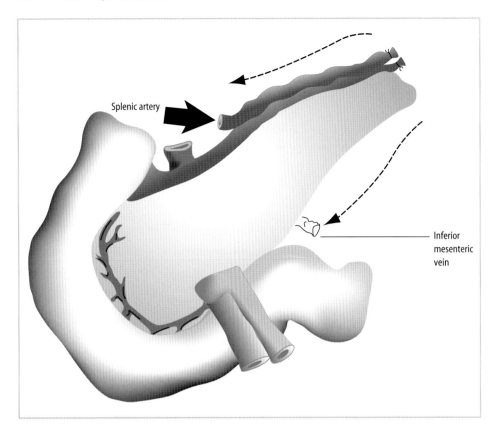

Figure 5.5

3. Excess tissue along the superior and inferior aspect of the body of the pancreas is then ligated. Along the superior border of the pancreas, care should be taken to not injure the splenic artery (solid black arrow) (Figure 5.5). The orifice of the splenic artery is visualized at the medial aspect of the upper border of the body, and tagged with a stitch for easy identification. At the inferior border of the body, the medial aspect is marked by the inferior mesenteric vein (blue arrow), which should be ligated (Figure 5.6).

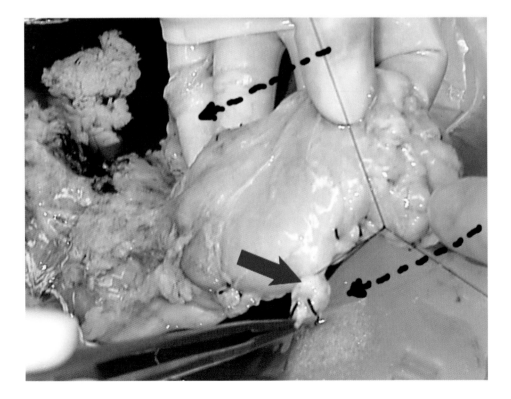

Figure 5.6

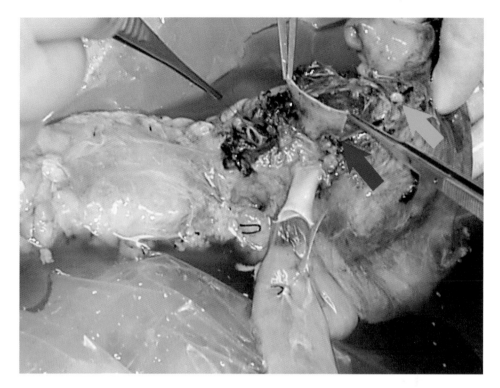

Figure 5.7

4. The head of the pancreas is then approached from its posterior aspect. The common bile duct (green arrow) is identified and suture ligated. The portal vein (blue arrow) is identified and dissected free for a short distance to allow for easier anastomosis in the recipient (Figure 5.7).

5. Similarly, the superior mesenteric artery (yellow arrow) is mobilized by dissecting and ligating the surrounding ganglion tissue (Figure 5.8). Care should be taken not to carry the dissection too close to the pancreatic parenchyma, for fear of injuring the

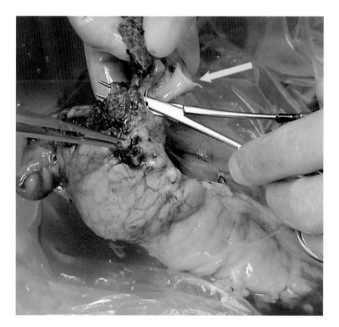

Figure 5.8

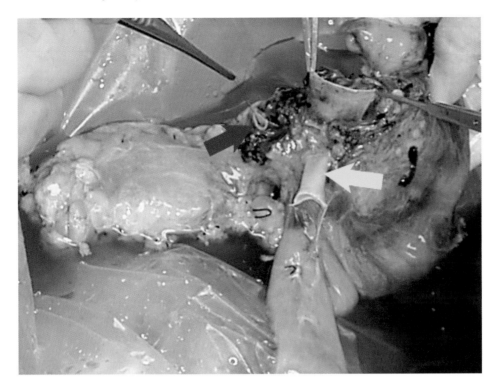

Figure 5.9

inferior pancreaticoduodenal artery. Similarly, excess tissue around the origin of the splenic artery (red arrow) is ligated (Figure 5.9).

6. The pancreas is then approached from its anterior aspect. Lymphatic and ganglion tissue along the superior aspect of the head are ligated. The proximal duodenal cuff staple line (which should be distal to the pylorus) is inverted with a running non-absorbable suture (Figure 5.10). Similarly, the long duodenal-jejunal segment distally is dissected off the pancreas. If a bladder-drained graft is planned, the duodenal cuff should be kept short to minimize metabolic losses. The excess bowel can then be divided and

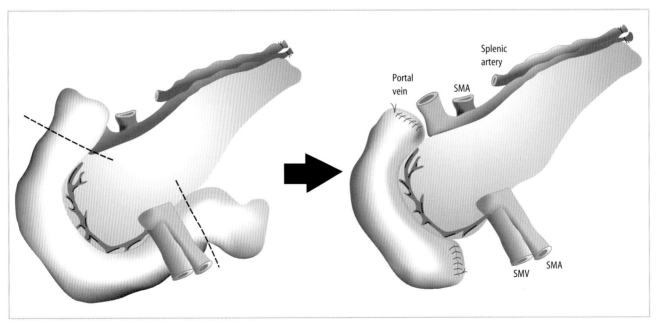

Figure 5.10

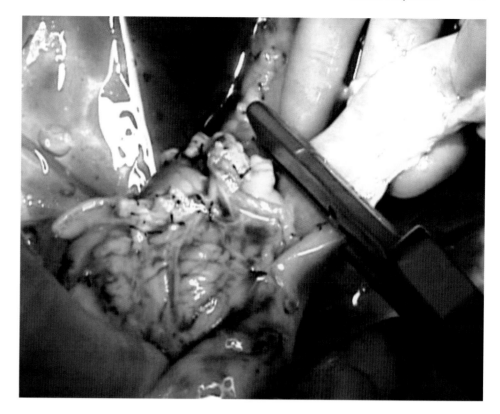

Figure 5.11

discarded using a stapling device; the staple line is oversewn (Figure 5.11). Alternatively, if the exocrine drainage anastomosis is to be done using a stapling device, the distal segment can be left long to allow for introduction of the stapler. (SMA, superior mesenteric artery; SMV, superior mesenteric vein.)

7. Again, looking at the pancreas from its anterior aspect, redundant tissue in the area of the root of the transverse mesocolon is ligated. Finally the root of the mesentery, which contains the superior mesenteric artery and vein (SMA and SMV) (black and gray arrows) is either serially ligated or divided with a vascular stapler (Figure 5.12). The staple line is then oversewn.

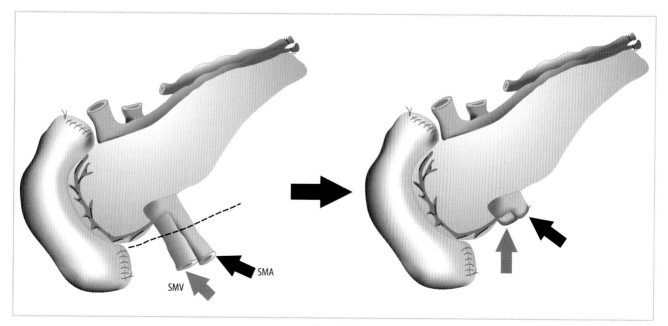

Figure 5.12

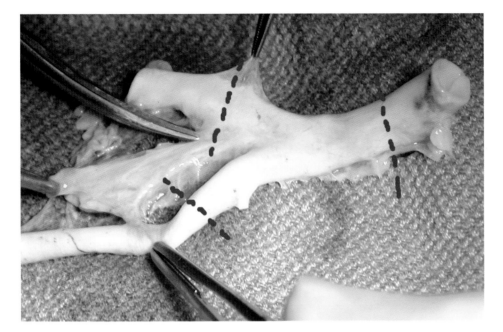

Figure 5.13

8. Preparations are now made to place the arterial Y graft onto the two arterial vessels to create one arterial orifice for anastomosis in the recipient. The distance between the superior mesenteric and splenic arteries is noted, and the donor iliac artery Y graft is trimmed to appropriate length (Figures 5.13 and 5.14).

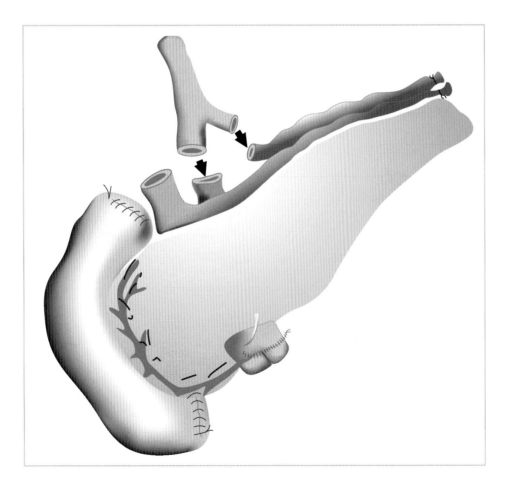

Figure 5.14

9. An end-to-end anastomosis is fashioned between the internal iliac artery stump of the Y graft and the splenic artery (red arrow) of the pancreas graft (Figure 5.15). The external iliac artery limb of the Y graft should then be cut to appropriate length so that it lies next to the superior mesenteric artery (yellow arrow) without any redundancy.

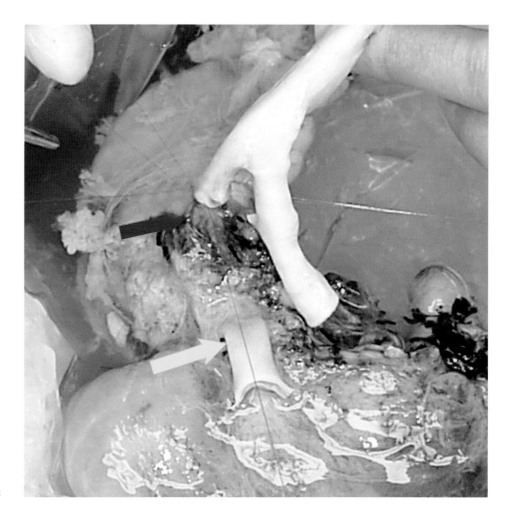

Figure 5.15

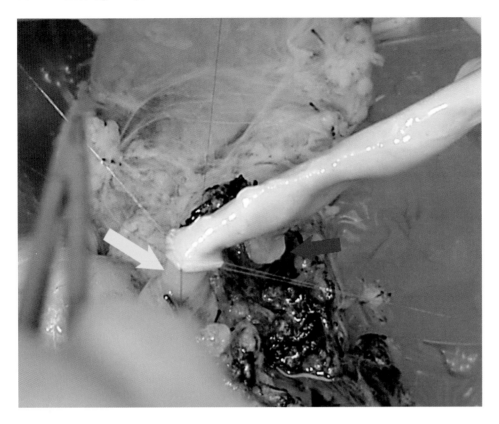

Figure 5.16

10. The end of the external iliac artery of the Y graft is then anastomosed to the superior mesenteric artery (yellow arrow), again in an end-to-end fashion (Figure 5.16).

11. The pancreas graft is now ready for implantation (Figure 5.17).

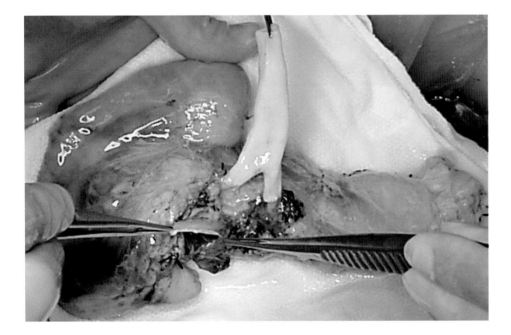

Figure 5.17

Simultaneous Pancreas Kidney (SPK): Systemic/Enteric Drainage

A pancreas transplant is most commonly performed in conjunction with a simultaneous kidney transplant (Figure 5.18). The pancreas is often drained into the systemic circulation, usually by connecting the portal vein of the graft to the iliac vein of the recipient. This drains the endocrine secretions into the systemic circulation. The exocrine secretions can then be managed by connecting the donor duodenum to the recipient bladder or the bowel. Alternatively, the portal vein of the graft can be drained into the portal circulation, by connecting to the superior mesenteric vein or a large tributary of the vein. Exocrine secretions are then drained into the recipient's bowel, as the pancreas will generally not reach the bladder when drained into the portal circulation.

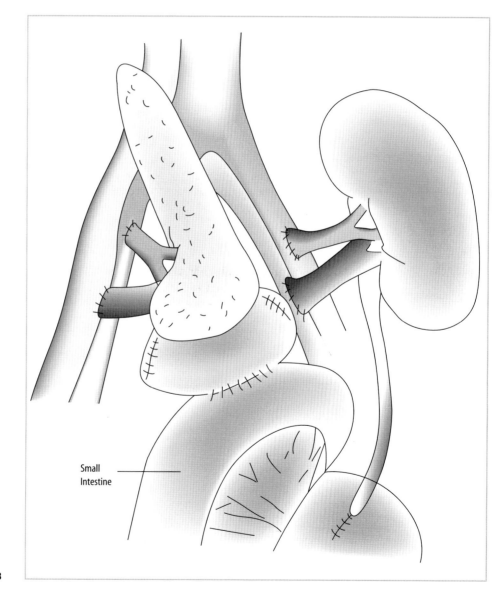

Small Intestine

Figure 5.18

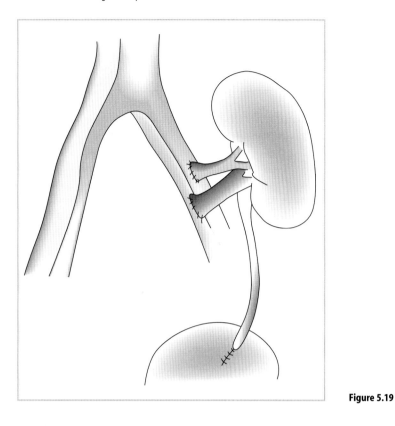

Figure 5.19

a) Surgical Procedure

1. The initial part of the operation usually involves implantation of the kidney. If there is concern regarding prolonged ischemia of the pancreas graft, then this organ can be implanted first, followed by the kidney. In either case, a long midline incision is performed, and the kidney is placed on the left-sided iliac vessels (Figures 5.19 and 5.20).

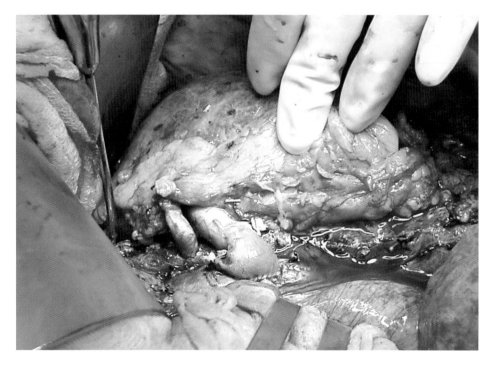

Figure 5.20

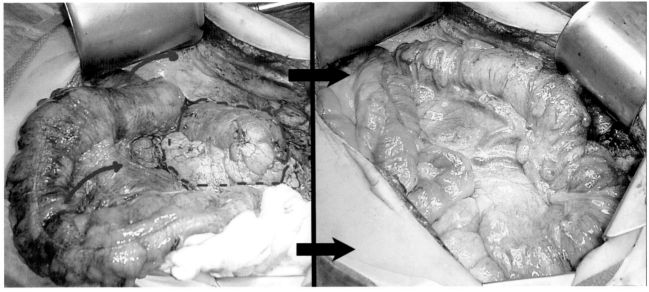

Figure 5.21

2. The sigmoid colon is returned to its position, where it drapes over and covers the kidney (broken blue lines) (Figure 5.21).

3. The retractors are then repositioned in preparation for the dissection of the right-sided iliac vessels. The cecum and right colon are mobilized to the left (solid arrows) to expose the right iliac vessels and to make space for the pancreas graft (Figure 5.22).

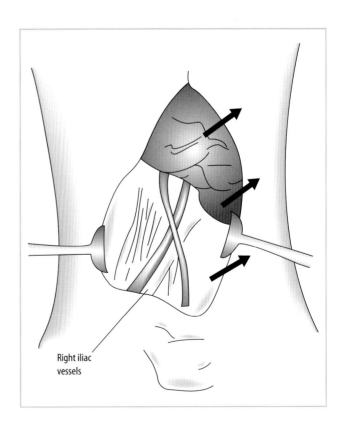

Right iliac
vessels

Figure 5.22

4. A good length of the common iliac, external iliac, and internal iliac arteries is dissected out in preparation for the arterial anastomosis (Figure 5.23). The distal common iliac artery is the preferred site for implantation of the artery (blue mark).

5. The right iliac vein is then completely mobilized (broken blue line), and all the pelvic branches (yellow arrow) of this vein should be divided to allow for the vein to be

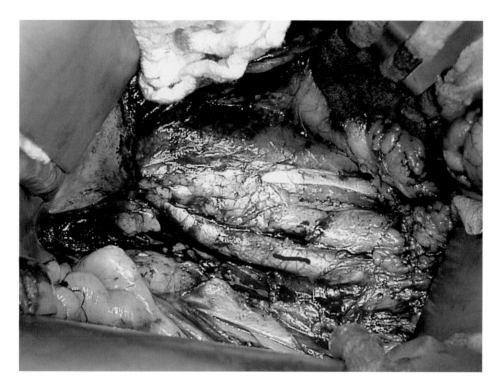

Figure 5.23

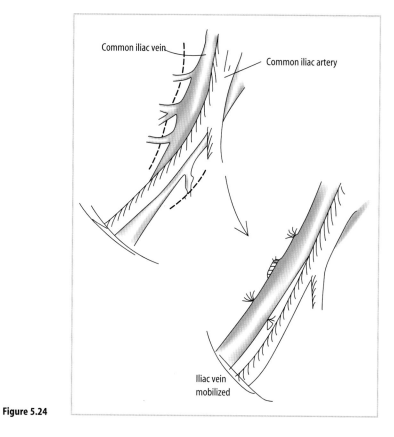

Figure 5.24

in a more superficial location (Figures 5.24 and 5.25). Dividing the branches also allows the vein to be lateral to the artery, which is the correct orientation when the pancreas graft is oriented such that the duodenum is pointing toward the recipient's pelvis. It is wise to suture ligate the stumps of these branches from the main right iliac vein (Figure 5.25) to prevent ligature slippage and troublesome bleeding.

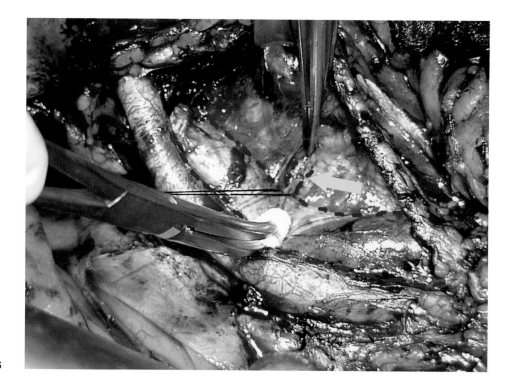

Figure 5.25

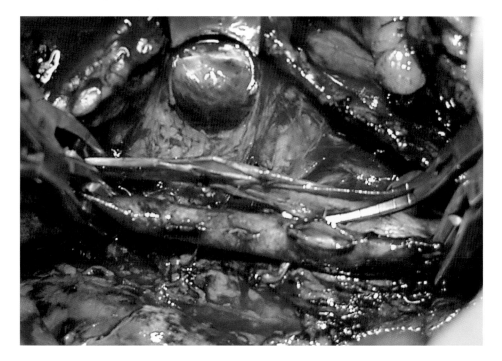

Figure 5.26

6. Clamps are placed on the iliac artery and vein, proximally and distally, and the sites for the venous and arterial anastomosis are determined. Arteriotomy and venotomy are made, and stay sutures are placed (Figure 5.26).

7. The venous anastomosis is performed first, usually using a "4-stitch" technique, to create an end-to-side anastomosis. Care should be taken to ensure that there is no twisting of the vein or that it is left too long (Figure 5.27).

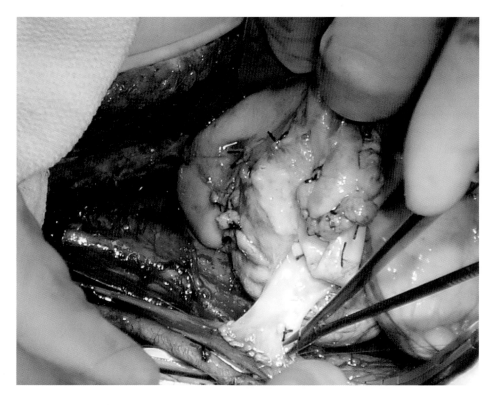

Figure 5.27

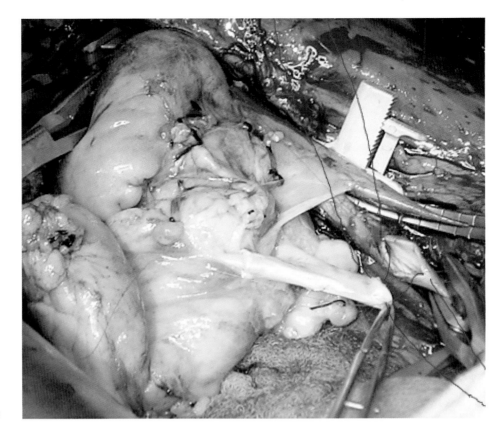

Figure 5.28

8. The arterial Y graft is then trimmed to appropriate length and anastomosed to the common iliac artery, again using a "4-stitch" technique (Figures 5.28 and 5.29).

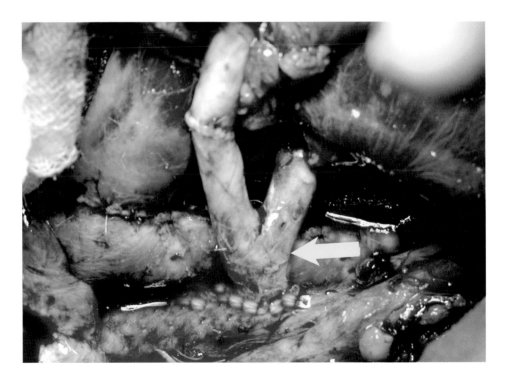

Figure 5.29

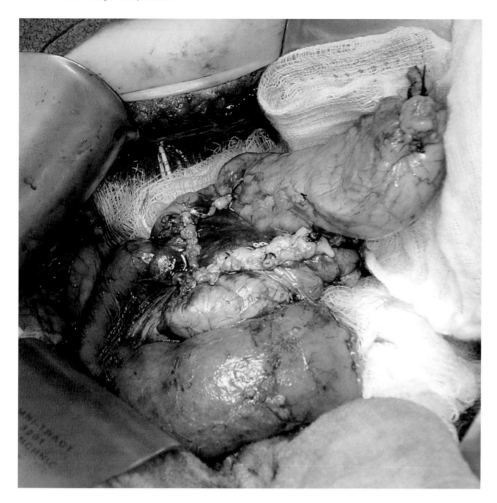

Figure 5.30

9. The clamps are removed and the pancreas allowed to reperfuse (Figure 5.30). The graft should be inspected carefully at this point to control any bleeding.

10. The exocrine secretions can then be drained by connecting the donor duodenum to the bladder or bowel of the recipient. The latter is generally preferred because of a

lower incidence of metabolic and urinary tract problems. However, if there is any concern regarding the donor duodenum, or if ischemia time has been long, a bladder anastomosis is always safer. The bowel anastomosis can be performed either to a Roux-en-Y limb or just simply to the side of the bowel. The site should be fairly proximal to prevent future diarrhea. However, it is more important to choose the portion of the bowel that reaches the donor duodenum without tension. The bowel anastomosis can be performed in a hand-sewn fashion or with a stapler. With a hand-sewn technique, a two-layer anastomosis is done, using a nonabsorbable suture for the outer layer and an absorbable suture for the inner layer. Both layers can be performed with a simple running suture technique. The outer layer of the back wall is placed first after carefully aligning the donor duodenum (blue arrow) and recipient small bowel (yellow arrow) (Figure 5.31).

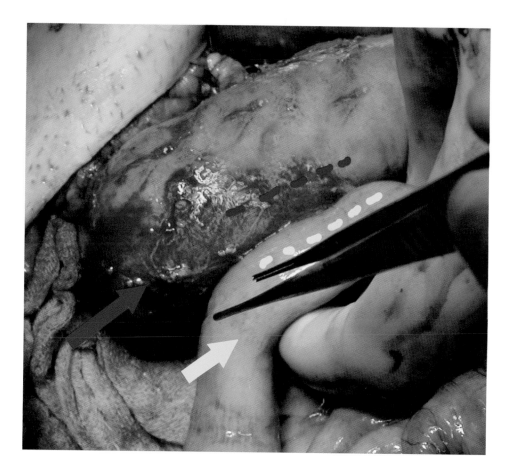

Figure 5.31

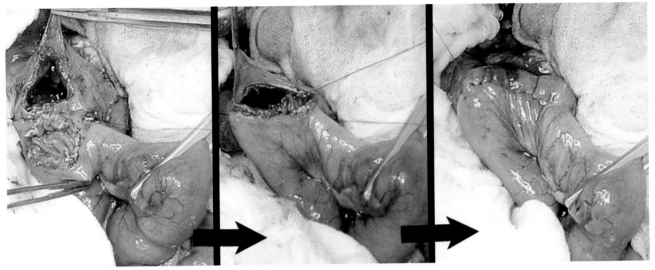

Figure 5.32

11. The duodenum and side of the bowel are opened for a corresponding length. The inner layer of the back wall is performed. The anastomosis is completed by performing the two layers of the anterior wall (Figure 5.32).

Simultaneous Pancreas Kidney: Portal/Enteric Drainage

A. Osama Gaber and Hosein Shokouh-Amiri

The major differences between the portal pancreas operation and other pancreas transplant procedures are related to the location of the portal anastomosis in the recipient, the orientation of the pancreas, and the need to traverse the small bowel mesentery for the arterial anastomosis. The location and size of the portal vein are of utmost importance, as they determine the venous outflow from the transplant pancreas. We have learned through experience that in some patients, portal anastomosis of the donor portal vein is not advisable because of the small size of the portal tributaries. In cases where the superior mesenteric vein or its branches are small or too deeply located in a thickened mesentery, it is preferable to use systemic placement of the gland to the interior vena cava (IVC) or the iliac veins. The orientation of the gland is also important as the donor-to-recipient anastomosis has to be constructed parallel to the axis of the vein to prevent distorting the recipient vein if one attempts to construct a perfectly vertical anastomosis. Since the bowel anastomosis fixes the vein in position, the location of that anastomosis should be chosen so as not to rotate the venous anastomosis, which could increase the risk of venous thrombosis. Finally, the arterial anastomosis site should be chosen in such a way as to prevent redundancy of the arterial conduit, particularly in the donor external and internal iliac limbs. Because the pancreas is a low-flow organ, these vascular considerations are important in preventing arterial or venous thrombosis. In addition, since the majority of portal pancreas transplants are drained enterically, there is no need to keep the duodenal segment short, and a generous duodenal segment helps increase the total amount of flow into the gland and reduces the thrombosis risk.

The operation is generally performed by an intraperitoneal approach through a midline incision (Figure 5.33). In rare cases with extensive intraperitoneal adhesions, a retroperitoneal dissection of the superior mesenteric vein can be performed and then a peritoneal window is constructed to ensure utilization of the peritoneal surface in absorption of potential pancreatic surface leaks and prevent retroperitoneal fluid collections.

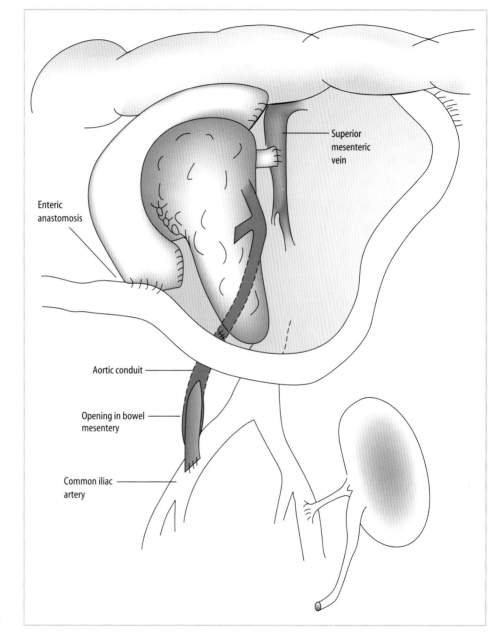

Figure 5.33

a) Surgical Procedure

Bench Preparation of the Pancreas

Preparation of the pancreas for the portal procedure follows the same steps as in other pancreas transplant procedures: closure of the bowel ends over the staple lines, removal of retroperitoneal tissue from around the superior mesenteric artery, ascertaining hemostasis at the cut edge of the mesenteric edge overlying the uncinate process, dissection of the portal vein to ensure adequate length for anastomosis, and construction of the arterial conduit for a single donor-recipient anastomosis. The donor portal vein should be redundant over the pancreatic surface to prevent tethering of the venous anastomosis following gland perfusion. The arterial conduit is usually constructed with a segment of the common iliac and its external and internal branches. Whenever possible, the external and internal iliac branches of the arterial conduit should be shortened such as to traverse the majority of the distance between the pancreatic blood vessels and the recipient iliac artery by the straight, and less likely to kink, common iliac artery of the donor (Figure 5.34).

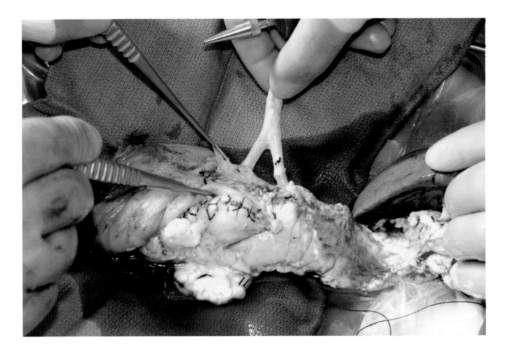

Figure 5.34

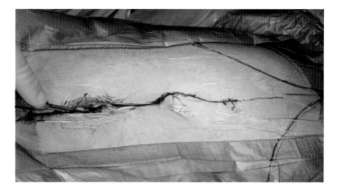

Figure 5.35

Recipient Operation

1. With the patient in the supine position, a midline incision extending from the xyphoid to the pubic symphysis is made (Figure 5.35). It is generally necessary to divide the falciform ligament of the liver. A thorough abdominal exploration is then performed to ascertain the absence of anatomic or pathologic anomalies that could affect the procedure.

2. The transverse colon is then reflected upward and out of the incision and wrapped in warm moist towels on the skin surface. Abdominal retractors are then placed on both sides of the wound. Bowel loops are packed in the left lateral gutter and inferiorly in the pelvis, stretching the mesenteric root. This exposes the recipients' duodenal loop, ligament of Trietz, and the uncinate process. The superior mesenteric vein (blue arrow) with its tributaries can be seen under the thin peritoneal covering of the root of the mesentery (Figure 5.36).

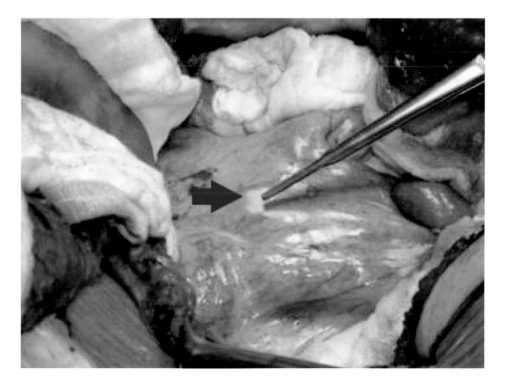

Figure 5.36

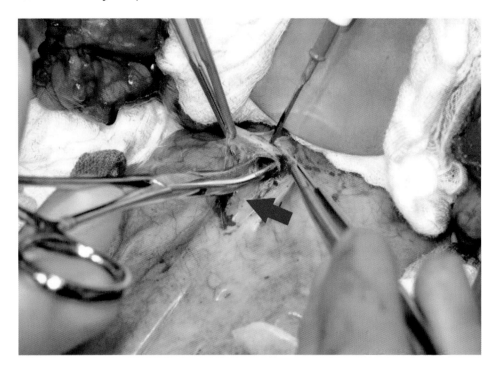

Figure 5.37

3. The peritoneum overlying the vessels is cut with the scissors or the electrocautery making sure to continuously separate the superior mesenteric vein (blue arrow) by gently teasing it away from the peritoneal membrane to prevent its injury (Figure 5.37). The dissection is carried in the root of the mesentery until the vein is well exposed for a distance of about 4 to 5 inches and the venous tributaries are dissected. Using minimal traction, the posterior aspect of the vein is exposed to ensure the absence of any tributaries that could cause bleeding during the anastomosis. The main vein and all its tributaries are then encircled with thin vessel loops.

4. It is important during the dissection around the vein (blue arrow) to look for lymphatic tributaries and ligate larger lymph channels whenever possible to avoid the development of postoperative lymph leaks (Figure 5.38). Small venous tributaries can be

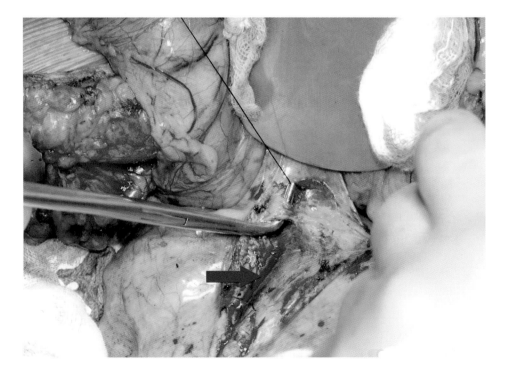

Figure 5.38

ligated on the vein side and electrocoagulated on the mesenteric side. Care should be exercised to avoid electrocoagulating both ends, so as to prevent postoperative bleeding from the small branches. Following completion of the dissection it is not uncommon for the vein to be in spasm and have a reduced diameter. In such cases, it is best to remove all vessel loops, proceed with dissection of the iliac vessels, and decide at a later point whether the vein size permits portal anastomosis.

5. Exposure of the iliac vessels is generally done on the right side except in cases where a prior kidney has been done on the right; here one could use the left side. The packing of the bowel loops is removed and the retractor is adjusted to provide maximum exposure on the right side. Mobilization of the right colon and the small intestinal mesentery is undertaken (Figure 5.39). The right colon and intestines are then wrapped in a large towel and reflected upward and to the left. The sigmoid colon is also covered by moist towels and retracted to the left.

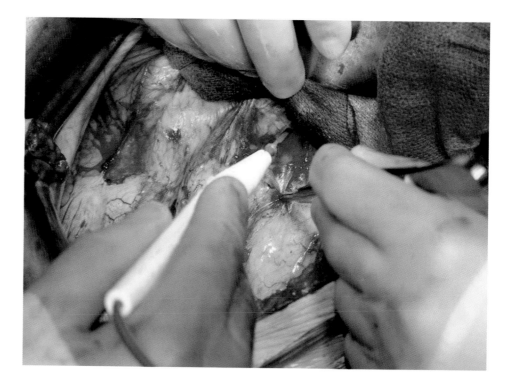

Figure 5.39

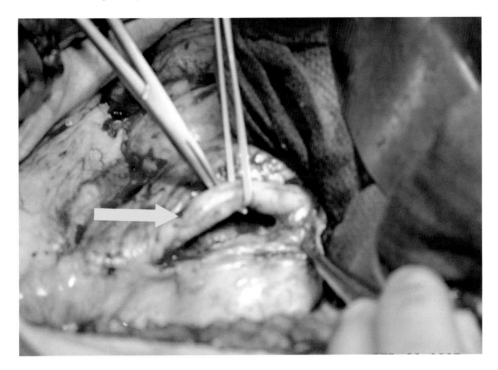

Figure 5.40

6. The retroperitoneum is then opened after identification of the ureter and the gonadal vessels. These structures are gently swept medially and dissection is carried on top of the common iliac artery. The common iliac artery (yellow arrow) is exposed from the aorta to the beginning of the external iliac (Figure 5.40). Gentle palpation ensures that there are no hard calcifications that could prevent performing a safe anastomosis. In patients with calcification, the external iliac could be dissected, or alternatively one could use the recipient aorta. Since occlusion for the arterial anastomosis is generally done by a large side-biting C-clamp, one has to dissect enough of the common iliac vein to ensure safe placement of the vascular clamp.

7. The bowel loops are then brought back into their anatomic position and the bowels are packed as during the portal vein dissection, maintaining the right-sided traction to avoid repositioning retractors between the venous and arterial anastomosis.

8. Once the decision is made (based on the size of the portal tributary) to proceed with portal placement, the next step is to decide on the location, size, and direction of the anastomosis. We prefer to place the anastomosis distal to a large tributary. Our preference is based on a theoretical concern that clotting of the venous anastomosis could propagate upward into the portal circulation with catastrophic results on bowel venous drainage. Although this has never been reported, we still favor having flow proximal to the anastomotic site. The recipient superior mesenteric vein (blue arrow) is controlled either by traction on the vessel loops or by small bulldog clamps (Figure 5.41). An anterior venotomy is then performed, taking care to avoid injury of the back wall of the soft vessel, particularly if a posterior branch necessitates placement of a posterior clamp.

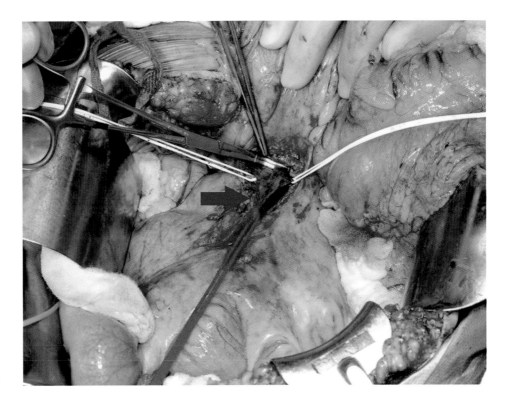

Figure 5.41

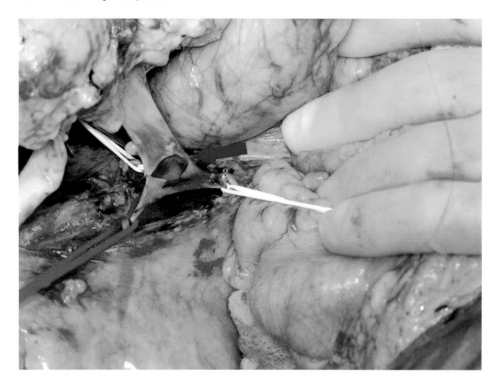

Figure 5.42

9. The allograft pancreas is then wrapped in two white towels with ice slush overlying its surface. Venous anastomosis (blue arrow) is performed using 6.0 Prolene in a running fashion (Figure 5.42). The surgeon's side is completed first, and then the assistant has the benefit of the traction on the back wall afforded by ligation of the back wall stitch in the middle of the anastomosis.

10. Once both sides of the venous anastomosis are completed, a bulldog clamp is placed on the donor portal vein and recipient's portal flow is restored (Figure 5.43). The venous anastomosis (blue arrow) is inspected and any suture line bleeding is dealt with.

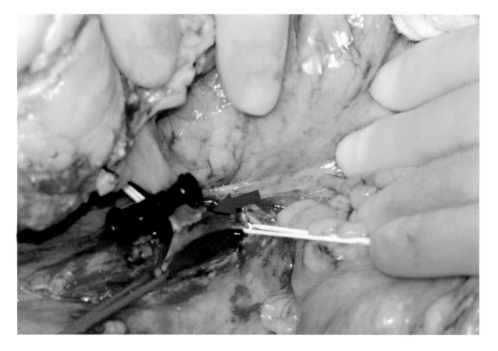

Figure 5.43

11. The site of the anastomosis on the iliac artery is then visualized by elevation of the right colon and the root of the mesentery. The arterial conduit (blue arrow) is also visualized, and the point at which the conduit traverses the mesentery is chosen so as to achieve the shortest, most vertical path for the conduit to the artery. The electro-cautery is used to incise the mesentery, and a curved vascular clamp is passed on top of the recipient iliac artery through the root of the mesentery. The arterial conduit is then adjusted to remove any possible rotation, and the donor common iliac artery is passed though the defect in the root of the mesentery to the site of the arterial anastomosis (Figure 5.44).

12. The right colon and small intestine are again wrapped in a moist towel and moved upward and to the left, exposing the dissected retroperitoneum. The recipient iliac artery is then occluded with a large C-clamp. The arterial conduit (blue arrow) is then shortened to appropriate length and beveled for the anastomosis. The recipient arteriotomy (yellow arrow) is created with a No. 11 blade and fashioned with a 4.8-mm aortic punch. A 5.0 Prolene suture is used to create the end-to-side arterial anastomosis

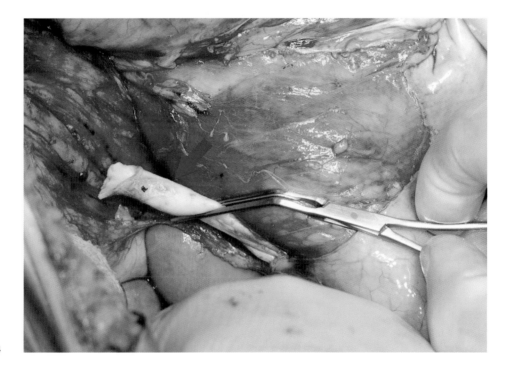

Figure 5.44

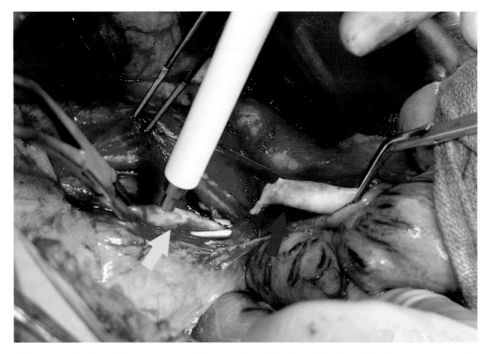

Figure 5.45

(Figure 5.45). Once the anastomosis is completed, the bowel is brought down to anatomic position, the portal anastomosis is exposed, and the bulldog clamp occluding the donor portal vein is removed, allowing, venous revascularization of the graft. In the absence of venous bleeding, the mesentery is lifted upward, allowing exposure of the arterial anastomosis, and the arterial clamp is removed, completing revascularization of the transplant pancreas. A quick inspection of the pancreas is necessary at this point to clamp and ligate any bleeders from the surface. Once hemostasis is achieved, the gland is wrapped in a warm towel and bowel anastomosis is started.

13. Enteric drainage is to a Roux-en-Y limb or a side-to-side anastomosis of the transplant duodenum to an adjoining bowel loop. Regardless of the technique used, the recipient bowel loop used in the anastomosis should be redundant enough to avoid rotation of the pancreas. We prefer hand-sewn, double layer (silk and PDS) bowel anastomosis (Figure 5.46).

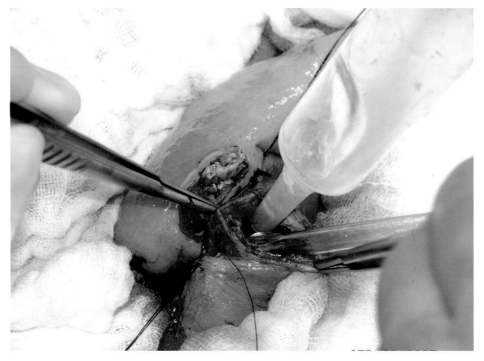

Figure 5.46

14. After placement of the posterior silk layer, bowel occlusion clamps are placed on the recipient bowel and the electrocautery is used to open both the recipient bowel and donor duodenum. Once the duodenal segment is opened, contents are cultured and the segment irrigated copiously with antibiotics. Following completion of the bowel anastomosis (Figure 5.47), the abdominal cavity is irrigated and all contaminated instruments are handed off the field. If a Roux-en-Y limb has been used, the side-to-side bowel anastomosis is completed prior to handing off the contaminated instruments. In these cases it is important to close the mesenteric gap created by mobilizing the bowel for the intestinal anastomosis to prevent internal herniation. Once bowel work is completed and following abdominal irrigation, the spleen is excised followed by a final careful inspection of the pancreas to ensure appropriate hemostasis.

15. When a kidney transplant is to be performed, the retractors are then moved to allow maximum exposure on the left side. We prefer creating a retroperitoneal pocket by dissecting the peritoneum off the abdominal wall muscles. This allows complete closure of the retroperitoneal space around the kidney at the time of closure. In larger individuals, however, accessing the vessels from behind the sigmoid colon mesentery achieves good exposure of the iliac vessels for kidney placement.

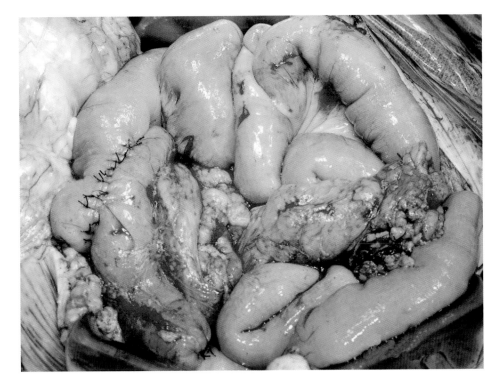

Figure 5.47

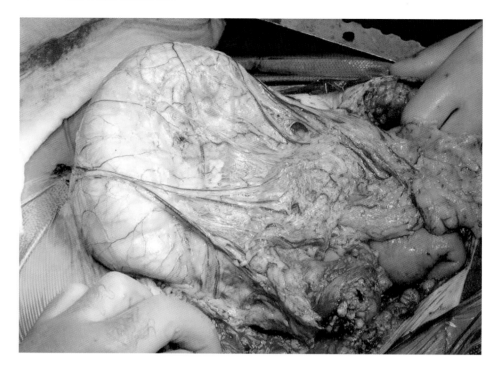

Figure 5.48

Technical Points

1. If possible, we prefer to wrap the pancreas with the omentum (Figure 5.48). This requires mobilizing some of the omentum off the transverse colon but serves to keep bowel loops separable from the pancreas in the case of reoperative therapy.

2. We attempt to bring the tail of the pancreas up to the abdominal wall by stitching some of the ligated splenic vessels to the peritoneum on one side of the incision. One has to be careful, however, of pancreatic rotation, and one should favor allowing the pancreas to choose its own axis.

Acknowledgments

The authors acknowledge the expert assistance of Dr. Mohammad Shokouh-Amiri for preparation of the illustrations and Mrs. Shaherah Rankins-Amos for assistance with manuscript preparation.

Isolated Pancreas Transplant: Bladder Drainage

Isolated pancreas transplants can be either in the form of a pancreas after kidney transplant (PAK) or a pancreas transplant alone (PTA). A PAK procedure is usually performed once the recipient has adequately recovered from the kidney transplant. A pancreas transplant alone (PTA) may be performed for the diabetic patient without renal failure but with significant problems with glucose control (e.g., ketoacidosis, hypogylcemic unawareness, etc.) or evidence of secondary organ damage (i.e., neuropathy). The majority of isolated pancreas grafts are drained into the bladder. This has the advantage of allowing for urine amylase monitoring, which can act as a surrogate marker for rejection – a decrease in urine amylase values indicating pancreatic graft dysfunction. Drainage to the bowel is, however, more physiologic and not associated with problems such as urethritis, hematuria, dehydration, and acidosis. As rejection rates decrease, enteric drainage is becoming a more widely used option, even for PTA and PAK transplants.

An intraperitoneal approach is preferred, with a midline incision in the lower abdomen. The preference is to place the pancreas in the right iliac fossa, with the head and duodenum pointing downwards (Figure 5.49). One then has the option of either bladder or enteric drainage. If the right iliac vessels have already been used, the pancreas can be placed on the left side, or higher in the abdomen with portal/enteric drainage.

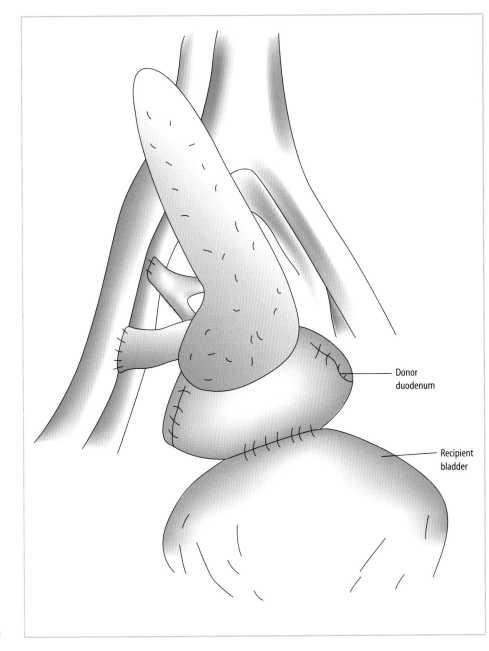

Donor
duodenum

Recipient
bladder

Figure 5.49

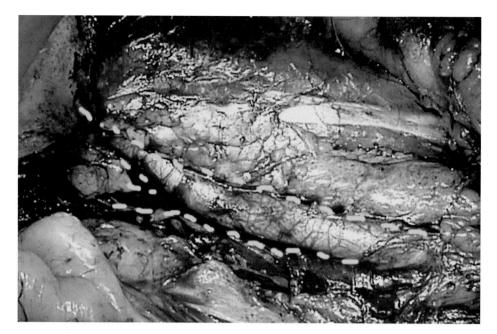

Figure 5.50

a) Surgical Procedure

1. The start of the procedure is exactly as described for the pancreas portion of the simultaneous pancreas kidney transplant. After a midline incision, the cecum is mobilized and the iliac vessels are identified. The external iliac artery, internal iliac artery, and common iliac artery (broken yellow line) are all isolated and encircled. The arterial anastomosis is ideally placed on the common iliac artery (Figure 5.50).

2. The iliac vein is completely mobilized with division and suture ligation of all hypogastric branches (Figure 5.51). This allows the iliac vein to be placed in a more superficial location lateral to the iliac artery, which is the correct orientation of the portal vein and Y graft of the pancreas graft when it is placed in its position with the duodenal cuff next to the recipient bladder. This only applies if the pancreas is being placed on the right side. If the pancreas is to be placed on the left side, the iliac vein should be positioned medial to the iliac artery.

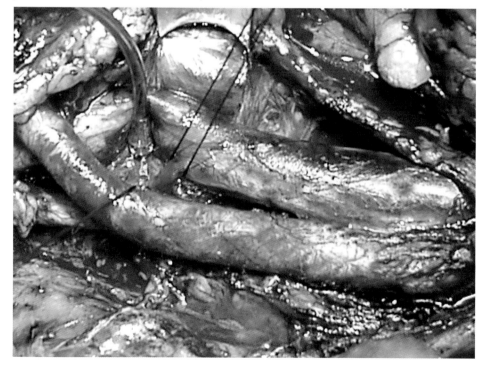

Figure 5.51

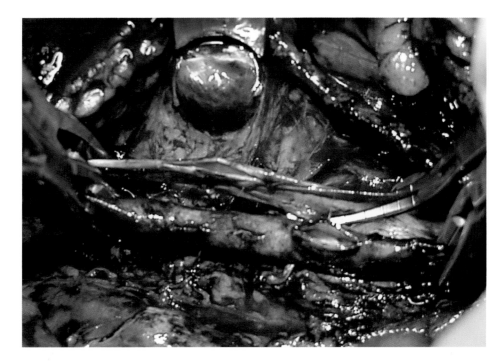

Figure 5.52

3. Clamps are placed proximally and distally on the iliac artery and vein. Appropriate marks are made for the position of the arteriotomy and venotomy. The venotomy should be placed just distal to the arteriotomy site, and if possible, the two should not overlap in position (Figures 5.52 and 5.53).

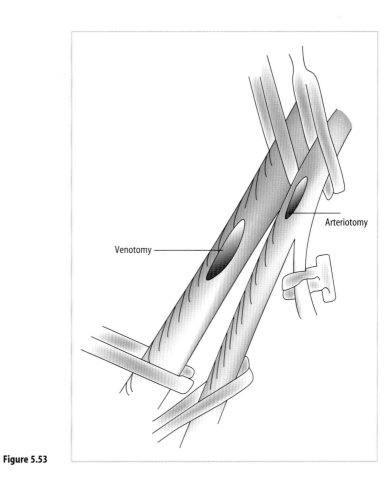

Venotomy

Arteriotomy

Figure 5.53

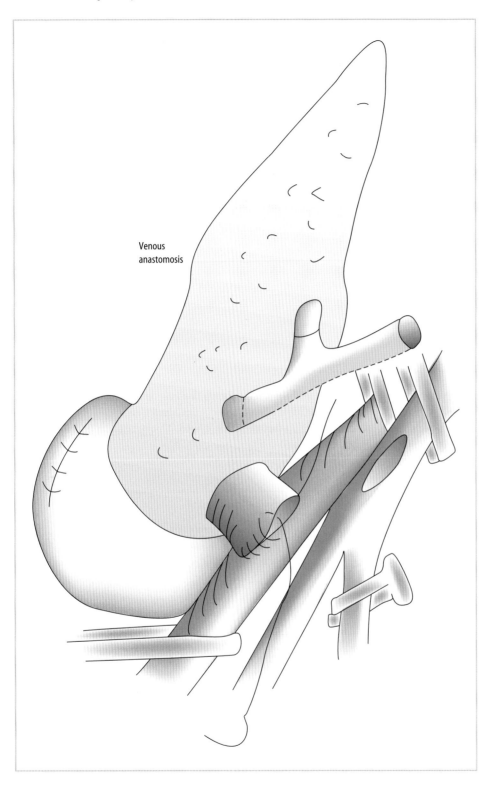

Venous
anastomosis

Figure 5.54

4. The venous anastomosis is usually performed first, creating an end-to-side anastomosis between the end of the portal vein and the side of the iliac vein (Figure 5.54).

5. The Y graft is trimmed to appropriate length so that there is not undue redundancy, and the arterial anastomosis is performed, again in and end-to-side fashion (Figure 5.55).

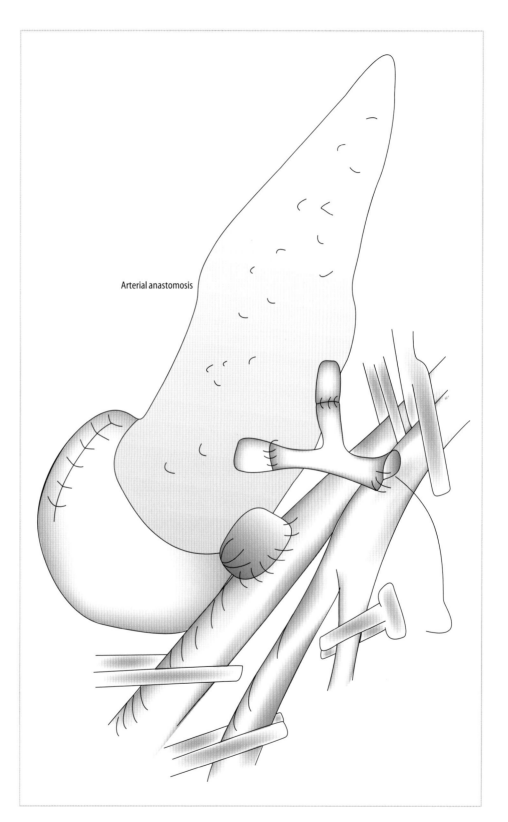

Arterial anastomosis

Figure 5.55

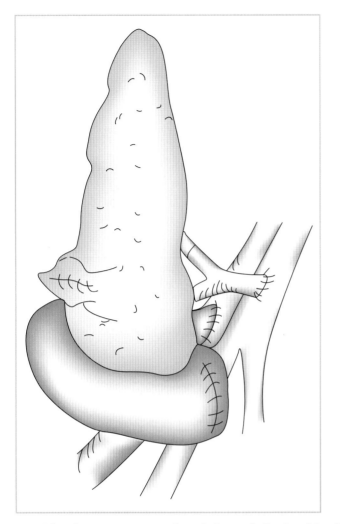

Figure 5.56

6. The clamps are removed, and the graft (broken blue line) is allowed to perfuse (Figures 5.56 and 5.57). Bleeding points are controlled using hemoclips or suture ligatures. The graft is inspected to make sure hemostasis is adequate and the anastomosis lies adequately, before proceeding with the bladder anastomosis.

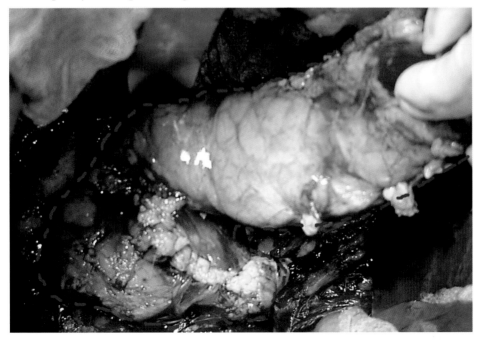

Figure 5.57

7. The bladder anastomosis is fashioned between the dome of the bladder (broken blue line) and the antimesenteric border of the duodenum (broken yellow line) (Figure 5.58). A two-layer hand-sewn anastomosis is fashioned using continuous nonabsorbable

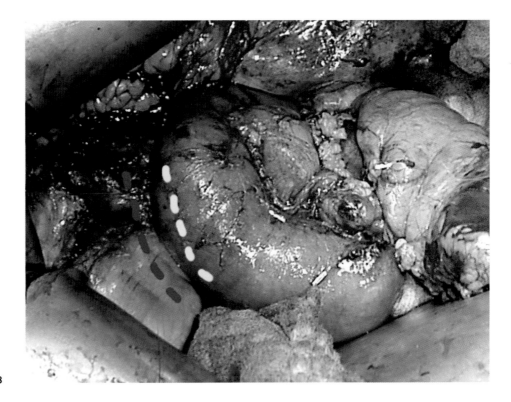

Figure 5.58

suture for the outer layer, and continuous absorbable suture for the inner layer. The posterior outer layer is performed first using a running nonabsorbable suture. Appropriate-sized openings are then made in the donor duodenum and recipient bladder (Figure 5.59).

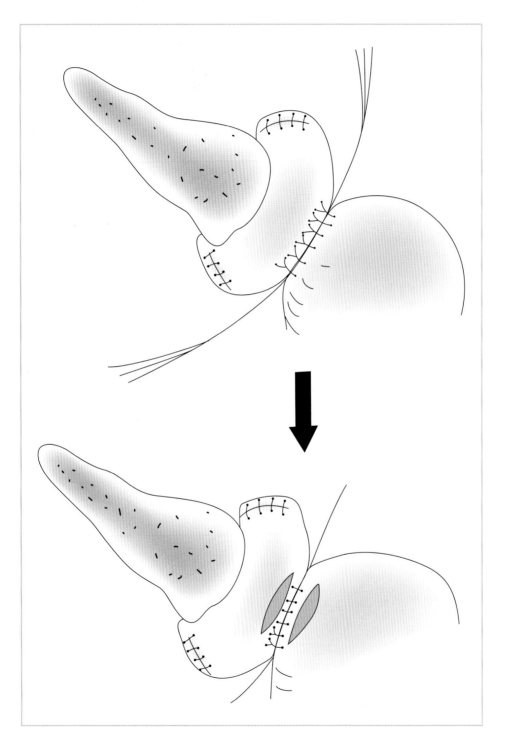

Figure 5.59

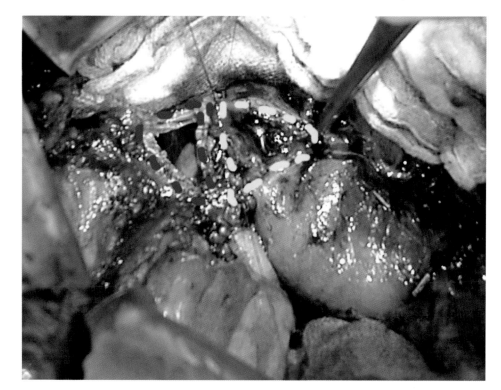

Figure 5.60

8. The inner layer of the back wall is then completed using an absorbable suture in a continuous manner (Figure 5.60). The inner layer of the anterior wall is then constructed in a similar fashion. The outer layer of the anterior wall is completed last, using a non-absorbable continuous or interrupted stitch (Figure 5.61).

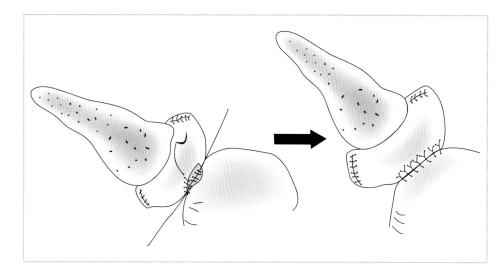

Figure 5.61

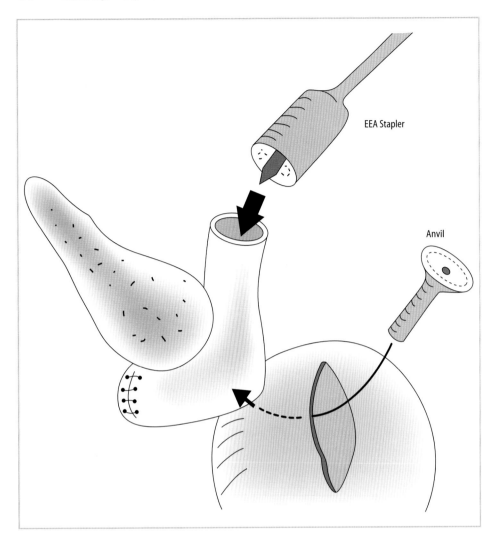

EEA Stapler

Anvil

Figure 5.62

9. Alternatively, this anastomosis can be done using a luminal stapling device. A cystotomy is made in the dome of the bladder and this is used to insert the anvil of the stapler into the posterior aspect of the bladder (Figure 5.62).

10. The stapler is inserted via the end of the distal duodenum of the graft, and the pin forced through the center of the antimesenteric border (Figure 5.63). It is connected to the anvil and fired. Excess donor duodenum is then trimmed using a linear stapling device.

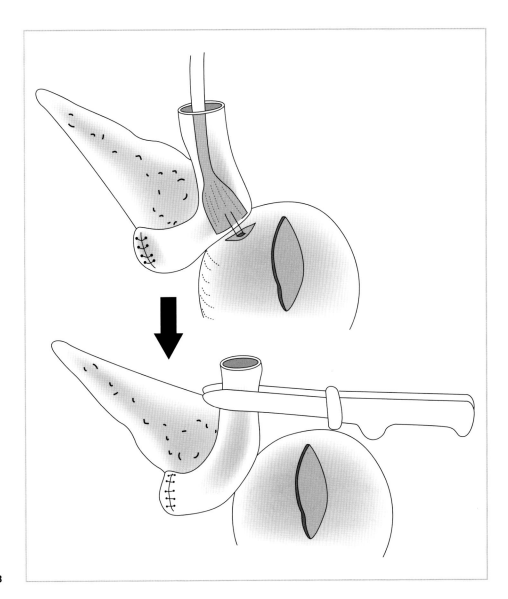

Figure 5.63

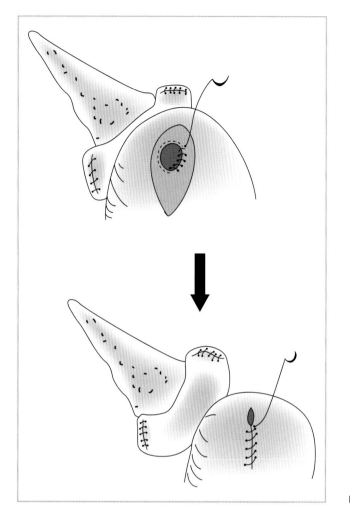

Figure 5.64

11. The staple line is oversewn for hemostasis, and the bladder is closed in two layers (Figure 5.64).

Pancreas Transplant from a Living Donor

Miquel Tan, Raja Kandaswamy, and
Rainer W.G. Gruessner

Although the pancreas was the first extrarenal organ to be successfully used from living donors (LDs), of the greater than 18,000 pancreas transplants performed since the 1960s, less than 1% have come from live donation. Several reasons account for the underuse of this resource, among them the potential morbidity of a distal pancreatectomy in an otherwise healthy donor and a higher technical failure rate compared to deceased donor transplants. In selected cases, however, LD pancreas transplantation may be an appropriate option. This includes high panel reactive antibody (PRA) recipients who are unlikely to receive a cadaver organ or uremic diabetics on the simultaneous cadaver pancreas-kidney (SPK) waiting list. This procedure may be performed either for an isolated pancreas transplant, or combined with a nephrectomy for an SPK transplant.

a) Donor Evaluation

It is crucial that all potential donors undergo a thorough preoperative evaluation. The purpose is twofold: first, to ensure that the donor is healthy enough to undergo the operation safely, and second, to ensure that the reduced pancreatic mass would be sufficient to maintain a normal metabolic state. The general health of the donor is best ascertained by a detailed history and physical examination, looking for evidence of cardiovascular, pulmonary, renal, and major gastrointestinal disease. This part of the workup is no different from the evaluation for any other general surgical patient undergoing a pancreatic resection.

Endocrinologic evaluation includes family history. Potential donors should be at least 10 years older than the age of onset of diabetes in the recipient (and the onset of diabetes in the recipient must have been at least 10 years pretransplant). In addition, for sibling donors, no family member other than the recipient should be diabetic. When these two criteria are met, donors are at no greater risk for diabetes than the general population, even if they are human leukocyte antigen (HLA) identical with the recipient. Potential donors should be asked about their alcohol intake. Female donors who have had previous pregnancies should be asked about gestational diabetes.

Metabolic studies are done to try to estimate islet cell mass and reserve in the potential donor. Tests that can be done include measurement of the hemoglobin A_{1c} (should be <6%), an oral glucose tolerance test (OGTT), insulin secretion in response to an intravenous glucose tolerance test (IVGTT), and an arginine stimulation test.

Lastly, some radiologic assessment of the vascular anatomy should be done. This step is more important if the kidney is to be procured also, as the vascular anatomy of the splenic artery is fairly constant in comparison to the renal arteries. An invasive arteriogram is no longer necessary to obtain this information as current CT or magnetic resonance imaging (MRI) provides adequate information with regard to the renal and splenic vessels.

The surgical procedure for removal of the pancreas with or without a kidney can be done either as an open or laparoscopic procedure. Initially the removal of the distal pancreas from a living donor was done via an open operative procedure. While this can be done safely, it does involve a significant recovery time for the donor. The advent of laparoscopic technology provides a viable alternative to the traditional open approach. This has been demonstrated most clearly with laparoscopic donor nephrectomy, which has rapidly become the procedure of choice for kidney donation because of reduced hospital stay and more rapid convalescence. Cosmetically, it is more appealing to potential donors compared to the traditional flank incision required for open nephrectomy. Laparoscopic nephrectomy is equivalent to the open procedure in terms of donor safety and quality of allograft. Laparoscopic techniques have rapidly been applied to other organ systems including the pancreas. Laparoscopic distal pancreatectomies have been described for treatment of a variety of pathologic states and appear to be safe with the additional benefit of reduced hospital costs and accelerated postoperative recovery. The technique of open and laparoscopic live donor pancreatectomy is subsequently described.

b) Surgical Procedure

Open Technique

1. A midline incision is preferred. If the kidney is to be removed, it is generally removed first. The right or left kidney can be used, depending on the vascular anatomy. The preference is to use the left kidney (because of concurrent partial mobilization of the pancreas, greater length of the renal vein, and lack of liver mobilization). The splenocolic ligament should be preserved, if possible, as it may carry collateral blood vessels to the spleen. The kidney is removed once the dissection is complete.

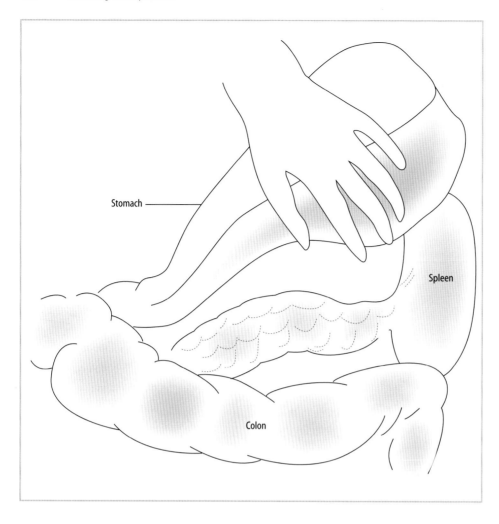

Stomach

Spleen

Colon

Figure 5.65

2. Procurement of the distal pancreas begins by dividing the gastrocolic ligament, starting medially and advancing laterally to the margin of the spleen (Figure 5.65). Care should be taken to preserve the gastroepiploic artery and the short gastric vessels in order to diminish the likelihood of devascularizing the spleen. The retroperitoneal attachments of the spleen are not disturbed, and the spleen is not mobilized. The stomach can then be retracted superiorly, and the inferior margin of the distal pancreas is mobilized.

3. A peritoneal incision is made over the tail of the pancreas at its junction with the spleen. The pancreas is gently dissected off the splenic surface. The splenic vessels are then identified, and the main trunks of both the splenic artery and vein divided proximal to the splenic branches (again, preserving collateral blood vessels supplying the spleen) (Figure 5.66).

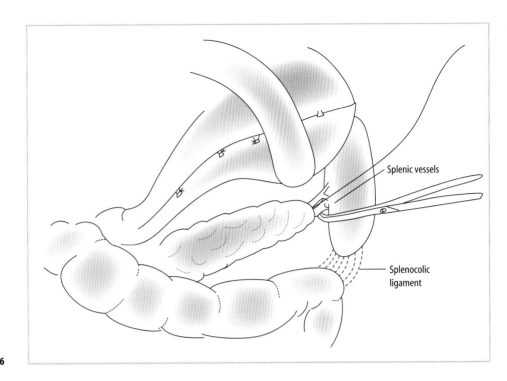

Figure 5.66

4. The superior margin of the pancreas is then mobilized, retaining the splenic artery and vein in continuity with the body and tail of the pancreas. As the pancreas is elevated from its bed and retracted medially, the confluence of the inferior mesentery vein (IMV) as it joins the splenic vein can be seen. The location of this confluence varies; it can be very close to the superior mesenteric vein (SMV)–splenic vein junction. Once the IMV is divided, the pancreas can be mobilized further to the surgical neck. The portal vein is identified at the confluence of the SMV and splenic vein. As the pancreas continues to be rotated medially, the splenic artery is isolated at its origin off the celiac trunk and encircled with a vessel loop (Figure 5.67).

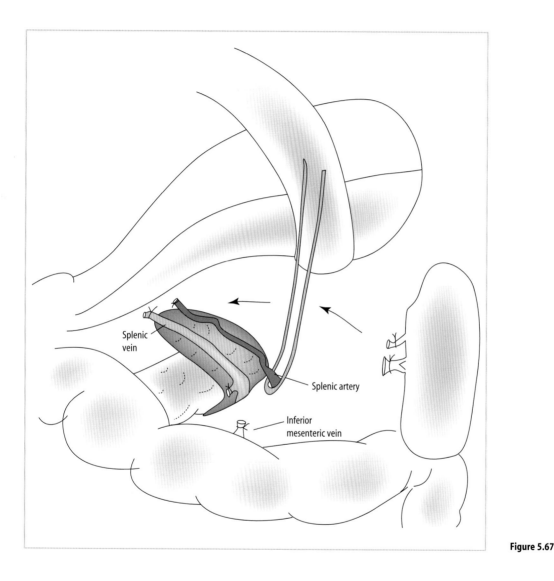

Figure 5.67

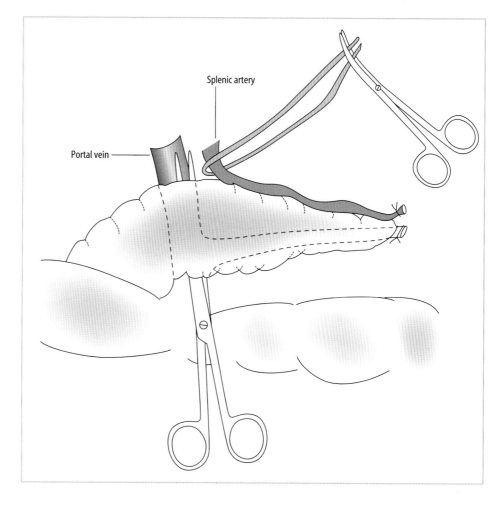

Splenic artery

Portal vein

Figure 5.68

5. The avascular plane between the pancreas and portal vein is bluntly dissected to define the narrowest portion of the pancreas (i.e., the neck) (Figure 5.68). This will be the site for division of the pancreas (broken blue line) (Figure 5.69), lying just anterior to the portal vein at the point of junction with the splenic vein (blue arrow).

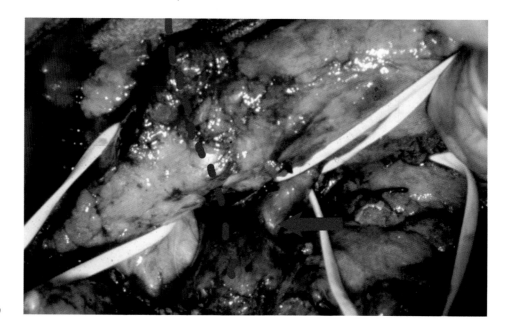

Figure 5.69

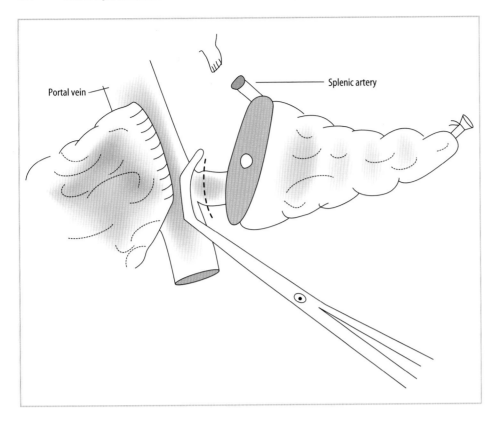

Figure 5.70

6. The pancreatic neck can then be divided using multiple 4.0 silk ligatures. Both ends of the pancreatic duct should be identified. The proximal end can be oversewn, and the distal duct tacked with a fine suture for identification. At this point, the segmental pancreas graft is ready for removal. Clamps are placed on the splenic artery and the splenic vein at its junction with the portal vein (Figure 5.70). After dividing the vessels and removing the graft, the vascular stumps are oversewn closed.

7. The recipient operation is not very different from its deceased donor counterpart. A lower abdominal midline incision is used. If a kidney graft is to be implanted, it should be placed on the left side. The pancreas graft should be placed on the right side if possible, because of the more superficial location of the vessels on this side. In preparation for the pancreas graft implantation, all branches of the iliac vein, including the hypogastric, should be divided (allowing the vein to lie in a more superficial location). To allow for an "artery-lateral-to-the-vein" alignment (opposite of positioning for deceased donor transplant), it is useful to divide the internal iliac artery. Doing so gives a better lie to the graft after it is implanted and decreases the chances of the graft artery kinking. The donor splenic artery can then be anastomosed end-to-side to the external or common iliac artery (yellow arrow); the splenic vein is anastomosed end to side to the iliac vein (blue arrow) (Figure 5.71).

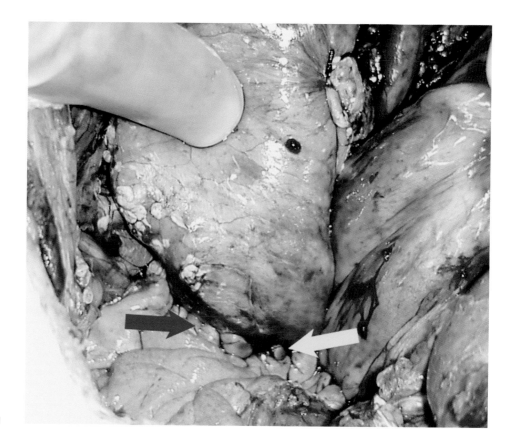

Figure 5.71

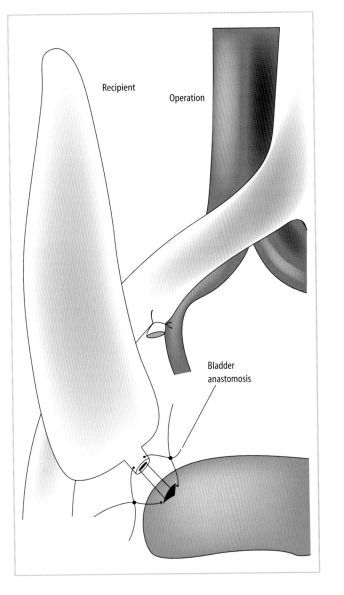

Recipient

Operation

Bladder
anastomosis

Figure 5.72

8. Pancreatic exocrine secretions can be managed by a number of techniques. If the pancreatic duct is of adequate size, a direct anastomosis between the duct and bladder mucosa can be constructed with interrupted 7.0 absorbable sutures (Figure 5.72). If the duct is small and the diameter of the cut edge of the pancreas is small, then an invagination technique can be used. The pancreas graft is invaginated into the bladder using one internal layer of 4.0 absorbable sutures and one external layer of interrupted 4.0 nonabsorbable sutures. Doing so obviates the need for a tedious duct-to-mucosa anastomosis, but it could create problems from exposure of pancreatic tissue to urine. The pancreatic duct may also be drained enterally, using a Roux-en-Y limb of distal bowel.

Laparoscopic Technique

1. After induction of general anesthesia, the patient is placed in a modified right lateral decubitus position to allow the patient to be rotated from a left-side-up position (for the nephrectomy) to a supine position (for the distal pancreatectomy). For patients undergoing a distal pancreatectomy alone, the patient is kept in the supine position.

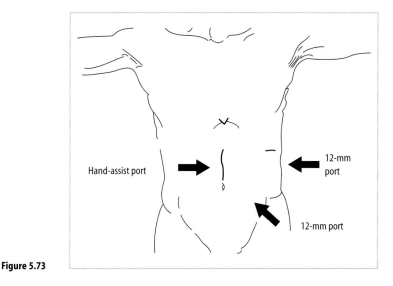

Figure 5.73

If a left nephrectomy is to be performed at the same time, the patient is placed in right lateral decubitus position. The operative table is then flexed to 45 degrees to open up the left subcostal space to facilitate dissection of the kidney. A 6-cm midline incision is then made either supra- or periumbilically depending on the patient's body habitus. A donor with a longer torso would require the incision to be placed in a supraumbilical position so that the surgeon's hand can reach both the kidney and pancreas. A Gelport® (Applied Medical, Rancho Santa Margarita, CA) or HandPort® (Smith and Nephew Inc., Andover, MA) device is placed in the midline incision to allow for hand assistance. Using standard laparoscopic equipment, a 12-mm port is placed at the level of the umbilicus along the lateral edge of the left rectus for insertion of a 30-degree camera. After pneumoperitoneum is established, a second 12-mm port is inserted in the left mid-abdomen in the plane of the anterior axillary line (Figure 5.73). This allows insertion of ultrasonic shears, laparoscopic scissors, and any other needed instrumentation. The surgeon and assistant stand on the patient's right side during the nephrectomy (Figure 5.74). The assistant moves to the patient's left side during the pancreatectomy. Mobilization of the left colon, ureter, and left gonadal vein, as well as dissection of the kidney is described in detail elsewhere.

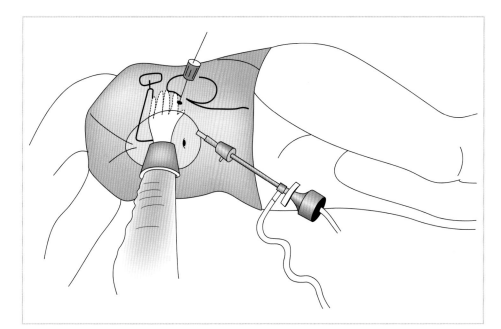

Figure 5.74

2. After removal of the kidney, the donor is then rotated to a supine position with reverse Trendelenburg to help move the transverse colon away from the operative field. The partially dissected inferior margin of the pancreas is mobilized using ultrasonic shears and electrocautery. The IMV is identified, ligated with hemoclips, and divided near its insertion into the splenic vein. The tail of the pancreas is then encircled by making a hole in the avascular plane along the superior margin of the pancreatic tail and passing a finger along the underside and posterior aspect of the pancreas. The tail is encircled with a vessel loop to facilitate atraumatic anterior retraction of the pancreas (Figure 5.75). The posterior surface of the pancreas is then freed from its retroperitoneal

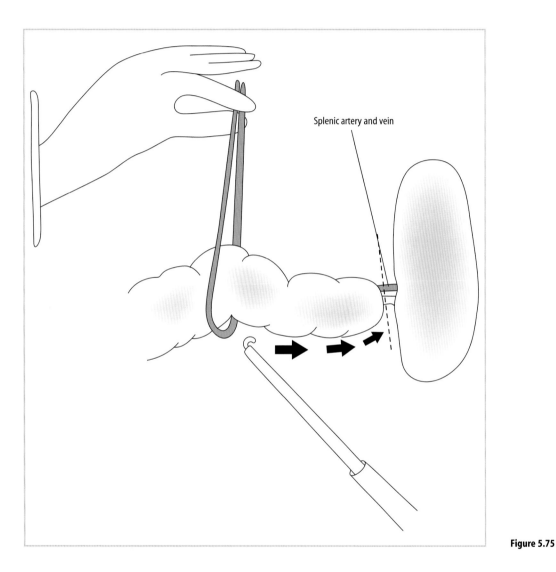

Splenic artery and vein

Figure 5.75

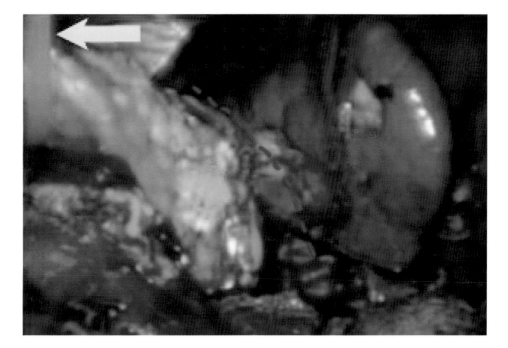

Figure 5.76

attachments using electrocautery. The splenic artery and vein are identified in the hilum of the spleen and individually ligated and divided using a 35-mm vascular stapler, allowing the pancreas to be lifted from its bed and retracted medially (broken blue line) (Figure 5.76). Care should be taken not to disturb the short gastric vessels and right gastroepiploic artery, as this constitutes the main remaining blood supply to the spleen.

3. With the splenic vessels divided distally and the pancreas retracted medially, its posterior aspect can be visualized. The splenic vein (blue arrow) and the splenic artery (yellow arrow) can be seen running along the posterior aspect of the pancreas (Figure 5.77).

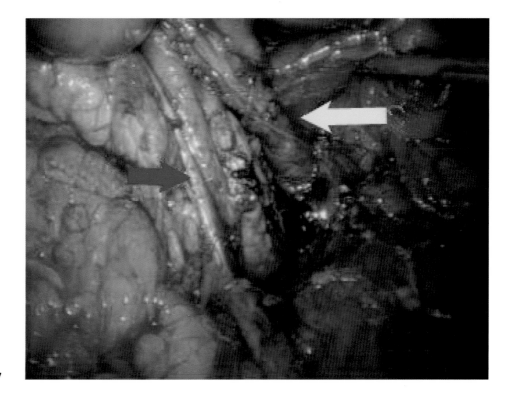

Figure 5.77

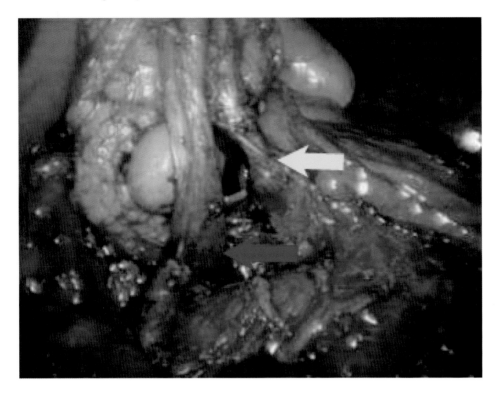

Figure 5.78

4. The splenic vein is mobilized circumferentially near its junction with the superior mesenteric vein (blue arrow). Likewise, the splenic artery is mobilized just as it branches off the celiac axis (yellow arrow) (Figure 5.78).

5. Heparin (30 units/kg) is administered intravenously prior to ligation of the vessels. Two clips are applied to the splenic artery just distal to the celiac axis (yellow arrow) (Figure 5.79). The splenic artery is then divided with laparoscopic scissors. The splenic vein can be divided at its junction with the SMV, either using clips or a stapling device (blue arrow).

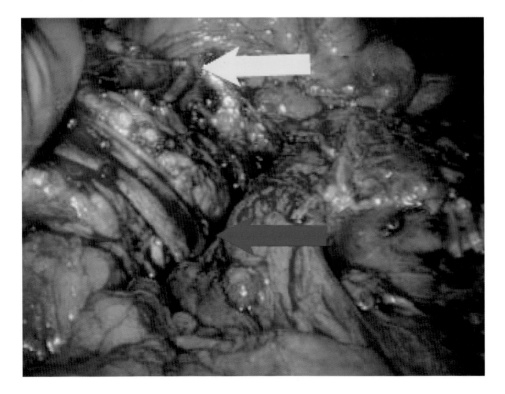

Figure 5.79

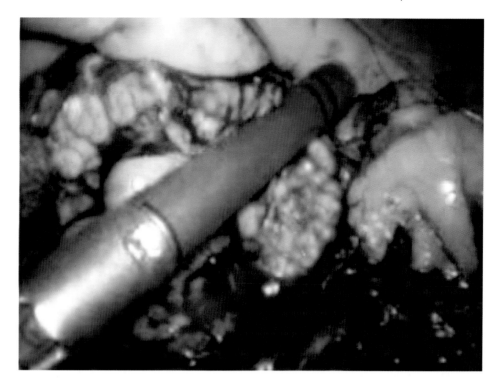

Figure 5.80

6. A linear cutting stapler device is used to transect the pancreatic neck (Figure 5.80). The distal pancreatic segment is then extracted by hand through the midline incision and passed off to the recipient team to be flushed immediately with cold University of Wisconsin solution.

7. The staple line (green arrow) of the pancreatic remnant is carefully inspected (Figure 5.81) and oversewn intracorporeally with 4–0 polypropylene suture to achieve hemostasis and prevent leakage of the pancreatic duct. The vascular stumps of the splenic artery (yellow arrow) and vein (blue arrow) are carefully inspected to make sure there is no bleeding. After irrigation, a drain is placed near the pancreatic remnant. The spleen should be reexamined at this point to assess its viability. Closure is then performed.

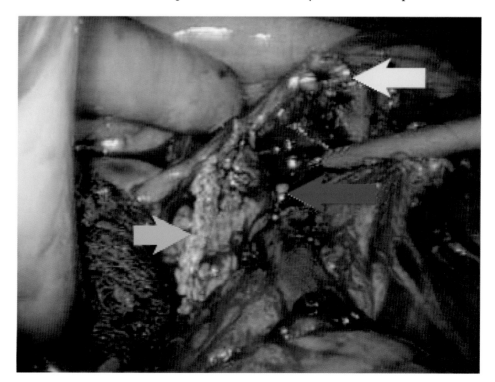

Figure 5.81

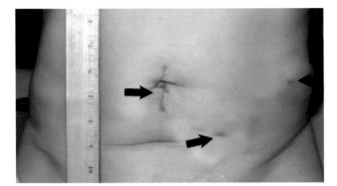

Figure 5.82

8. The pancreas and kidney graft can then be implanted in the recipient, similarly to as described previously for the open approach.

9. The appearance of the incisions at 2 weeks after surgery in the donor is shown (Figure 5.82).

Surgical Complications After Pancreas Transplant

The incidence of surgical complications after pancreas transplant has decreased significantly over the last 10 years. Nonetheless, surgical complications remain very common in pancreas transplant recipients, with an incidence nearly two- to threefold higher compared to kidney transplant recipients. While the most common cause of pancreas graft loss is an immunologic failure, the second most common reason is a surgical complication leading to technical failure of the graft. There are several reasons why the pancreas is more prone to surgical complications. Unlike the kidney, which receives a high volume of blood, the pancreas is a low-flow organ, hence predisposing it to thrombosis. The gland is predisposed to inflammation, which likely is a result of preservation injury to the organ, and presents clinically as pancreatitis. A significant amount of lymphatic tissue and ganglion tissue with numerous small blood vessels surrounds the pancreas, resulting in a high risk of bleeding after reperfusion. Finally, the graft duodenum is a contaminated viscus, which tolerates prolonged cold ischemia poorly, hence predisposing to the complications of leaks and infections. However, improvements in surgical techniques, better preservation techniques, and improved prophylaxis regimens have all helped to decrease the complication rate. Potential complications after pancreas transplant include the following:

a) Thrombosis

The incidence of thrombosis after pancreas transplant, including thrombosis of the portal vein or arterial Y graft, is between 5% and 8%. Risk factors for thrombosis include torsion or kinking of the vessels (which may occur if the Y-graft or portal vein is left too long), prolonged preservation time, donor obesity, or atherosclerotic disease in the donor vessels. Thrombosis most commonly occurs within the first week posttransplant, and is heralded by an increase in blood glucose levels, an increase in insulin requirements, or a decrease in urine amylase levels. Venous thrombosis is also characteristically accompanied by hematuria (for bladder-drained grafts), tenderness and swelling of the graft, and ipsilateral lower extremity edema. Urgent diagnosis is important to try to avoid further complications associated with a potentially necrotic pancreas. An ultrasound should be the initial test. If no flow is seen, the patient is explored and graft pancreatectomy is performed.

b) Hemorrhage

Postoperative bleeding may be minimized by meticulous intraoperative control of bleeding sites. Although hemorrhage may be exacerbated by anticoagulants and antiplatelet drugs, their benefits seem to outweigh the risks. Bleeding is a much less significant cause (<1%) of graft loss than is thrombosis (5% to 8%). Significant bleeding is treated by immediate reexploration.

c) Pancreatitis

Most cases of graft pancreatitis occur early on, are self-limited, and are probably due to ischemic preservation injury. Clinical manifestations may include graft tenderness, fever, and hyperamylasemia. Treatment consists of intravenous (IV) fluid replacement and fasting the recipient. Sometimes early pancreatitis may be very severe, with partial necrosis of the graft; this is usually an indication for graft pancreatectomy. Graft pancreatitis can also occur late (months or years after transplant) and may be caused by reflux into the allograft duct in recipients with bladder drainage, direct trauma to the pancreas, or cytomegalovirus (CMV) infection. Reflux is treated by urinary catheter drainage, and occasionally conversion to enteric drainage; CMV infections are treated with ganciclovir.

d) Urologic Complications

Urologic complications are almost exclusively limited to recipients who undergo bladder drainage. Hematuria is not uncommon in the first several months posttransplant, but it is usually transient and self-limiting. Bladder calculi may develop, due to exposed sutures or staples along the duodenocystostomy, which may serve as a nidus for stone formation. Recurrent urinary tract infections commonly occur concurrently. Treatment consists of cystoscopy with removal of the sutures or staples. Urinary leaks are most commonly from the proximal duodenal cuff or the duodenal anastomosis to the bladder and typically occur during the first several weeks posttransplant. Small leaks can be successfully managed by prolonged (for at least 2 weeks) Foley catheter drainage; larger leaks require surgical intervention. Other urinary complications include chronic refractory metabolic acidosis due to bicarbonate loss, persistent and recurrent urinary tract infections, and urethritis. Along with recurrent hematuria, these complications are the major indications for converting patients from bladder drainage to enteric drainage of exocrine secretions. Eventually, 15% to 20% of recipients who undergo initial bladder drainage require conversion to enteric drainage. For this reason, the recent trend has been to perform enteric drainage at the time of the transplant. Enteric drainage is associated with significantly fewer urinary tract infections and urologic complications, but this approach obviates the use of urinary amylase determinations, which are a sensitive indicator of pancreatic allograft rejection.

e) Infections

Infections remain a significant problem after pancreas transplantation. Most common are superficial wound infections. Deep intraabdominal infections may also be seen and are often related to graft complications such as leaks. Thanks to appropriate perioperative antimicrobial regimens (for prophylaxis against gram-positive bacteria, gram-negative bacteria, and yeast), the incidence of significant infections has decreased, although it remains approximately 10% and is associated with significant morbidity and mortality. Thus, should serious intraabdominal infection occur, whether or not associated with the above-described complications, reexploration and graft removal must be strongly considered, with concurrent reduction in immunosuppressive drug therapy.

f) Leaks

A leak may occur from the graft duodenum to bladder or bowel anastomosis. It may also occur from the proximal or distal duodenal cuff. The incidence is between 3% and 5%, and does not differ significantly between bladder- and enteric-drained grafts. Clinical presentation, however, may be quite different in these two scenarios. Patients with enteric-drained grafts and a leak generally present with severe pain and generalized peritonitis, as the enteric contents are leaking into their abdominal cavity. With significant intraabdominal contamination, graft salvage is usually not possible and removal of the graft is the best option. With bladder drainage, leaks do not usually present with such severe symptoms, and graft salvage is usually possible.

g) Minimizing Surgical Complications

Several steps can be taken to minimize surgical complications after pancreas transplant. Broadly, these steps can be separated into the following three categories:

1. Proper donor and recipient selection
2. Meticulous surgical techniques
3. Careful postoperative care

Donor selection plays a very important role in minimizing surgical complications. Donors with a body mass index greater than 30 generally have a pancreas with significant fatty infiltration. This predisposes to bleeding and deep infections after transplant. Cold ischemia of the graft should be minimized as much as possible, as prolonged preservation is associated with an increased risk for leaks and thrombosis. Ultimately, careful examination of the pancreas at the time of procurement and during the benching process is the best indicator of whether a pancreas should be used or not. Careful benching of the cadaver pancreas also plays a major role in minimizing complications. The spleen should be removed without damaging the tail of the pancreas. Large clumps of fat and lymphatic tissue should not be left on the gland, as they often are poorly perfused posttransplant, and serve as a nidus for infection. Care should be taken not to devascularize the proximal and distal ends of the graft duodenum. Finally, careful attention should be paid to the arterial Y graft, ensuring that it is placed properly on the vessels without significant redundancy.

The care of the recipient early after transplant also may impact on surgical complications. Use of low-dose heparin or some other variant is likely helpful in diminishing the incidence of graft thrombosis. While the risk of bleeding is increased with the use of anticoagulation, this rarely is severe enough to result in loss of the graft. Lastly, the routine use of antibacterial and antifungal prophylaxis for a short time after transplant likely plays a role in diminishing the incidence of posttransplant infections.

Selected Readings

1. Boggi U, Vistoli F, Signori S, et al. A technique for retroperitoneal pancreas transplantation with portal-enteric drainage. Transplantation 2005;79(9):1137–1142.
2. Gaber AO, Shokouh-Amiri H, Grewal HP, Britt LG. A technique for portal pancreatic transplantation with enteric drainage. Surg Gynecol Obstet 1993;177(4):417–419.
3. Gaber AO, Shokouh-Amiri MH, Hathaway DK, et al. Results of pancreas transplantation with portal venous and enteric drainage. Ann Surg. 1995;221(6):613–622; discussion 622–624.
4. Gruessner RWG, Kandaswamy R, Denny R. Laparoscopic simultaneous nephrectomy and distal pancreatectomy from a live donor. J Am Coll Surg 2001;193(3):333.
5. Gruessner RWG, Kendall DM, Drangstveit MB, Gruessner AC, Sutherland DER. Simultaneous pancreas-kidney transplantation from live donors. Ann Surg 1997;226(4):471.
6. Gruessner RWG, Leone JP, Sutherland DER. Combined kidney and pancreas transplants from living donors. Transplant Proc 1998;30:282.

7. Gruessner AC, Sutherland DER. Pancreas transplant outcomes for United States (US) and non-US cases as reported to the United Network for Organ Sharing (UNOS) and the International Pancreas Transplant Registry (IPTR) as of October 2002. Clin Transplant 2002:41.

8 Gruessner AC, Sutherland DE. Pancreas transplant outcomes for United States (US) and non-US cases as reported to the United Network for Organ Sharing (UNOS) and the International Pancreas Transplant Registry (IPTR) as of June 2004. Clin Transplant 2005;19(4):433–455.

9. Gruessner RWG, Sutherland DER. Simultaneous kidney and segmental pancreas transplants from living related donors – the first two successful cases. Transplantation 1996;61:1265.

10. Gruessner RWG, Sutherland DER, Drangstveit MB, Bland BJ, Gruessner AC. Pancreas transplants from living donors: short- and-long-term outcome. Transplant Proc 2001;33:819.

11. Jacobs SC, Cho E, Foster C, Liao P, Bartlett ST. Laparoscopic donor nephrectomy: the University of Maryland 6-year experience. J Urol 2004;171(1):47.

12. Kercher KW, Heniford BT, Matthews BD, et al. Laparoscopic versus open nephrectomy in 210 consecutive patients: outcomes, cost, and changes in practice patterns. Surg Endosc 2003;17(12):1889.

13. Leventhal JR, Deeik RK, Joehl RJ, et al. Laparoscopic live donor nephrectomy – is it safe? Transplantation 2000;70(4):602.

14. Martin X, Petruzzo P, Dawahra M, et al. Effects of portal versus systemic venous drainage in kidney-pancreas recipients. Transplant Int 2000;13(1):64–68.

15. Philosophe B, Farney AC, Schweitzer EJ, et al. Superiority of portal venous drainage over systemic venous drainage in pancreas transplantation: a retrospective study. Ann Surg 2001;234(5):689–696.

16. Reddy KS, Stratta RJ, Shokouh-Amiri MH, Alloway R, Egidi MF, Gaber AO. Surgical complications after pancreas transplantation with portal-enteric drainage. J Am Coll Surg 1999;189(3):305–313.

17. Schweitzer EJ, Wilson J, Jacobs S, et al. Increased rates of donation with laparoscopic donor nephrectomy. Ann Surg 2000;232(3):392.

18. Sharara AI, Dandan IS, Khalifeh M. Living-related donor transplantation other than kidney. Transplant Proc 2001;33:2745.

19. Stratta RJ, Gaber AO, Shokouh-Amiri MH, et al. A prospective comparison of systemic-bladder versus portal-enteric drainage in vascularized pancreas transplantation. Surgery 2000;127(2):217–226.

20. Sutherland DER, Najarian JS, Gruessner RWG. Living versus cadaver pancreas transplants. Transplant Proc 1998;30:2264.

21. Tan M, Kandaswamy R, Gruessner RWG. Laparoscopic donor distal pancreatectomy for living donor pancreas transplantation. Am J Transplant 2005;5(8):1966–1970.

22. Troppmann C, Gruessner AC, Sutherland DE, Gruessner RW. [Organ donation by living donors in isolated pancreas and simultaneous pancreas-kidney transplantation]. Zentralbl Chir 1999;124(8):734.

23. Ueno T, Oka M, Nishihara K, et al. Laparoscopic distal pancreatectomy with preservation of the spleen. Surg Laparosc Endosc Percutan Tech 1999;9(4):290.

24. Vezakis A, Davides D, Larvin M, McMahon MJ. Laparoscopic surgery combined with preservation of the spleen for distal pancreatic tumors. Surg Endosc 1999;13.

6

Liver Transplantation

Abhinav Humar and William D. Payne

Standard Procedure
a) Preoperative Evaluation
b) Surgical Procedure
c) Postoperative Care
d) Results
Benching the Liver from a Deceased Donor
a) Surgical Procedure
Adult Cadaver Liver Transplant
a) Surgical Procedure
Deceased Donor Split-Liver Transplant: Adult/Pediatric Recipients
Hasan Yersiz and John F. Renz
a) Surgical Procedure
Deceased Donor Split-Liver Transplant: Adult/Adult Recipients
a) Selection Criteria
b) Technical Aspects
c) Ethics of Splitting
d) Split Potential
e) Surgical Procedure
Living-Donor Liver Transplant: Pediatric Recipient
a) Donor Procedure
b) Recipient Procedure
Living-Donor Liver Transplant: Adult Recipient
a) Donor Procedure
b) Recipient Procedure
Surgical Complications After Liver Transplant
a) Hemorrhage
b) Hepatic Artery Complications
c) Portal Vein Complications
d) Biliary Complications
e) Wound Complications
f) Primary Nonfunction

Standard Procedure

The field of liver transplantation has undergone remarkable advances in the last two decades. An essentially experimental procedure in the early 1980s, a liver transplant is now the treatment of choice for patients with acute and chronic liver failure. Patient survival at 1 year posttransplant has increased from 30% in the early 1980s to more than

85% at present. The major reasons for this dramatic increase include refined surgical and preservation techniques, better immunosuppressive protocols, more effective treatment of infections, and improved care during the critical perioperative period. Yet a liver transplant remains a major undertaking, with the potential for complications affecting every major organ system.

The history of liver transplantation began with experimental transplants performed in dogs in the late 1950s. The first liver transplant attempted in humans was in 1963 by Thomas Starzl. The recipient was a 3-year-old boy with biliary atresia, who unfortunately died of hemorrhage. The first successful liver transplant was in 1967, again by Starzl. Yet, for the next 10 years, liver transplants remained essentially experimental, with survival rates well below 50%. Still, advances in the surgical procedure and in anesthetic management continued to be made during that time. The major breakthrough for the field came in the early 1980s, with the introduction and clinical use of the immunosuppressive agent cyclosporine. Patient survival dramatically improved, and liver transplant was soon being recognized as a viable therapeutic option for patients with liver failure. Results continued to improve through the 1980s, thanks to ongoing improvements in immunosuppression, in critical care management, in surgical technique, and in preservation solutions. The late 1980s and 1990s saw a dramatic increase in the number of liver transplants. However, there was an even greater increase in the number of patients waiting for a transplant, which in turn increased waiting times, as well as mortality rates while waiting.

The longer time and higher mortality rates on the deceased-donor liver waiting list led to the development of innovative surgical techniques, such as split-liver transplants and living-donor liver transplants. Initially, these new techniques were mainly applied to pediatric patients because of the difficulty associated with finding appropriate size-matched organs for them. However, as the number of adults on the waiting list grew, these techniques started to be applied for adult recipients as well. The use of living-donor liver transplants progressed at an even more rapid pace in countries where the concept of deceased-donor organ donation was not widely accepted.

a) Preoperative Evaluation

A liver transplant is indicated for liver failure, whether acute or chronic. Liver failure is signaled by a number of clinical symptoms (e.g., ascites, variceal bleeding, hepatic encephalopathy, malnutrition) and by biochemical liver test results that suggest impaired hepatic synthetic function (e.g., hypoalbuminemia, hyperbilirubinemia, coagulopathy). The cause of liver failure often influences its presentation. For example, patients with acute liver failure generally have hepatic encephalopathy and coagulopathy, whereas patients with chronic liver disease most commonly have ascites, gastrointestinal bleeding, and malnutrition.

A host of diseases are potentially treatable by a liver transplant. Broadly, they can be categorized as acute or chronic, and then subdivided by the cause of the liver disease. Chronic liver diseases account for the majority of liver transplants today. The most common cause in North America is chronic hepatitis, usually due to hepatitis C, less commonly to hepatitis B. Chronic alcohol abuse accelerates the process, especially with hepatitis C. Chronic hepatitis may also result from autoimmune causes, primarily in women; it can present either acutely over months or insidiously over years. Alcohol often plays a role in end-stage liver disease secondary to hepatitis C, but it may also lead to liver failure in the absence of that viral infection.

Cholestatic disorders (primary biliary cirrhosis, primary sclerosing cholangitis, and biliary atresia) also account for a significant percentage of transplant candidates with chronic liver disease. A variety of metabolic diseases can result in progressive, chronic liver injury and cirrhosis, including hereditary hemochromatosis, α_1-antitrypsin deficiency, and Wilson's disease.

Hepatocellular carcinoma (HCC) may be a complication of cirrhosis from any cause, most commonly with hepatitis B, hepatitis C, hemochromatosis, and tyrosinemia. Patients with HCC may have stable liver disease, but are not candidates for hepatic resection because of the underlying cirrhosis; they are best treated with a liver transplant. The best transplant candidates are those with a single lesion less than 5 cm in size, or with no more than three lesions, the largest no greater than 3 cm in size. Beyond this, the tumor recurrence rates after transplant may be quite high.

Acute liver disease, more commonly termed fulminant hepatic failure, is defined as the development of hepatic encephalopathy and profound coagulopathy shortly after the onset of symptoms, such as jaundice, in patients without preexisting liver disease. The most common causes include acetaminophen overdose, acute hepatitis B, various drugs and hepatotoxins, and Wilson's disease; often, however, no cause is identified. Treatment consists of appropriate critical care support, giving patients time for spontaneous recovery. The prognosis for spontaneous recovery depends on the patient's age (those younger than 10 and older than 40 years have a poor prognosis), the underlying cause, and the severity of liver injury (as indicated by degree of hepatic encephalopathy, coagulopathy, and kidney dysfunction).

The simple presence of chronic liver disease with established cirrhosis is not an indication for a transplant. Some patients have very well compensated cirrhosis with a low expectant mortality. Patients with decompensated cirrhosis, however, have a poor prognosis without transplant. The signs and symptoms of decompensated cirrhosis include hepatic encephalopathy, ascites, spontaneous bacterial peritonitis, portal hypertensive bleeding, hepatorenal syndrome, and severe debilitation with muscle wasting.

Once it is decided that a liver transplant is clinically indicated, it is important to ensure that there are no contraindications to transplant. There are no specific age limits for recipients; their mean age is steadily increasing. Patients must have adequate cardiac and pulmonary function. Coronary artery disease is uncommon in liver transplant candidates, but those with cirrhosis may develop significant hypoxia and pulmonary hypertension; those with severe hypoxemia or with right atrial pressures greater than 60 mm Hg rarely survive a liver transplant. Other contraindications, as with other types of transplants, include uncontrolled systemic infection and malignancy. Those HCC patients with metastatic disease, obvious vascular invasion, or significant tumor burden are not good transplant candidates. Patients with other types of extrahepatic malignancy should be deferred for at least 2 years after completing curative therapy before a transplant is attempted. Currently, the most common contraindication to a liver transplant is ongoing substance abuse. Before considering patients for a transplant, most centers require a documented period of abstinence, demonstration of compliant behavior, and willingness to pursue a chemical dependency program.

b) Surgical Procedure

The surgical procedure is divided into three phases: pre-anhepatic, anhepatic, and post-anhepatic. The pre-anhepatic phase involves mobilizing the recipient's diseased liver in preparation for its removal. The basic steps include isolating the supra- and infrahepatic vena cava, portal vein, and hepatic artery, and then dividing the bile duct. Given existing coagulopathy and portal hypertension, the recipient hepatectomy may be the most difficult part of the procedure. The anesthesia team must be prepared to deal with excessive blood loss.

Once the above structures have been isolated, vascular clamps are applied. The recipient's liver is removed, thus beginning the anhepatic phase. This phase is characterized by decreased venous return to the heart because of occlusion of the inferior vena cava and portal vein. Some centers routinely employ a venovenous bypass (VVB) system during this time: blood is drawn from the lower body and bowels via a cannula in the common femoral vein and portal vein, and returned through a central venous cannula in the upper body. Potential advantages of bypass include improved hemodynamic stability, reduction of bleeding from an engorged portal system, and avoidance of elevated venous pressure in the renal veins. However, many centers do not routinely use VVB or selectively reserve it for patients who demonstrate hemodynamic instability with a trial of caval clamping.

With the recipient liver removed, the donor liver is anastomosed to the appropriate structures to place it in an orthotopic position. The suprahepatic caval anastomosis is performed first, followed by the infrahepatic cava and the portal vein. The portal and caval clamps may be removed at this time. The new liver is then allowed to reperfuse. Either before or after this step, the hepatic artery may be anastomosed.

With the clamps removed and the new liver reperfused, the post-anhepatic phase begins, often characterized by marked changes in the recipient's status. The most dramatic changes in hemodynamic parameters usually occur on reperfusion, namely hypotension and the potential for serious arrhythmia. Severe coagulopathy may also develop because of the release of natural anticoagulants from the ischemic liver or because of active fibrinolysis. Both ε-aminocaproic acid and aprotinin have been used prophylactically to prevent fibrinolysis and decrease transfusion requirements. Electrolyte abnormalities, most commonly hyperkalemia and hypercalcemia, are often seen after reperfusion; they are usually transient and respond well to treatment with calcium chloride and sodium bicarbonate. After reperfusion, the final anastomosis is performed, establishing biliary drainage. The recipient's remaining common bile duct (choledochoduodenostomy) or a loop of bowel (choledochojejunostomy) may be used.

Several variations of the standard operation have been described. With the "piggyback technique," the recipient's inferior vena cava is preserved, the infrahepatic donor cava is oversewn, and the suprahepatic cava is anastomosed to the confluence of the recipient hepatic veins. With this technique, the recipient's cava does not have to be completely cross-clamped during anastomosis—thus allowing blood from the lower body to return to the heart uninterrupted, without the need for VVB. The piggyback technique has many potential advantages, including improved hemodynamic stability, improved kidney perfusion, and avoidance of the complications possible with VVB. However, no good randomized studies have yet demonstrated the superiority of one technique over the other.

Another important variation of the standard operation is a partial transplant, either a living-donor transplant or a deceased-donor split-liver transplant. Both have developed in response to the donor shortage, and are gaining in popularity. Usually, in living-donor liver transplants for pediatric recipients, the left lateral segment or left lobe is used; for adult recipients, the right lobe is used. Split-liver transplants from deceased donors involve dividing the donor liver into two segments, each of which is subsequently transplanted.

c) Postoperative Care

The immediate postoperative care for liver recipients involves (1) stabilizing the major organ systems (e.g., cardiovascular, pulmonary, renal); (2) evaluating graft function and achieving adequate immunosuppression; and (3) monitoring and treating complications directly and indirectly related to the transplant. This initial care should generally be performed in an intensive care unit (ICU) setting, because recipients usually require mechanical ventilatory support for the first 12 to 24 hours. The goal is to maintain adequate oxygen saturation, acid–base equilibrium, and stable hemodynamics. Continuous hemodynamic monitoring is important to ensure adequate perfusion of the graft and vital organs. Hemodynamic instability early posttransplant is usually due to fluid imbalance, but ongoing bleeding must first be ruled out. Instability may also be secondary to the myocardial dysfunction that is often seen early in the reperfusion phase, but that may persist into the early postoperative period. Such dysfunction is characterized by decreased compliance and contractility of the ventricles. The usual treatment is to optimize preload and afterload and to use inotropic agents such as dopamine or dobutamine if necessary.

Fluid management, electrolyte status, and kidney function require frequent evaluation. Most liver recipients have an increased extravascular volume but a reduced intravascular volume. Attention should be given to the potassium, calcium, magnesium, phosphate, and glucose levels. Potassium may be elevated because of poor kidney function, a residual perfusion effect, or medications. Diuretics may be required to remove excess fluid acquired intraoperatively, but they may result in hypokalemia. Magnesium levels should be kept above 2 mg/dL to prevent seizures, and phosphate levels between 2 and 5 mg/dL for proper support of the respiratory and alimentary tracts. Marked hyperglycemia, which may be secondary to steroids, should be treated with insulin. Hypoglycemia is often an indication of poor hepatic function.

A crucial aspect of postoperative care is to repeatedly evaluate graft function. In fact, doing so begins intraoperatively, soon after the liver is reperfused. Signs of hepatic function include good texture and good color of the graft, evidence of bile production, and restoration of hemodynamic stability. Postoperatively, hepatic function can be assessed using clinical signs and laboratory values. Patients who rapidly awaken from anesthesia and whose mental status progressively improves likely have a well-functioning graft. Laboratory indicators of good graft function include normalization of the coagulation profile, resolution of hypoglycemia and hyperbilirubinemia, and clearance of serum lactate. Adequate urine production and good output of bile through the biliary tube (if present) are also indicators of good graft function. Serum transaminase levels will usually rise during the first 48 to 72 hours posttransplant secondary to preservation injury, and then should fall rapidly over the next 24 to 48 hours.

Another important aspect of postoperative care is to monitor for any surgical and medical complications. The incidence of complications tends to be high after liver transplants, especially in patients who were severely debilitated pretransplant. Surgical complications related directly to the operation include postoperative hemorrhage and problems with the anastomoses.

d) Results

Patient and graft survival rates after liver transplants have improved significantly since the mid-1990s, with many centers now reporting graft survival rates of about 85% at 1 year. The main factors affecting short-term (within the first year posttransplant) patient and graft survival are the medical condition of the patient at the time of transplant and the development of early postoperative surgical complications. Severely debilitated patients, with numerous comorbid conditions such as kidney dysfunction, coagulopathy, and malnutrition, have a significantly higher risk of early posttransplant mortality. Such patients are more likely to develop surgical and medical complications (especially infections) and are unable to tolerate them. The national U.S. data shows that for 2001, patient survival at 1 year was 86.4%, and graft survival 80.2%.

Long-term survival rates (after the first year posttransplant) depend more on the cause of the underlying liver disease and on the presence or absence in the recipient of risk factors for other medical problems (especially cardiovascular risk factors). Generally, from 1 to 10 years posttransplant, survival curves slowly decline. Roughly half of the deaths in this time period are due to events not related to the underlying liver disease (e.g., myocardial infarctions, cerebrovascular accidents, and trauma). The other half of the deaths, however, are related to complications either of the underlying liver disease (e.g., recurrence) or of immunosuppression (e.g., infection or malignancy).

The original cause of liver failure has a definite impact on long-term survival rates. Primary biliary cirrhosis in adults and biliary atresia in children are generally associated with a better long-term outcome, because recurrence of these diseases in the transplanted liver is rare. But recipients with HCC or hepatitis C usually have poorer long-term outcome, because these diseases may recur posttransplant.

Benching the Liver from a Deceased Donor

Similar to the kidney or pancreas, benchwork of the cadaver liver is an important part of the operative procedure. The basic steps involved include careful inspection of the liver, removal of attached diaphragm, dissection of the infra- and suprahepatic cava, and dissection of the hilar structures (common bile duct, portal vein, and hepatic artery).

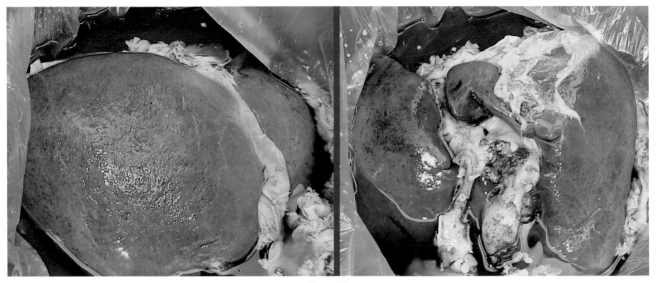

Figure 6.1

a) Surgical Procedure

1. All aspects of the liver are carefully inspected to evaluate for steatosis and areas of trauma (Figure 6.1). Biopsy may be warranted if the appearance is abnormal.

2. Starting first with the posterior aspect of the liver, the retrohepatic cava (broken blue line) is visualized and excess retroperitoneal tissue is removed. It helps to have the assistant place his/her finger in the cava during this step (Figure 6.2). The adrenal vein (blue arrow) and any lumbar veins are identified and ligated, and the adrenal gland (broken yellow line) is removed.

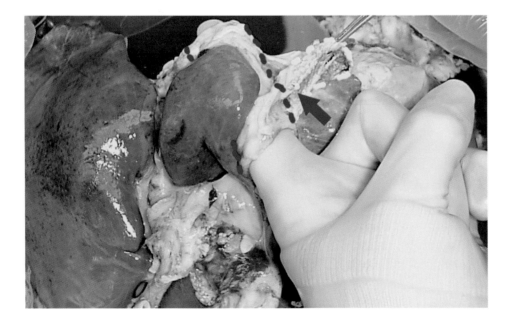

Figure 6.2

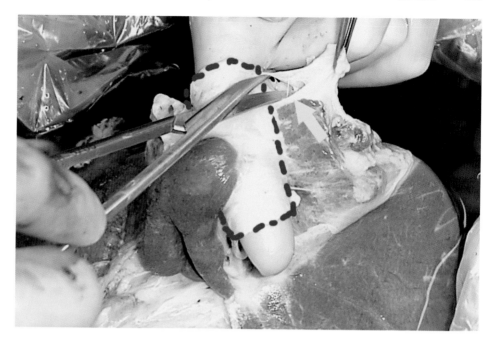

Figure 6.3

3. Diaphragm attached to the right and left lobe is dissected free and discarded. Phrenic vein branches (yellow arrow) should be identified and ligated (Figure 6.3).

4. The cava can be inspected and probed from the inside to ensure that all phrenic branches (black arrow) and the adrenal vein (gray arrow) have been ligated (Figure 6.4).

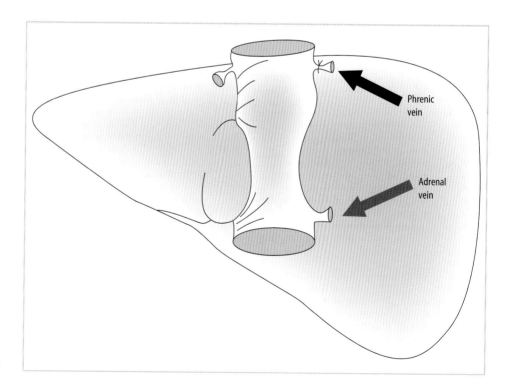

Phrenic
vein

Adrenal
vein

Figure 6.4

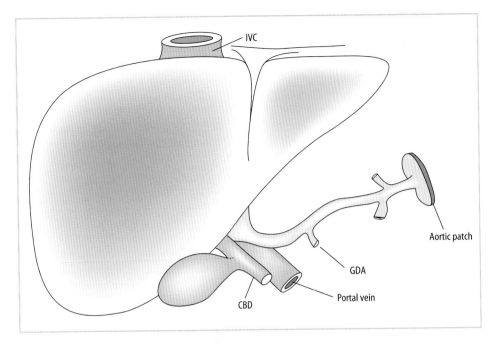

Figure 6.5

5. The hilum is inspected and the common bile duct, hepatic artery, and portal vein identified (Figures 6.5 and 6.6). The portal vein (blue arrow) is dissected free distally in the hilum until the bifurcation is seen. The arterial blood supply (yellow arrow) is inspected for variations. An aortic patch is made and excess tissue is removed from the patch to the gastroduodenal artery (GDA). Branches not going to the liver are oversewn.

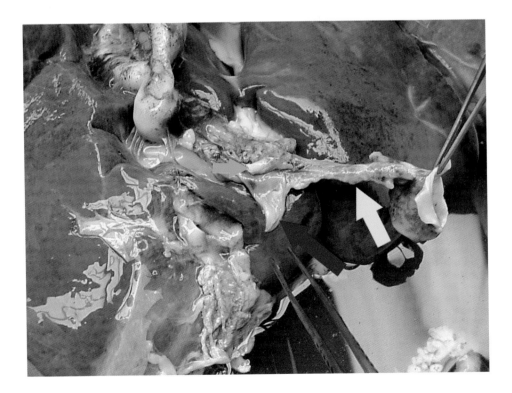

Figure 6.6

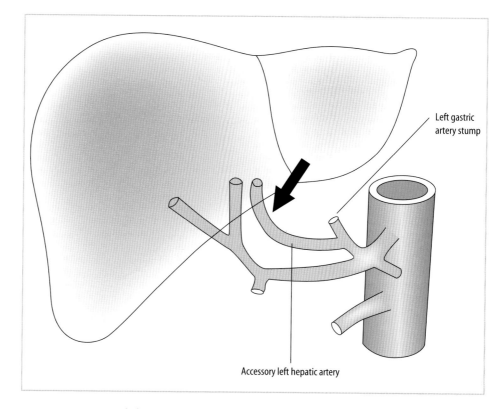

Figure 6.7

6. An accessory left hepatic artery (HA) usually arises from the left gastric artery, a branch of the celiac axis (Figure 6.7). Generally no reconstruction is required. The accessory left HA is traced from its origin to the liver, and branches not going to the liver are ligated.

7. An accessory right HA usually arises from the superior mesenteric artery (SMA), and passes behind the common bile duct. It should be dissected free from its origin to distally until there is an adequate length. It can then be reconstructed by mobilizing it and anastomosing to either the stump of the splenic artery (SA) (Figure 6.8b), or the

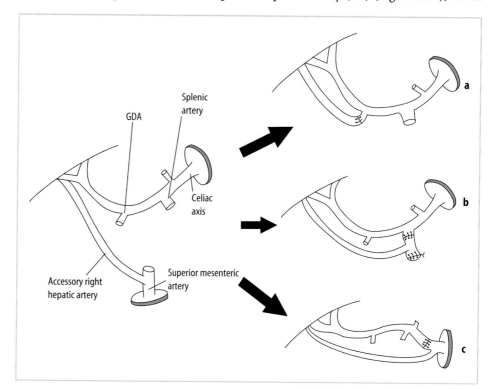

Figure 6.8

gastroduodenal artery (GDA) (Figure 6.8a), or by anastomosing the common hepatic artery itself onto the stump of the SMA (Figure 6.8c).

8. If a caval replacement technique is planned, the inferior vena cava is left open at both ends (Figure 6.9a). If a standard piggyback technique is planned, the infrahepatic cava is closed with a running stitch (Figure 6.9b). A small corner of this closure is left open to allow for later flushing of the liver once the anastomoses are completed. If a side-to-side cavaplasty is planned for outflow reconstruction, both the supra- and infrahepatic caval openings are closed and a venotomy is made in the middle of the cava, along its posterior aspect (Figure 6.9c).

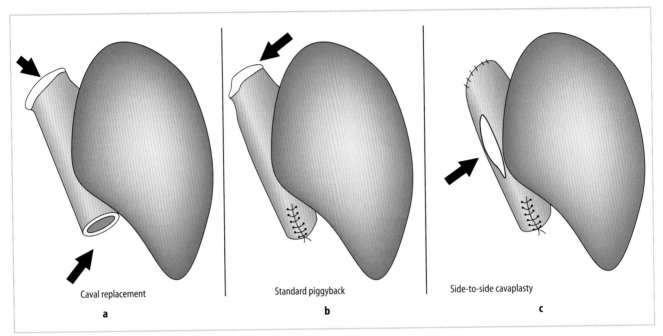

Caval replacement

a

Standard piggyback

b

Side-to-side cavaplasty

c

Figure 6.9

Adult Cadaver Liver Transplant

a) Surgical Procedure

1. The patient is placed in the supine position with both arms abducted. A bilateral subcostal incision, which can be extended in the midline toward the xiphoid, is made (Figure 6.10). One of the groins (black arrow) should also be prepped if systemic bypass is later contemplated. The axillary vein can be used to shunt the blood back to the heart when on bypass, but our preference is to cannulate the internal jugular vein percutaneously (gray arrow).

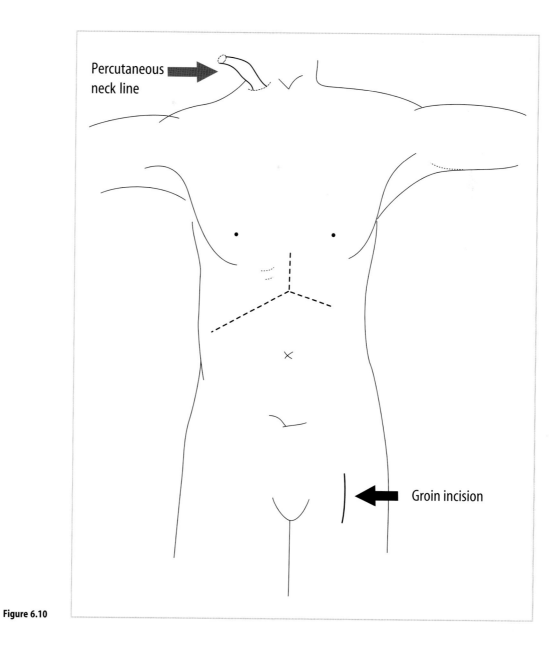

Figure 6.10

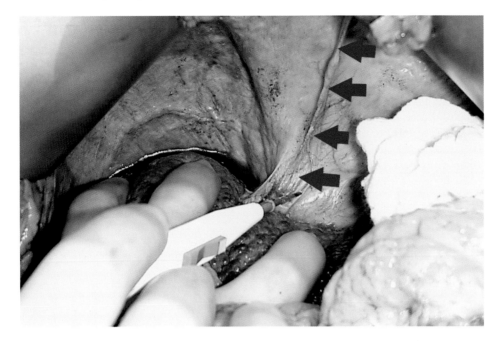

Figure 6.11

2. The operation begins with the removal of the diseased liver. The teres ligament is divided between ligatures; the liver is retracted inferiorly and the falciform ligament (blue arrows) divided with the electrocautery (Figure 6.11).

3. The left triangular ligament is divided (broken black line), stopping medially at the left hepatic vein (black arrow) (Figure 6.12).

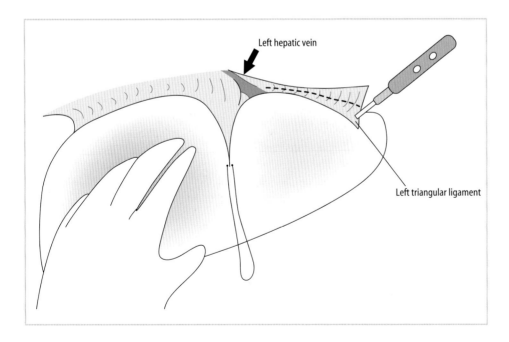

Left hepatic vein

Left triangular ligament

Figure 6.12

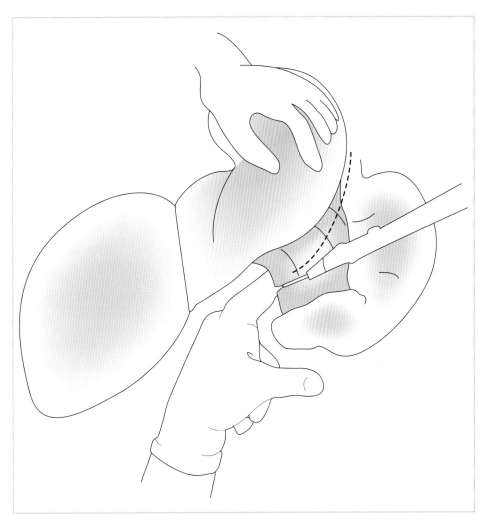

Figure 6.13

4. The gastrohepatic ligament is divided from the edge of the hepatic hilum superiorly to the edge of the left hepatic vein (Figures 6.13 and 6.14). Care should be taken to appropriately ligate an accessory left hepatic artery if present.

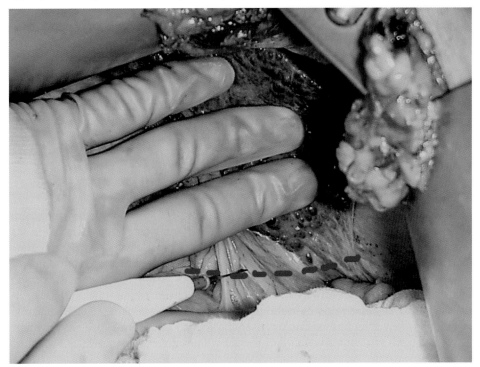

Figure 6.14

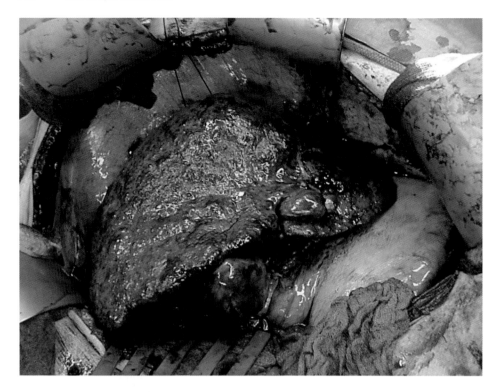

Figure 6.15

5. The self-retaining retractors can then be inserted to allow for wide exposure of the upper quadrant (Figure 6.15). Good retraction of the rib cage is an essential part of the procedure. An upper body retractor fixed to both sides of the bed provides good retraction of the rib cage, even in obese patients (Figure 6.16).

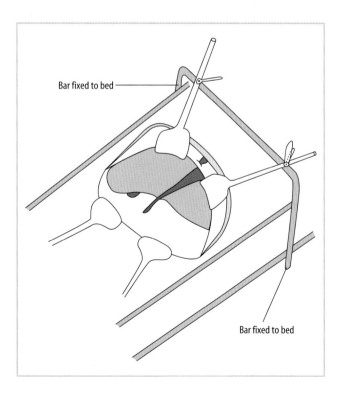

Bar fixed to bed

Bar fixed to bed

Figure 6.16

6. The hilar dissection is then commenced, starting high in the hilum, close to the liver (broken blue line) (Figure 6.17). Because of portal hypertension, there may be significant bleeding from small vessels and other tissues. The cautery and careful ligation are important to try to minimize bleeding.

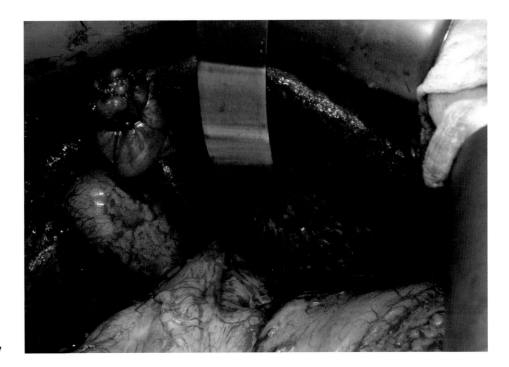

Figure 6.17

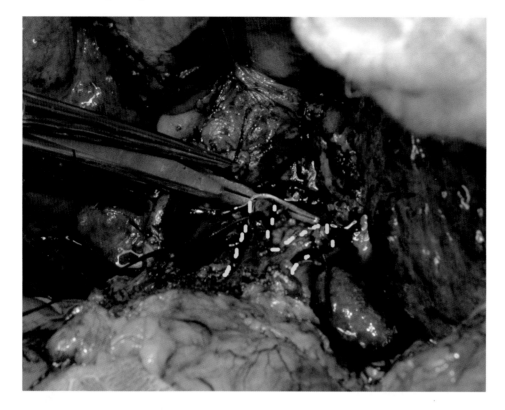

Figure 6.18

7. The common hepatic artery is isolated first, and traced distally to the left and right branches (Figure 6.18). These are individually divided to allow for later creation of a patch for the arterial anastomosis (Figure 6.19).

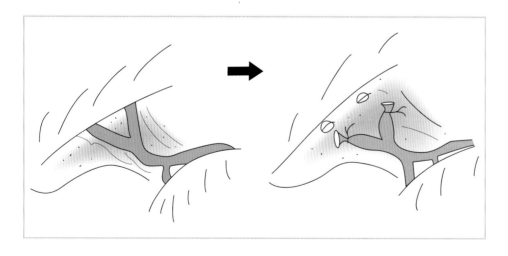

Figure 6.19

8. If the artery is small at this level, it should be traced further proximally beyond the gastroduodenal artery (yellow arrow) (Figure 6.20). The gastroduodenal artery can then be divided (broken yellow line) and a patch created for anastomosis using this bifurcation.

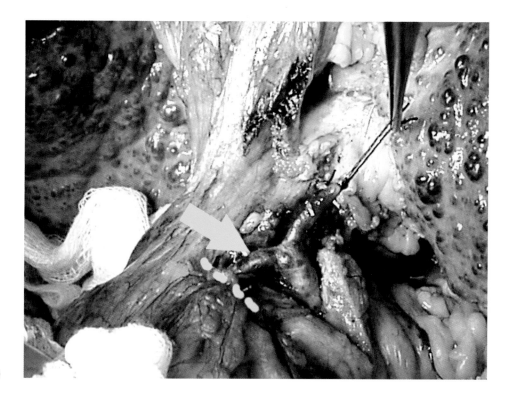

Figure 6.20

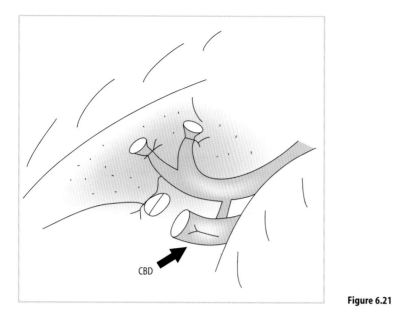

Figure 6.21

9. The common bile duct (CBD) (broken yellow line) is dissected free in the right edge of the hepatoduodenal ligament. The proximal end is ligated and the duct is divided, preserving some length on the distal portion that will be later used for anastomosis to the transplant duct (Figures 6.21 and 6.22). The distal end of the duct will require fine suture ligation of the accompanying biliary veins to control troublesome bleeding.

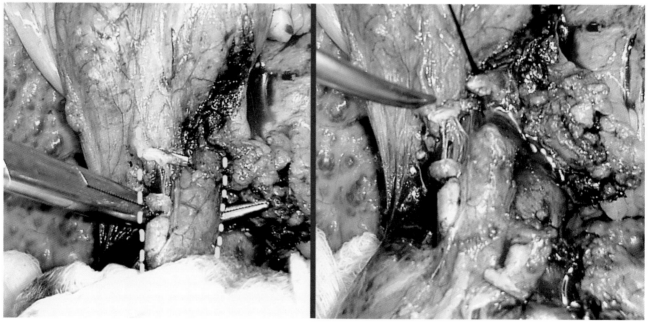

Figure 6.22

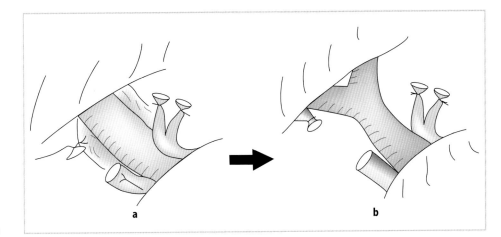

Figure 6.23

10. The portal vein is then identified lying in between and deep to the course of the common hepatic artery and the common bile duct. Once the portal vein is isolated and encircled (Figure 6.23a), all other structures in the hilum at that level (lymphatics, nodes, nerves) can be divided between ligatures or with cautery (Figure 6.23b). The portal vein is traced distally until the bifurcation is identified (Figure 6.24).

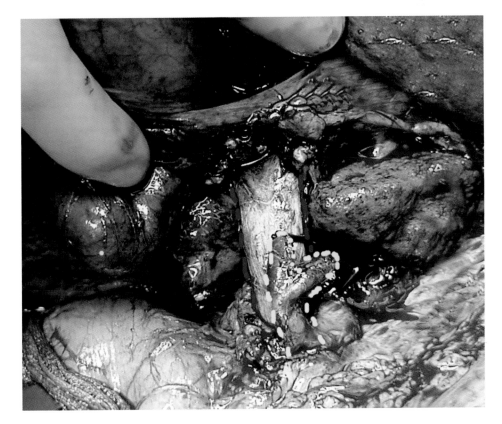

Figure 6.24

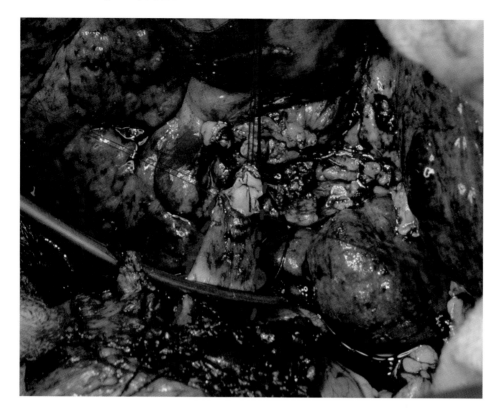

Figure 6.25

11. If a portal bypass is to be performed at this point, the portal vein (broken blue line) is clamped proximally with a vascular clamp, and divided as far distally as possible. The distal stump is oversewn or suture ligated (Figure 6.25).

12. A cannula is then placed in the portal vein and secured in place with a tie, which is tied around the distal portal vein (Figure 6.26) and then secured to the cannula.

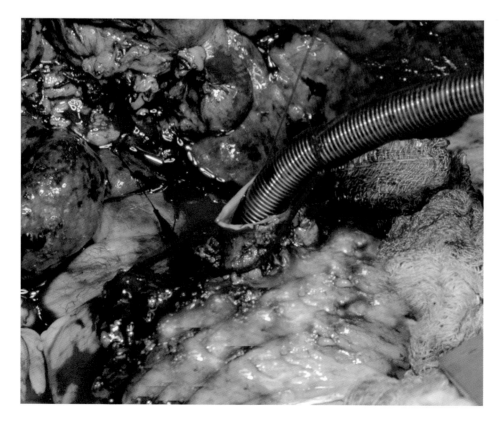

Figure 6.26

13. Systemic bypass can be performed by placing a cannula through the greater saphenous vein into the common iliac vein (Figure 6.27). This can be done through a groin incision.

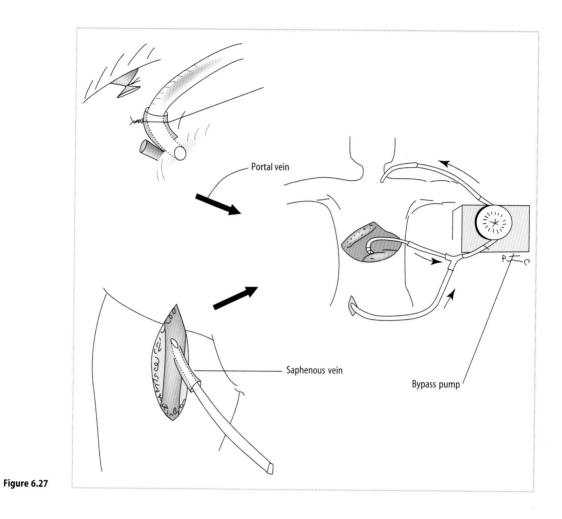

Portal vein

Saphenous vein

Bypass pump

Figure 6.27

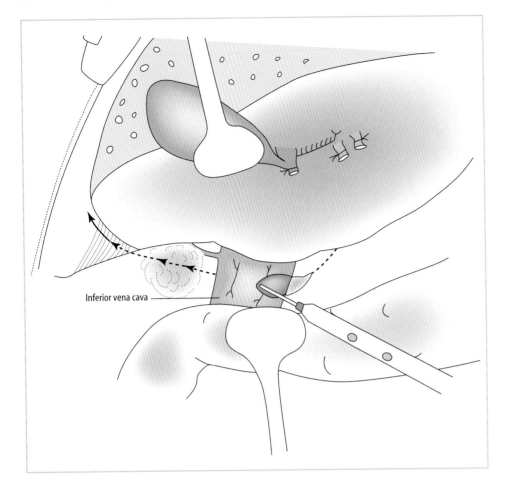

Figure 6.28

14. Mobilization of the liver is continued. The infrahepatic cava (broken blue line) is visualized by division of the peritoneum anterior to it with electrocautery (Figures 6.28 and 6.29). It can then be encircled (Figure 6.29). The adrenal branch (yellow arrow), if seen, should be divided when a caval replacement procedure is planned.

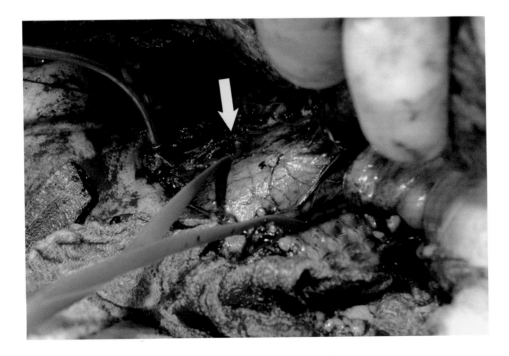

Figure 6.29

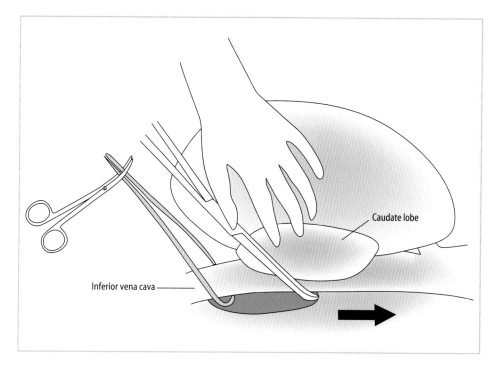

Caudate lobe

Inferior vena cava

Figure 6.30

15. The liver is then approached from the left side. With the left lobe retracted over to the right, dissection is continued from the infrahepatic cava superiorly along the margin of the left side of the inferior vena cava (Figure 6.30). Superiorly the dissection should extend to where the left phrenic vein enters the cava.

16. The left lobe is returned to its place and dissection is carried out further along the falciform ligament until the anterior aspect of the three hepatic veins is clearly visualized (Figure 6.31).

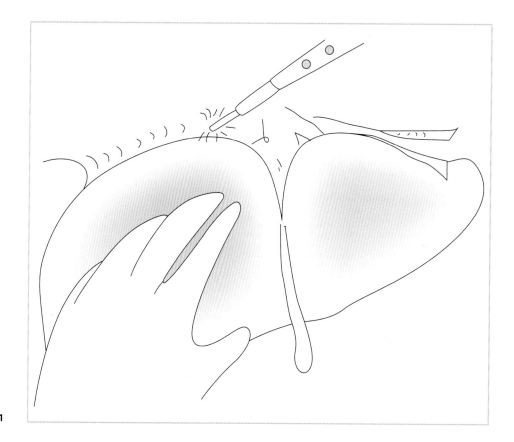

Figure 6.31

17. The liver and the right lobe are now rotated to the left, allowing for visualization and division of the right triangular ligament (Figure 6.32).

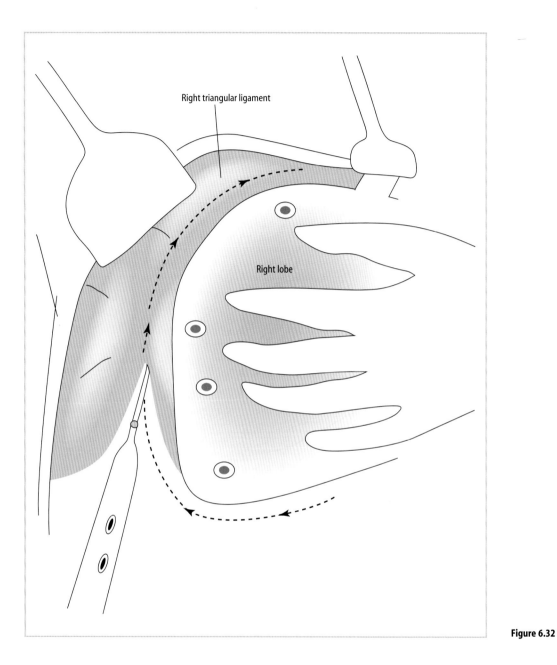

Figure 6.32

18. Continuing to rotate the liver to the left, the entire right lobe along its bare area is mobilized from the retroperitoneum (Figure 6.33). Care should be taken to stay close to the surface of the liver to avoid bleeding from enlarged retroperitoneal veins. The right lateral aspect of the retrohepatic cava should now be visible.

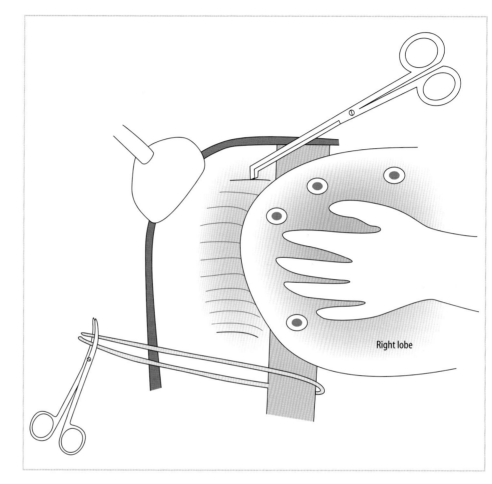

Figure 6.33

19. The suprahepatic cava can now be encircled and a plastic tubing or umbilical tape passed around it (Figure 6.34).

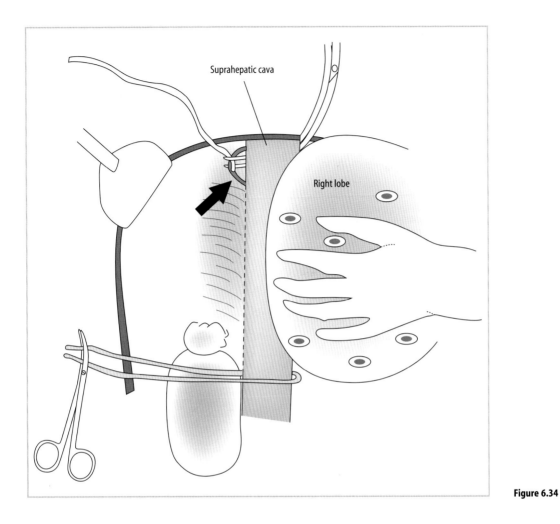

Figure 6.34

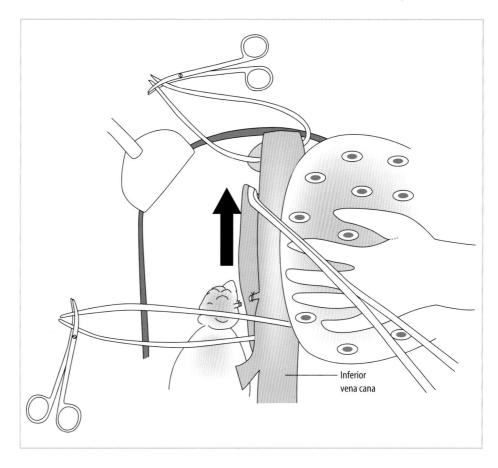

Inferior
vena cana

Figure 6.35

20. Finally, the posterior aspect of the cava is completely freed from its tissue attachments. The adrenal vein, if not already divided, should be ligated and divided (Figure 6.35).

21. Clamps are then placed on the supra- and infrahepatic cava; these structures are divided and the liver is removed (Figure 6.36). With the liver removed, the retroperitoneal area can be inspected for hemostasis. Once this is reasonably controlled, implantation of the graft can begin.

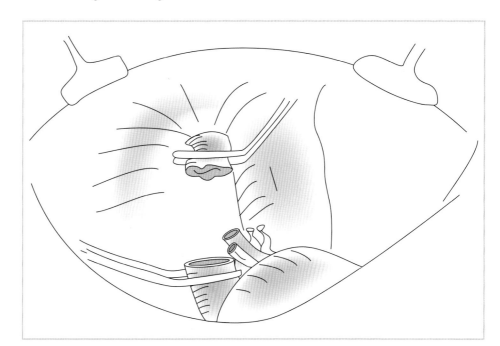

Figure 6.36

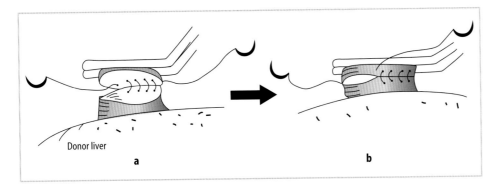

Donor liver

a

b

Figure 6.37

22. The suprahepatic caval anastomosis is then performed. The back wall is performed first using a vertical mattress type of suturing technique (Figure 6.37a), followed by an "over and over" stitch for the anterior wall (Figure 6.37b).

23. The infrahepatic caval anastomosis is performed next in a similar fashion (Figure 6.38a). A small corner in the anterior wall should be left open to wash blood and storage solution out of the liver at the "flushing" phase (Figure 6.38b).

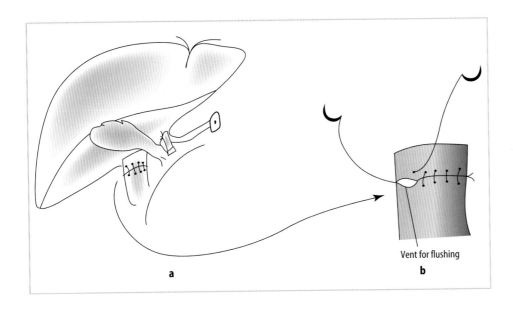

Vent for flushing

a

b

Figure 6.38

24. The hepatic arterial anastomosis can be performed next, or after the portal anastomosis and reperfusion of the liver are complete. The donor's proper hepatic artery can be sewn in an end-to-end fashion to the recipient's hepatic artery at the level of the right and left bifurcation, or at the level of the gastroduodenal artery. A bifurcation point is used for the arterial anastomosis so that the vessel can be opened up to create a patch around the main arterial vessel (Figure 6.39).

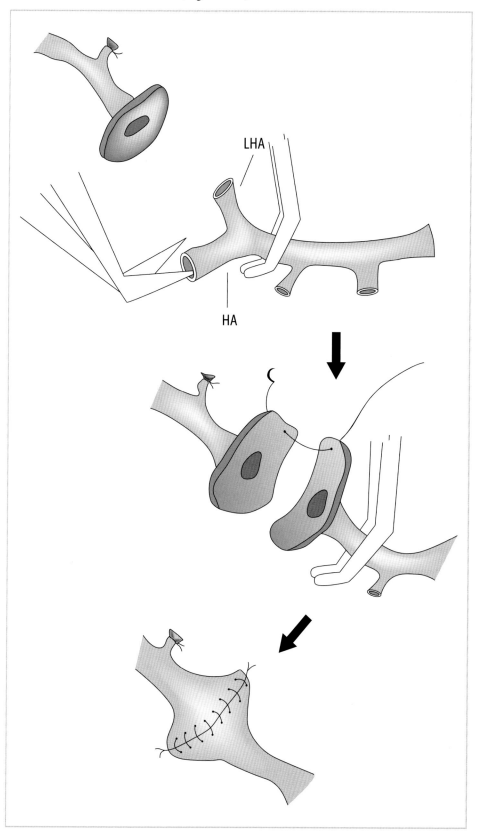

Figure 6.39

25. Finally the portal venous anastomosis is performed in an end-to-end continuous fashion. The ends are tied with an "air" knot (black arrow) of about 2 cm – this provides a "growth factor" for the vein, preventing narrowing when the vein fills with blood (Figure 6.40).

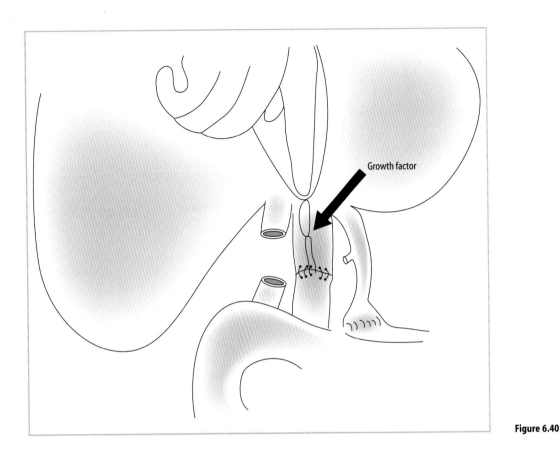

Figure 6.40

26. The graft is now ready to be flushed. The portal clamp is opened and 300 to 600 cc of blood is allowed to flush out via the small opening at the infrahepatic caval anastomosis (Figure 6.41). The opening for the flush is then closed, and all clamps are removed to allow the liver to perfuse with arterial and portal venous blood.

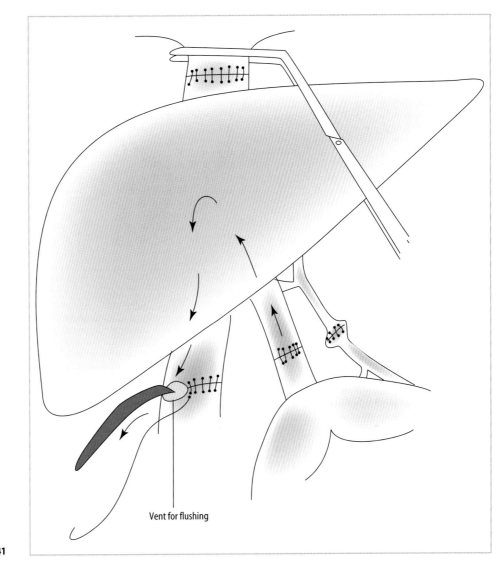

Vent for flushing

Figure 6.41

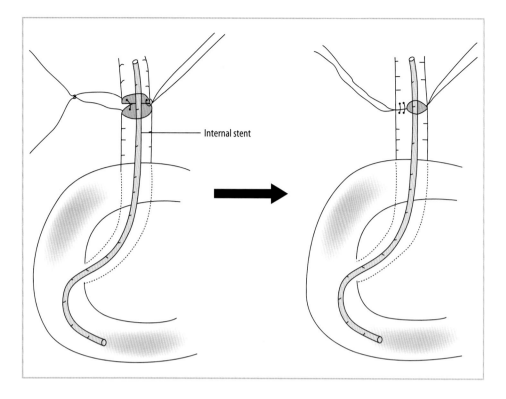

Figure 6.42

27. After any major bleeding points are controlled, the final anastomosis (the common bile duct, CBD) can be performed. The gallbladder is removed first. The donor CBD is anastomosed in an end-to-end fashion to the recipient CBD using interrupted absorbable sutures. The back wall is completed first, followed by the arterial wall. It is helpful to do this anastomosis over an internal stent (Figure 6.42).

28. Alternatively, if the recipient's distal common bile duct cannot be used (e.g., sclerosing cholangitis in recipient), biliary continuity can be restored with a hepaticojejunostomy to a Roux-en-Y bowel loop. The loop itself should be about 40 to 50 cm in length and should be brought up through the transverse mesocolon, such that it lies next to the donor bile duct without any tension (Figure 6.43).

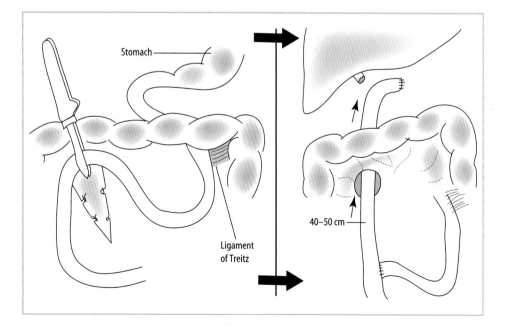

Figure 6.43

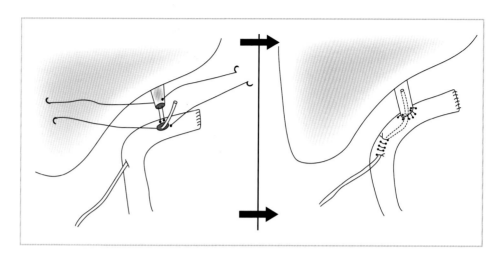

29. The bile duct is then sewn to a small opening created in the bowel using interrupted absorbable suture. The back wall is done first, followed by the anterior wall. It is helpful to place an external stent through this anastomosis, which is brought out through the Roux loop and then through the anterior abdominal wall (Figure 6.44).

Figure 6.44

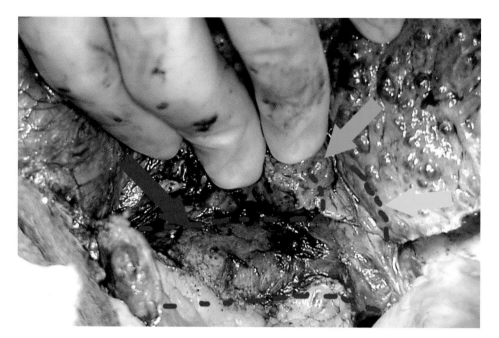

Figure 6.45

Standard "Piggyback" Technique

1. In a standard "piggyback" technique the retrohepatic cava of the recipient is preserved. The liver is mobilized completely off the underlying cava, leaving it attached by only the three main hepatic veins. This is done by first retracting the left lobe over to the right and mobilizing the caudate lobe (green arrow) from the cava (blue arrow) by division of any venous branches (Figures 6.45 and 6.46). It is easiest to start inferiorly and proceed superiorly, stopping at the lower border of the left hepatic vein (yellow arrow).

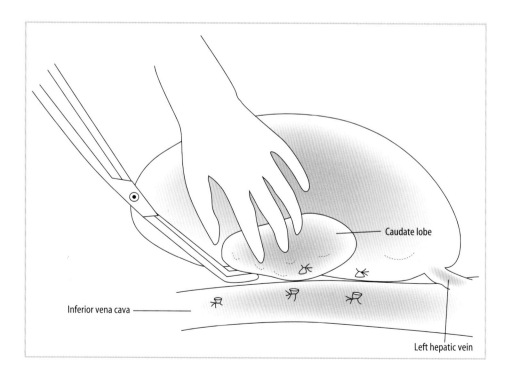

Figure 6.46

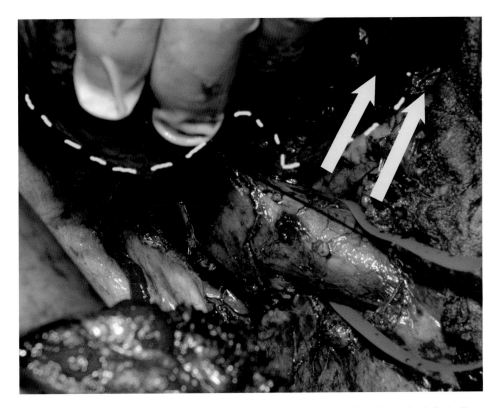

Figure 6.47

2. The liver (broken yellow line) is then retracted superiorly and to the left (yellow arrow), and the process is repeated from the right side (Figures 6.47 and 6.48). In this manner the liver is completely separated from the retrohepatic cava, leaving it attached by only the three main hepatic veins.

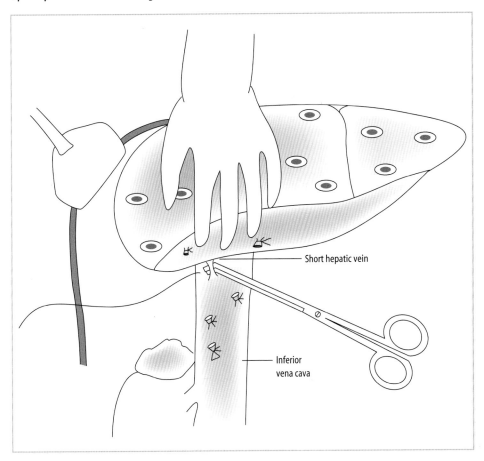

Figure 6.48

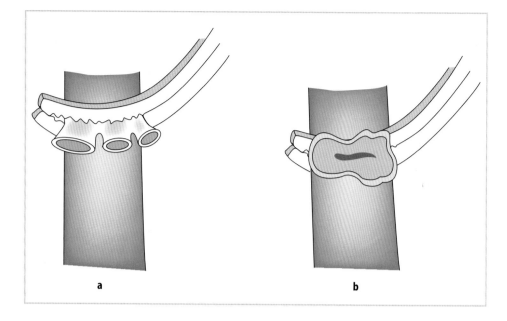

Figure 6.49

3. A clamp is then placed across the cava just distal to the junction with the three hepatic veins (Figure 6.49a). The cava is only partially occluded and venous return continues to the heart. The orifices of the three hepatic veins are then opened up together to create one common orifice (Figure 6.49b).

4. The suprahepatic cava of the donor is then sewn to the common orifice of the recipient hepatic veins (black arrow) (Figure 6.50a). Note the donor infrahepatic cava has already been sutured closed, except for a small opening in the corner to allow for later flushing (Figure 6.50b).

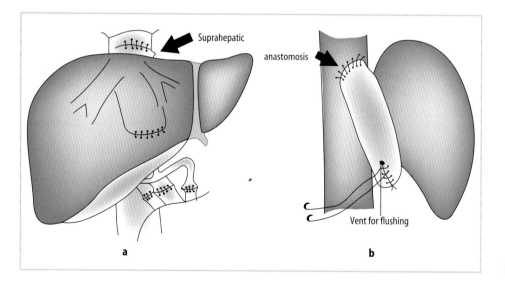

Figure 6.50

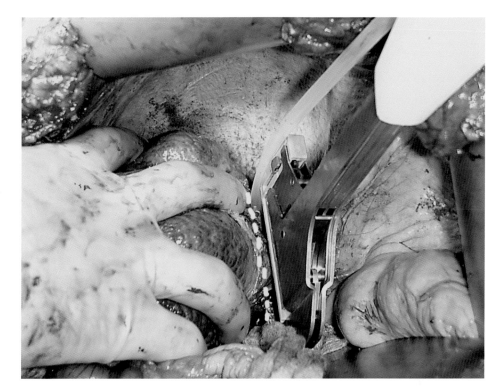

Figure 6.51

Side-to-Side Cavaplasty

1. In this modification of the piggyback procedure, the three hepatic veins of the recipient are simply sutured or stapled shut (Figure 6.51) and the diseased liver is removed by dividing the three hepatic veins beyond the staple line (broken yellow line) (Figure 6.52).

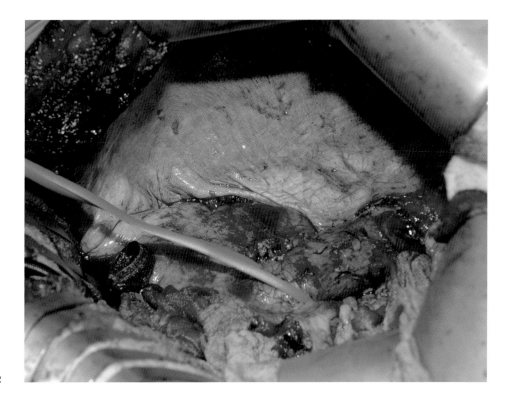

Figure 6.52

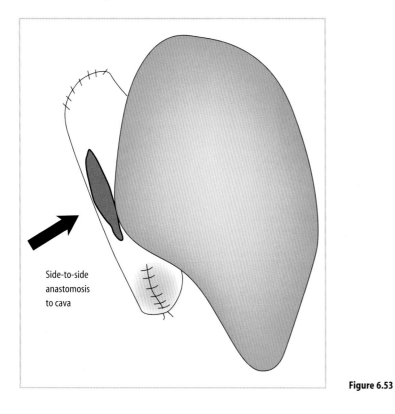

Side-to-side
anastomosis
to cava

Figure 6.53

2. The supra- and infrahepatic cava of the donor liver are sutured closed. A venotomy is made in the posterior aspect of the donor retrohepatic cava (Figure 6.53).

3. A corresponding venotomy is made on the anterior aspect of the recipient's retrohepatic cava, after application of a partially occluding clamp (Figure 6.54).

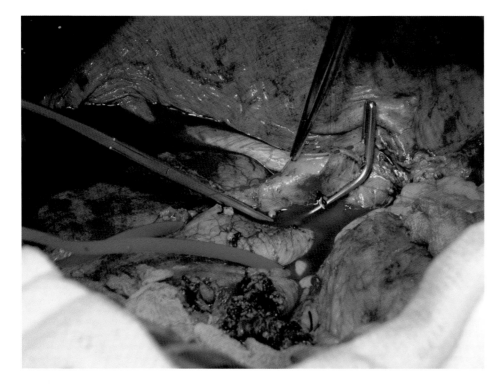

Figure 6.54

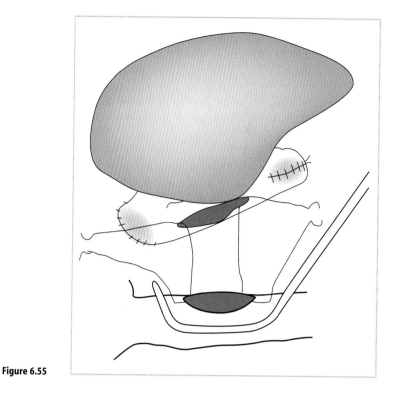

Figure 6.55

4. The anastomosis is then completed in a side-to-side fashion. This can be done by placing four corner sutures (Figure 6.55), and then sewing in a circumferential manner.

Deceased Donor Split-Liver Transplant: Adult/Pediatric Recipients

Hasan Yersiz and John F. Renz

One method to increase the number of liver transplants is to split the liver from a deceased donor into two grafts, which are then transplanted into two recipients. Thus, a whole adult liver from such a donor can be divided into two functioning grafts. The vast majority of split-liver transplants (SLTs) have been between one adult and one pediatric recipient. Usually the liver is split into a smaller portion (the left lateral segment, which can be transplanted into a pediatric recipient), and a larger portion (the extended right lobe, which can be transplanted into a normal-sized adult recipient). Results for pediatric recipients with SLTs have been very good, almost equivalent to those seen with whole-liver transplants. Benefits have included significant decreases in waiting-list times, decreased waiting-list mortality, and lower utilization of living donors.

Split-liver transplantation is an attractive alternative to living donation. Paramount to the success of SLT is careful donor and recipient selection. The SLT techniques have been restricted to ideal donors who are young, stable, and have had a relatively short period of hospitalization. The authors prefer the in situ technique over ex vivo dissection, as in situ dissection reduces cold ischemia, enhances identification of biliary and vascular structures, and reduces hemorrhage upon graft reperfusion. Comparison of living-donor, in situ, and ex vivo split-liver pediatric grafts confirmed a higher incidence of primary nonfunction among grafts prepared ex vivo versus in situ or living-donor techniques.

The technique described has been applied by our donor recovery teams at outside facilities during routine donor procurements without specialized equipment and simultaneous with additional organ (heart, lung, pancreas, kidney) procurements. Additional time is required for the procedure but this has not been an excessive burden provided adequate communication has occurred between donor teams. Furthermore, split-liver grafts have been successfully exported and shared between centers.

The current challenge within the transplant community is the formulation of public policy that will realize the greatest potential from a critically limited donor pool. Split-liver transplantation is an integral mechanism to achieve this goal; however, it is a technically demanding endeavor that requires additional logistic as well as personnel support. Broader application of split-liver transplantation, including extension of SLT to two adults from one adult cadaver graft, will only be realized after the liberalization of allocation policy as well as the provision of incentives for clinicians who choose to invest in this effort, since benefit will be derived by all potential candidates awaiting liver transplantation.

a) Surgical Procedure

1. Any technical description of split-liver transplantation must begin with acknowledgment of the anatomic classification of the liver described by Couinaud and refined by Bismuth. This anatomic system has been universally accepted by the transplant communities of Europe, Asia, and North America as the reference system for describing partial-organ liver grafts (Figure 6.56). This classification divides the liver into eight functional units, termed "segments." Individual segments each receive a hilar pedicle containing a portal venous branch, hepatic arterial branch, and a bile duct radicle with segmental drainage by individual venous branches. Hepatic parenchymal transection corresponds to "scissurae" or connective tissue planes that separate individual liver segments thereby reducing intraoperative blood loss and postresection parenchymal ischemia.

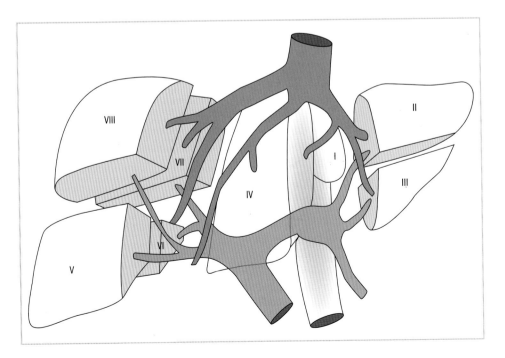

Figure 6.56

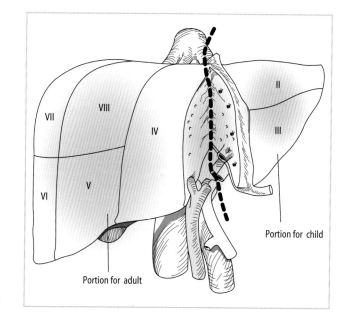

Figure 6.57

2. The technique described herein creates a Couinaud segment II/III graft, termed a left lateral segment graft, that produces an approximately 250-cc graft for pediatric recipients, and a Couinaud segment I, IV–VIII "trisegment" graft of approximately 1100 cc for transplantation of adult recipients (Figure 6.57).

3. Prior to the performance of SLT, the standard procedures of abdominal organ procurement including supraceliac and infrarenal aortic dissection as well as cannulation of the inferior mesenteric vein should be completed such that if the donor were to become unstable, the SLT could be aborted with rapid progression to aortic cannulation, cross-clamping, and organ cold perfusion. The dissection is initiated with division of the falci-form ligament and carried to the level of the diaphragm with identification of the hepatic veins. The left hepatic vein is isolated and encircled with a vessel loop (Figure 6.58).

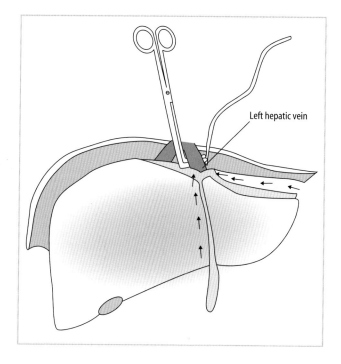

Figure 6.58

4. Preparation of the left lateral segment graft begins with hilar dissection at the base of the round ligament with isolation of the left hepatic artery and left portal vein branch. The left hepatic artery (yellow arrow) is encircled and dissection is carried throughout its entire length. Particular attention is devoted to the preservation of segment IV penetrating arteries (blue arrow) (Figure 6.59). If the segment IV artery arises high off the left hepatic artery and appears to provide significant arterial inflow, the authors recommend reanastomosis of the segment IV artery to the gastroduodenal origin.

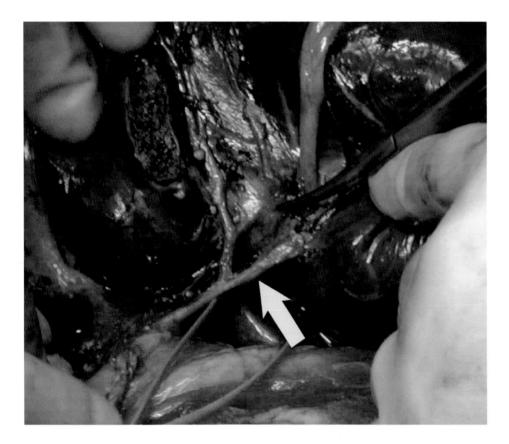

Figure 6.59

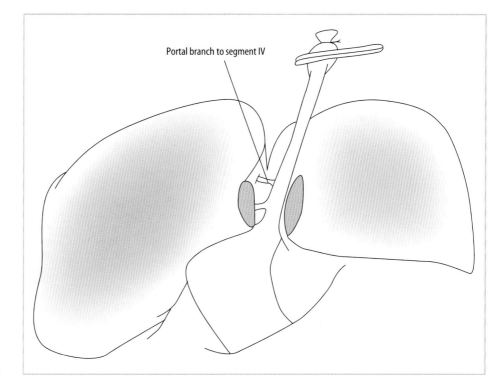

Portal branch to segment IV

Figure 6.60

5. Portal venous branches to segment IV are ligated and divided lateral to the umbilical fissure to isolate the entire left portal vein (Figure 6.60); however, portal venous branches to segment I are preserved as they originate from the main, not left, portal vein.

6. With total vascular control of the left lateral segment achieved, parenchymal transection is initiated with electrocautery by scoring the liver surface just to the right of the falciform ligament (Figure 6.61). The anterior liver parenchyma is divided by electrocautery between the left lateral segment and segment IV and carried to 1 cm above the left bile duct in the umbilical fissure. Small penetrating vessels and biliary radicles are suture ligated as required.

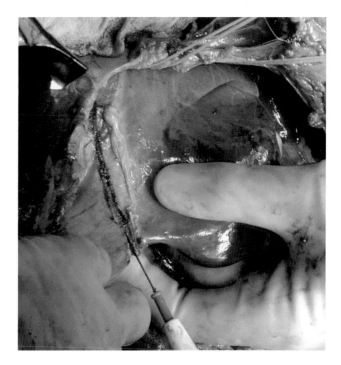

Figure 6.61

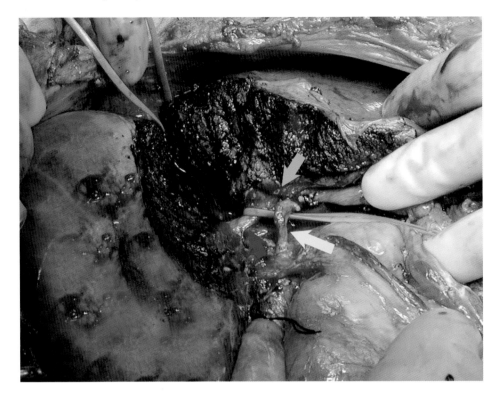

Figure 6.62

7. The remaining left hilar plate and bile duct are sharply transected with scissors close to the surface so as to preserve biliary drainage to segment IV. Intraoperative cholangiogram can be added to define anatomy. Upon completion of the dissection, the left lateral segment is separated from the remaining parenchyma with its own vascular pedicle and venous drainage (Figure 6.62). Organ procurement continues with perfusion and cooling of the donor organs.

8. Following perfusion, the left hepatic artery, the left portal vein, and the left hepatic veins are divided and the left bile duct is flushed with preservation solution prior to storage of the graft in cold solution (Figure 6.63).

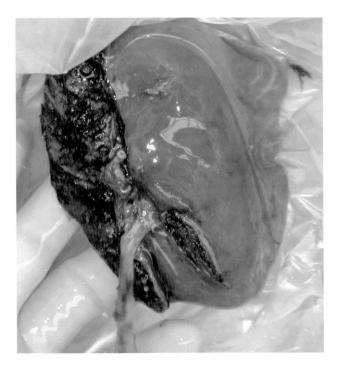

Figure 6.63

9. The right graft is removed in the usual fashion and stored in cold preservative solution (Figure 6.64).

10. Transplantation of the left lateral segment graft involves preservation of the native inferior vena cava. The right hepatic vein entrance to the vena cava is suture ligated as are the smaller accessory hepatic veins and the septum dividing the left, middle, and

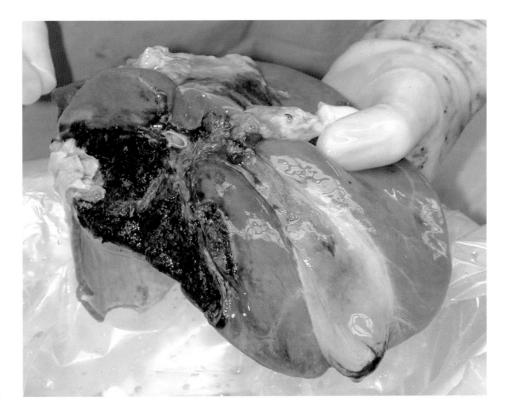

Figure 6.64

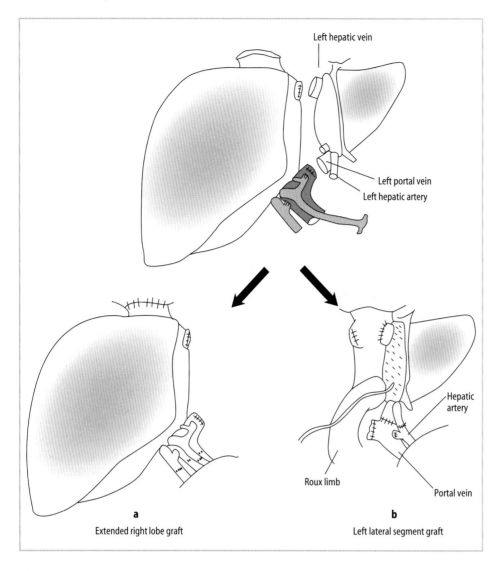

Left hepatic vein

Left portal vein

Left hepatic artery

Hepatic artery

Roux limb

Portal vein

a
Extended right lobe graft

b
Left lateral segment graft

Figure 6.65

right hepatic vein openings to the cava is divided to form a large common trunk for left hepatic venous anastomosis. Anastomosis of the portal vein is achieved either through an end-to-end or end-to-side fashion while the hepatic artery is anastomosed to the common hepatic artery or infrarenal aorta by an iliac artery interposition graft. Biliary drainage is achieved by a duct-to-duct or Roux-en-Y hepaticojejunostomy (Figure 6.65b). Transplantation of the extended right graft is done by standard techniques (Figure 6.65a).

Deceased Donor Split-Liver Transplant: Adult/Adult Recipients

The vast majority of SLTs have been performed between an adult and a pediatric recipient. The benefits for pediatric recipients have been tremendous, with a significant decrease in waiting times and mortality rates. Splitting an adult liver for pediatric recipients has no negative impact on the adult donor pool, but it does not increase it either. Yet adults now account for 96% of patients dying on the waiting list; in 1988, they accounted for only 70%. If SLTs are to have a significant impact on waiting-list time and mortality, they must be performed so that the resulting two grafts can also be used in two adult recipients.

Division of the liver at the falciform ligament will generate a left lateral segment that would be inadequate liver volume for the majority of adult recipients. Transection in the midplane of the liver divides it into the anatomic right lobe (60% of the liver) and the left lobe (40% of the liver); this will usually generate grafts of sufficient size for two adult recipients. The minimum amount of liver mass needed to sustain life immediately posttransplant is unclear. Some experience with living donor liver transplants suggests that a graft weight to recipient weight (GW/RW) ratio of 0.8% is the minimum. For deceased donors, the minimum amount of liver mass may also be influenced by such factors as donor hemodynamic stability and cold ischemic time.

a) Selection Criteria

Proper recipient and donor selection are crucial in ensuring a good outcome. A GW/RW ratio of close to 0.8% should likely be the minimum when selecting appropriate recipients. Graft size is not the only criterion in selecting donors and recipients. Donors should be medically ideal to minimize the risks of primary nonfunction, especially for left lobe recipients. Young, hemodynamically stable donors with normal liver function test results should be selected; with such donors, primary nonfunction for the recipients should be uncommon. Cold ischemic time should be minimized as much as possible in all SLT donors. For this reason, it is preferable to do the actual transection of the parenchyma in situ in the donor. Performing the split on the back table could add up to 2 to 3 hours of cold ischemia. Also, there is likely to be some warming of the liver on the back table, even if the split is being performed in a cold ice bath of University of Wisconsin solution. Performing the split in situ also has other advantages. Significantly less bleeding occurs when the organs are reperfused. Additionally, the two liver grafts can be assessed in the donor immediately after parenchymal transection and before vascular interruption, to ensure adequate perfusion and viability.

b) Technical Aspects

Several technical points need emphasis regarding the donor operation, which is very similar to a right lobe liver procurement from a living donor. The transection plane should stay to the right of the middle hepatic vein, so that this structure is retained with the left lobe. Segment IV makes up a crucial part of the left lobe, and hence the middle hepatic vein should be preserved with the left lobe to ensure that there is no congestion. Loss of the middle hepatic vein usually does not significantly affect drainage of segment V and VIII in the right lobe graft, as these segments drain adequately via the right hepatic vein. Regarding the dissection in the hilum, our preference has been to leave the full length of the hilar structures intact with the left lobe. The right-sided hilar structures are usually larger than the left-sided structures. Therefore, leaving the main vessels intact with the left lobe makes that transplant easier. One crucial technical point for the recipient operation is ensuring adequate venous outflow of the grafts to prevent congestion. Preserving the cava with the right lobe graft helps to maximize outflow by preserving all inferior hepatic veins. This also allows for back-table reconstruction of any segment V and VIII veins draining from the right lobe to the middle hepatic vein.

c) Ethics of Splitting

Surgical complications are probably more common in SLT (vs. whole graft) recipients, related to the cut surface of the liver, smaller vessels for anastomosis, and more complicated biliary reconstruction. Therefore, one important aspect of the recipient selection process is adequately informing the potential recipient of the splitting procedure and obtaining informed consent.

d) Split Potential

More data are needed to better define donor and recipient selection criteria, which are crucial to success. It is difficult to estimate how much impact adult SLTs will have on the donor pool. About 25% of all deceased donors in the United States are between 15 and 35 years of age. If many of these livers could be used for splits, the number of liver transplants could potentially increase by 20% to 25%, or by close to 1000. With better preservation techniques, more livers may be amenable to splitting. In the near future, this technique will likely become part of every major liver transplant center's repertoire, to provide the maximum advantage for their candidates on the waiting list.

e) Surgical Procedure

1. When splitting for two adults, the liver is split in its midplane, separating the anatomic right lobe (segments V, VI, VII, and VIII) from the anatomic left lobe (segments I, II, II, and IV). The cava and common bile duct are maintained with the right lobe graft, while the main portal vein and common hepatic artery are preserved with the left lobe graft (Figure 6.66).

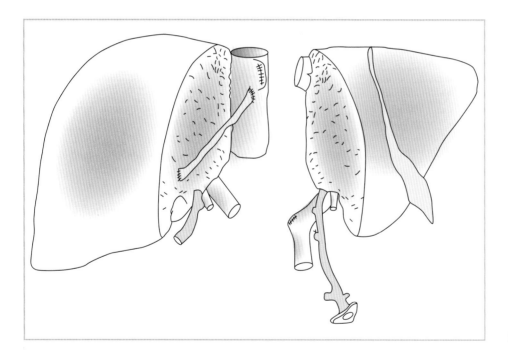

Figure 6.66

2. The liver is mobilized by division of the falciform and left ligaments. The common trunk of the left and middle hepatic vein (blue arrows) is encircled with an umbilical tape (Figure 6.67).

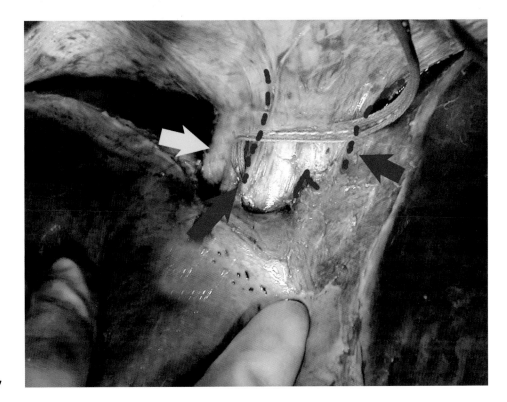

Figure 6.67

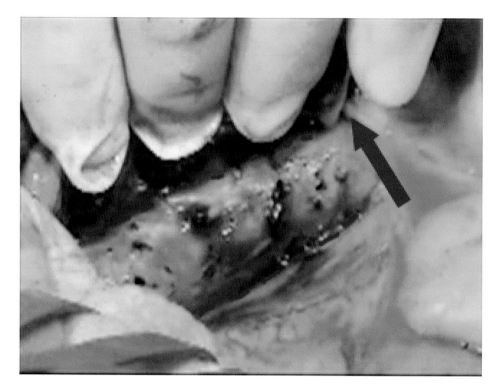

Figure 6.68

3. The left lobe including the caudate lobe is completely mobilized off the underlying cava (Figures 6.68 and 6.69).

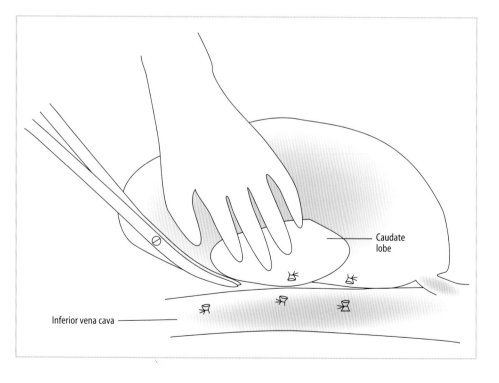

Caudate lobe

Inferior vena cava

Figure 6.69

4. The right hepatic artery (yellow arrow) and right portal vein are dissected free and mobilized (the gallbladder is removed first). The left hilar plate is taken down and the left hepatic duct (green arrow) in its extrahepatic portion is encircled (Figure 6.70). The line of planned transection through the hilum is (blue broken line) through the origin of the right portal vein and right hepatic artery, and at the junction of the left hepatic duct with the common hepatic duct.

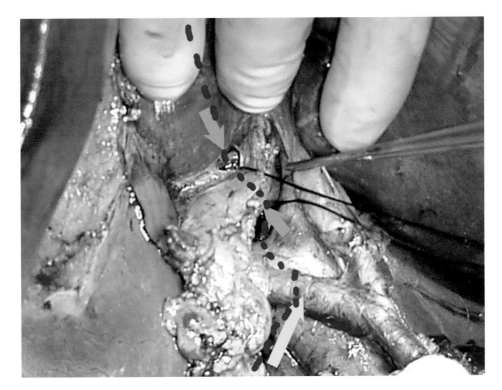

Figure 6.70

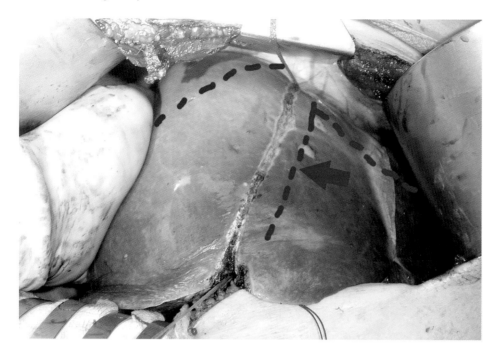

Figure 6.71

5. A line for parenchymal transection is drawn just to the right of the estimated course of the middle hepatic vein (blue arrow). The umbilical tape is passed around the left lobe to suspend it upward. Liver transection is then performed in situ (Figure 6.71).

6. After the parenchymal transection is complete, the two halves of the liver are inspected to make sure there is no significant vascular compromise of either portion (Figure 6.72). All organs are flushed with cold preservation solution in the usual manner.

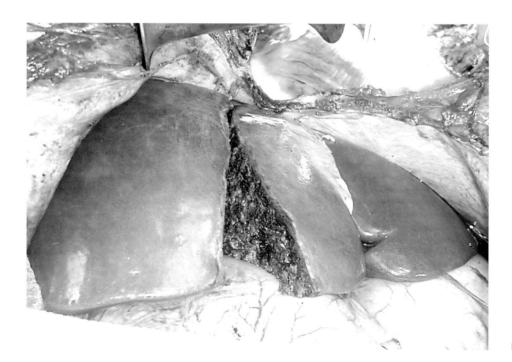

Figure 6.72

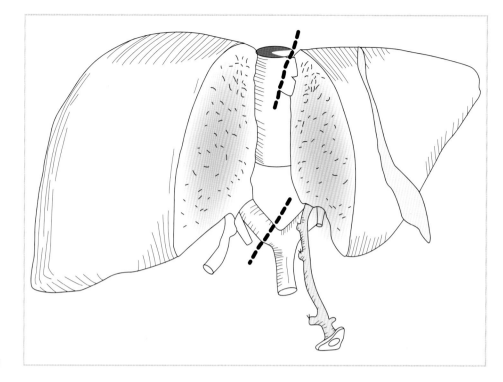

Figure 6.73

7. Final separation is done on the back table. The following structures are divided to completely separate the left and right lobes: the common junction of the middle and left hepatic vein (broken black line), the left hepatic duct at the junction with the right, the right hepatic artery, and the right portal vein close to its origin (broken blue line) (Figure 6.73).

8. Any large hepatic veins draining segment V or VIII (yellow arrow) into the middle hepatic vein are reconstructed with an appropriate sized vein graft. The right lobe is then ready for implantation (Figure 6.74).

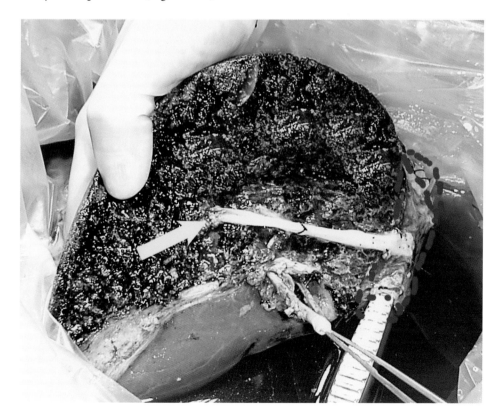

Figure 6.74

9. With the left lobe graft, the vascular stumps of the right portal vein and the right hepatic artery are oversewn; the graft is then ready for implantation. The outflow of the graft is based on the combined orifices of the middle and left hepatic veins (yellow arrow) (Figure 6.75).

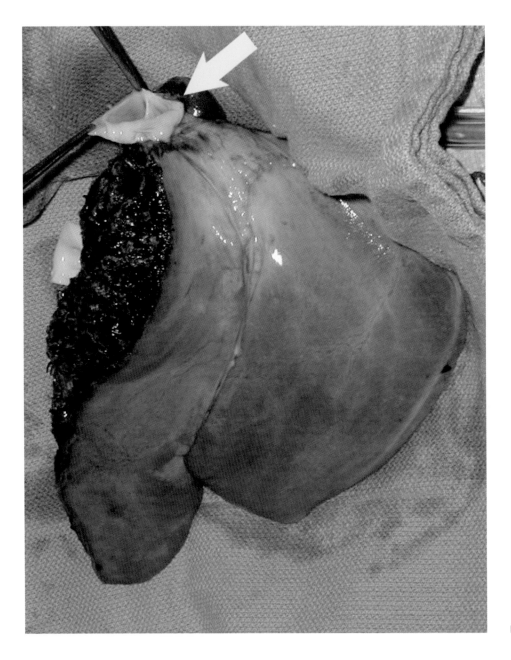

Figure 6.75

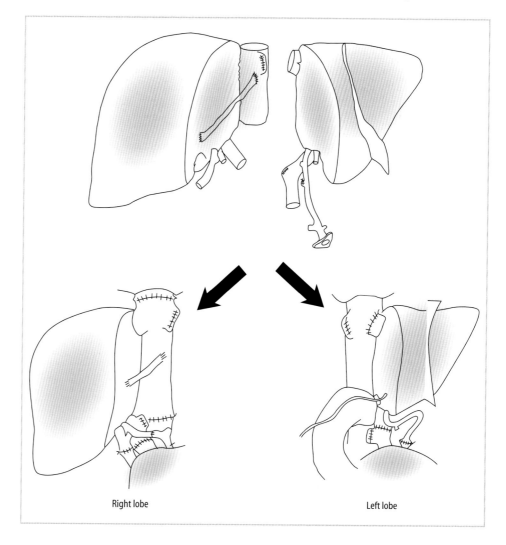

Right lobe   Left lobe

Figure 6.76

10. The grafts can then be implanted, usually with a piggyback procedure, though the right lobe can also be placed with a caval replacement procedure (Figure 6.76).

Living-Donor Liver Transplant: Pediatric Recipient

The greatest advantage of a living-donor liver transplant (LDLT) is that the patient avoids the waiting time associated with deceased donor organs. Over 15,000 people are now waiting for liver transplants in the U.S., but only 4500 transplants are performed every year. Roughly 25% of the candidates will die of their liver disease before having the chance to undergo a transplant. For those who do end up receiving a transplant from a deceased donor, the waiting time can be significant, resulting in severe debilitation. With an LDLT, this waiting time can be bypassed, allowing the transplant to be performed before the recipient's health deteriorates further. In areas of the world where deceased donor transplants are not performed, the advantages of LDLT are even more obvious.

A partial hepatectomy in an otherwise healthy donor is a significant undertaking, so all potential donors must be very carefully evaluated. Detailed medical screening must ensure that the donor is medically healthy, radiologic evaluation must ensure that the anatomy of the donor's liver is suitable, and a psychosocial evaluation is done to ensure that the donor is mentally fit and not being coerced. The decision to donate should be made entirely by the potential donor after careful consideration of the risks and of the potential complications, with no coercion from any individual.

For a pediatric recipient, usually the left lateral segment of the donor's liver (about 25% of the total liver) is removed. For a larger child, sometimes the left lobe is used. The operative procedure involves isolating the blood vessels supplying the portion of the liver to be removed, transecting the hepatic parenchyma, and then removing the portion to be transplanted. The operative procedure is in part very similar to that described for adult/pediatric cadaveric in-situ splits. The outflow of the graft is based on the left hepatic vein, while the inflow is based on the left hepatic artery and left portal vein (Figure 6.77).

The overall incidence of complications after living-donor liver donation ranges from 5% to 30%. There is also a small risk (<0.5%) of death. Bile duct problems are the most worrisome complication after donor surgery. Bile may leak from the cut surface of the liver or from the site where the bile duct is divided. That site may later become strictured. Generally, bile leaks resolve spontaneously with simple drainage. Strictures and sometimes bile leaks may require an endoscopic procedure and stenting. If the above measures fail, a reoperation may be required. Intraabdominal infections developing in donors are usually related to a biliary problem. Other complications after donor surgery may include

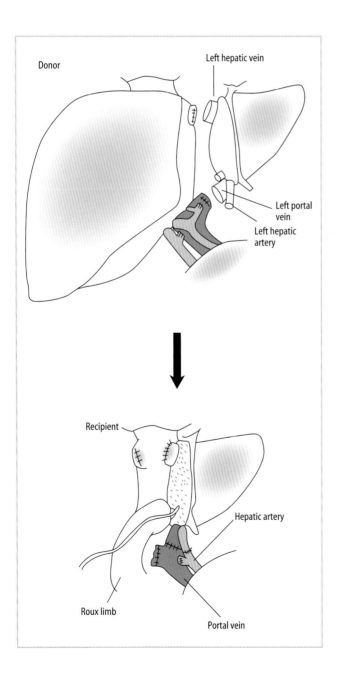

Figure 6.77

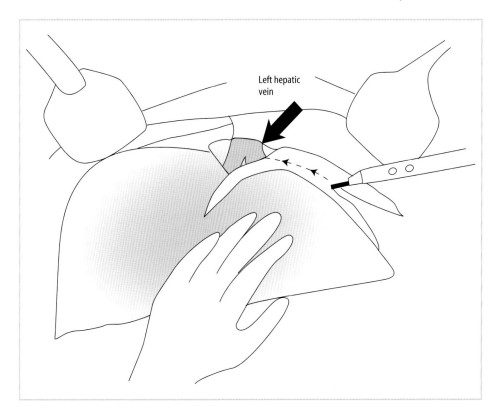

Figure 6.78

incisional problems such as infections and hernias. The risk of deep venous thrombosis and pulmonary embolism is the same as for other major abdominal procedures.

a) Donor Procedure

1. The abdomen is opened through a bilateral subcostal incision. The falciform ligament and left triangular ligaments are divided until the anterior aspect of the left hepatic vein (black arrow) is seen (Figures 6.78 and 6.79).

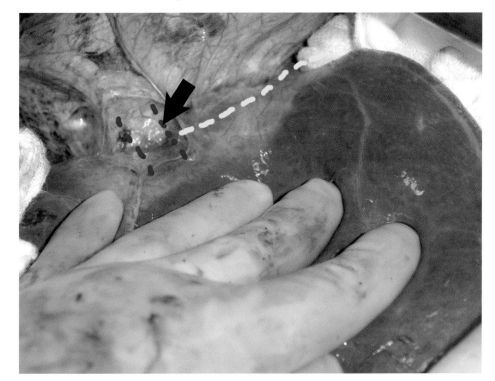

Figure 6.79

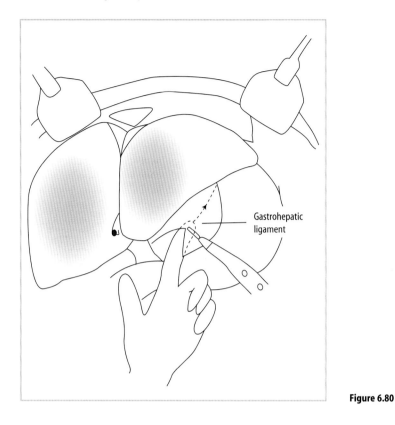

Figure 6.80

2. The left lateral segment is lifted up slightly and the gastrohepatic ligament is divided from the hilum posteriorly to the left hepatic vein superiorly (Figure 6.80).

3. The left hepatic vein (black arrow) can now be encircled with an umbilical tape (Figure 6.81).

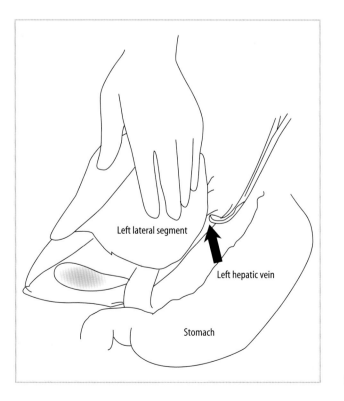

Figure 6.81

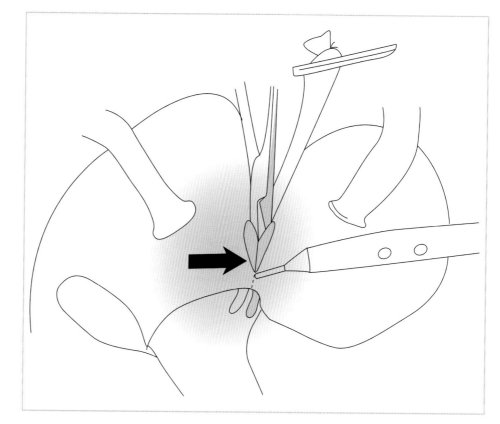

Figure 6.82

4. The bridge of liver tissue (black arrow) overlying the ligamentum teres and connecting the left lateral segment to segment IV is divided (Figure 6.82); this can usually be done with electrocautery.

5. The left hepatic artery (yellow arrow) is identified at the base of the ligamentum teres and traced distally to where it enters the liver, and proximally to the segment IV branch (Figure 6.83).

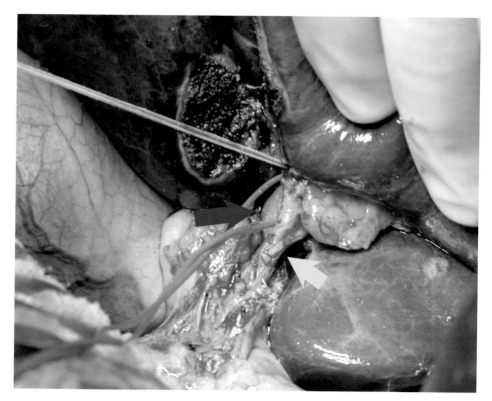

Figure 6.83

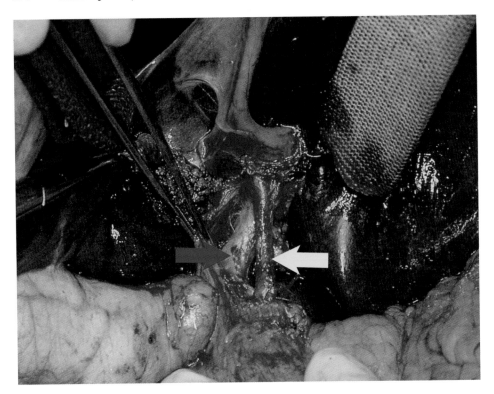

Figure 6.84

6. The left portal vein (blue arrow) can be identified and mobilized along its long extrahepatic course, lying slightly superior and posterior to the artery (yellow arrow) (Figures 6.84 and 6.85).

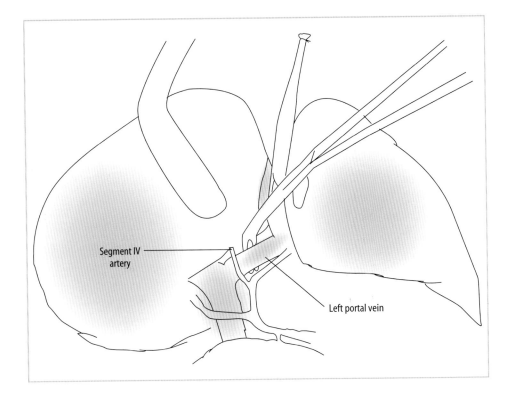

Segment IV artery

Left portal vein

Figure 6.85

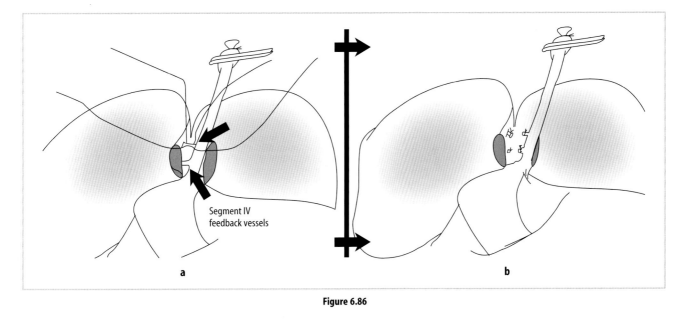

Figure 6.86

7. The falciform ligament is pulled to the left during this part, and "feedback vessels" (black arrow) of the portal vein going to segment IV can be identified (Figure 6.86a). These should be divided with suture ligation (Figures 6.86b and 6.87).

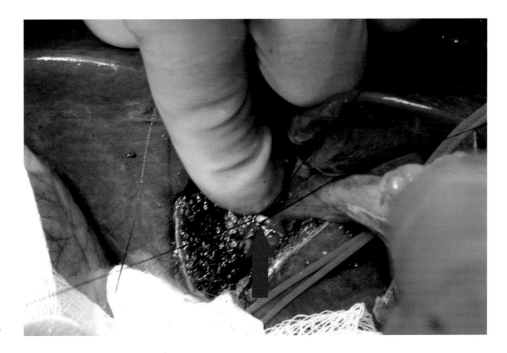

Figure 6.87

8. The umbilical tape previously passed around the left hepatic vein can be now brought around the left lateral segment itself, passing in the ligamentum groove, and anteriorly excluding the artery and vein going to the left lateral segment. Pulling on the two ends of the umbilical tape lifts up the portion of liver to be transected, giving a good guide for the plane of transection (Figure 6.88). This is known as the "hanging technique."

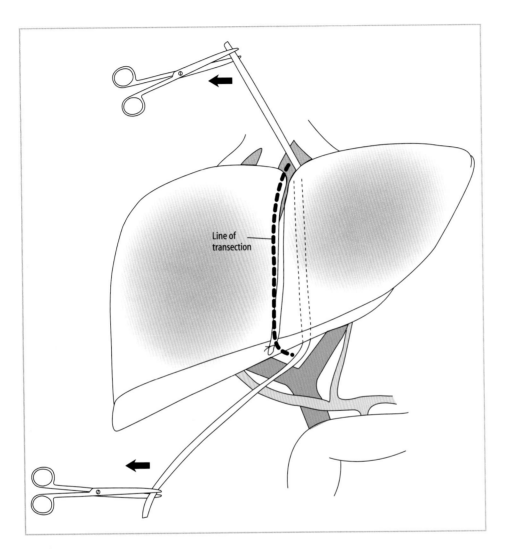

Line of transection

Figure 6.88

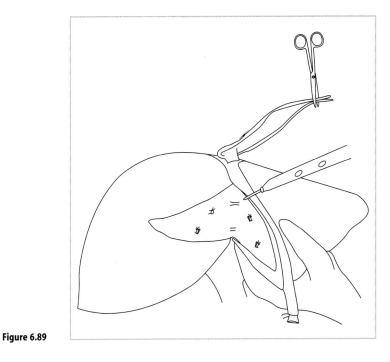

Figure 6.89

9. The parenchyma of the liver is then transected, staying just to the right of the falciform ligament (Figure 6.89).

10. As the parenchymal transection is continued, the biliary drainage from segment II and III will be encountered, just at the base of the lateral segment, superior to the vascular structures (Figure 6.90). This should be sharply transected.

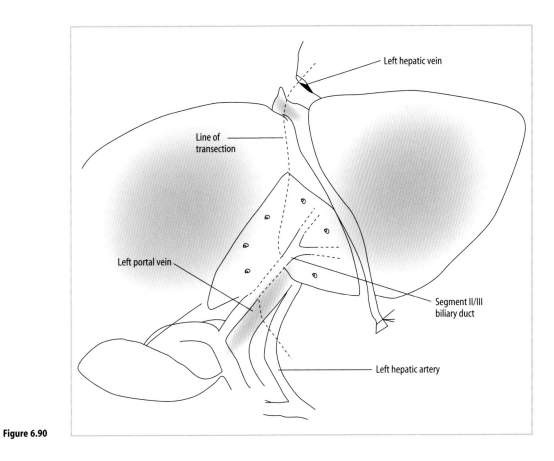

Figure 6.90

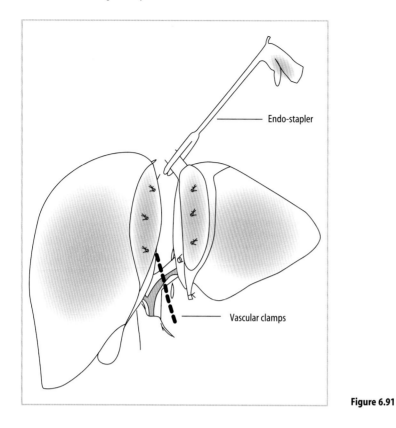

Endo-stapler

Vascular clamps

Figure 6.91

11. When the recipient team is ready, the graft can be removed by dividing the vascular structures (Figure 6.91). Clamps can be placed proximally on the left portal vein and left hepatic artery. The left hepatic vein is easiest taken with a laparoscopic stapling device.

12. The graft is flushed and given to the recipient team (Figure 6.92). The cut surface of the donor should be carefully inspected for any evidence of bleeding or bile leak. Once this is satisfactory, closure is performed.

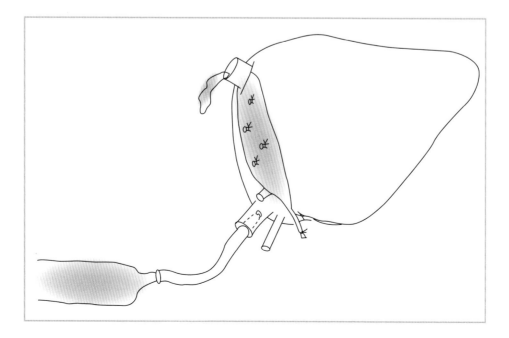

Figure 6.92

b) Recipient Procedure

1. A standard caval-preserving hepatectomy is performed while the donor team is procuring the left lateral segment graft.

2. Creation of a large, patulous, hepatic venous anastomosis is important to maximize outflow of the graft. This is best performed by isolating the cava between two clamps as shown. A large triangular opening is created on the anterior surface of the cava, usually at the site of the left and middle hepatic vein orifices (Figure 6.93).

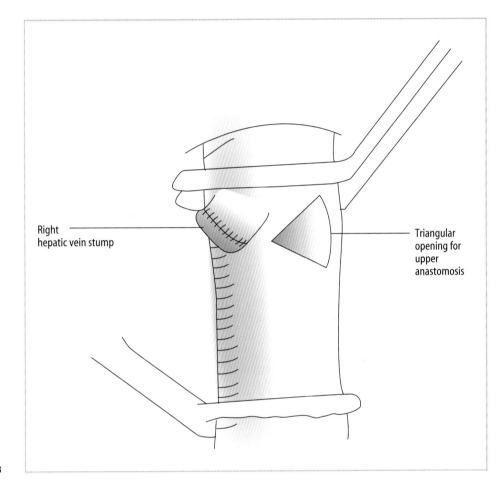

Right hepatic vein stump

Triangular opening for upper anastomosis

Figure 6.93

3. Three corner sutures are placed at the angles of the triangle and the corresponding locations on the donor hepatic vein (Figure 6.94a) (marking these locations on the donor vein with a marking pen prior to graft implantation is helpful to ensure proper orientation). The corner sutures are tied and the anastomosis completed with a running suture technique (Figures 6.94b). A small defect is left to allow for flushing of the graft.

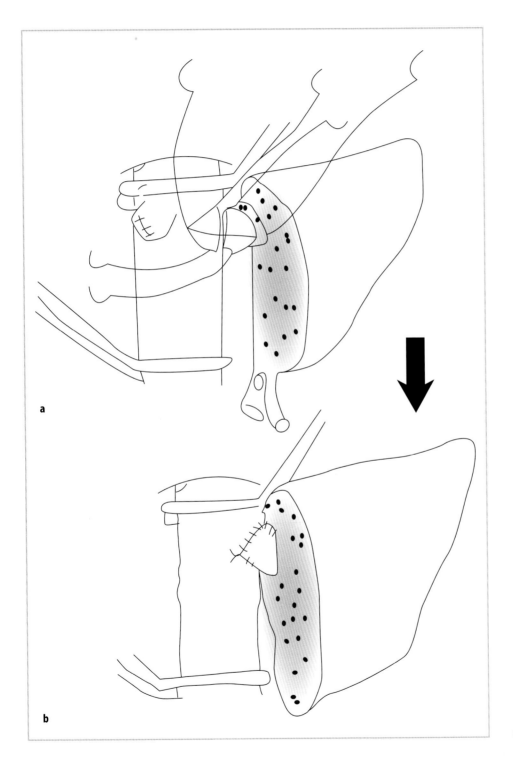

Figure 6.94

4. The portal venous anastomosis is completed next. Usually this can be done without the use of a jump graft. Correct orientation of the donor and recipient vein is important to ensure unobstructed flow.

5. The graft is then flushed to remove preservative solution from the graft. After flushing, the defect in the hepatic venous anastomosis is closed and the clamps removed.

6. The hepatic arterial anastomosis is completed next. Again, this can usually be done without the use of a "jump" graft (Figure 6.95). An operating microscope or high-powered loupes and fine interrupted sutures are helpful in creating this anastomosis.

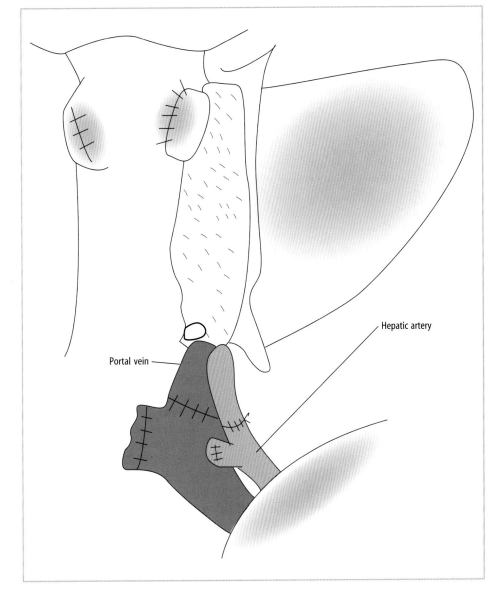

Figure 6.95

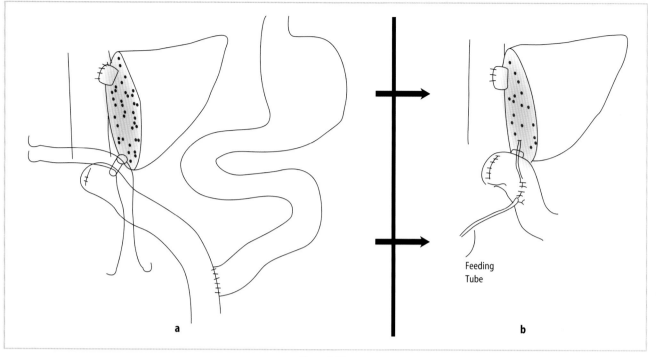

Feeding
Tube

Figure 6.96

7. A roux-en-Y loop is then created for the biliary anastomosis. The loop is brought up through a retrocolic opening, and placed adjacent to the bile duct(s), so that a tension-free anastomosis can be performed (Figure 6.96a). It is helpful to perform this anastomosis over a small feeding tube, which can be used as an external stent (Figure 6.96b).

Living-Donor Liver Transplant: Adult Recipient

The use of living donors for liver transplant has been of tremendous benefit for pediatric recipients and has resulted in a significant decrease in the waiting-list mortality rate for these patients. However, more than 90% of patients on the waiting list today are adults; the majority of deaths pretransplant occur in adults. Therefore, to have maximum impact on the waiting list, living donors also need to be utilized for adult recipients. For such recipients, a larger piece of the liver is required. The right lobe, the left lobe, and two left lobes from two donors have all been reported as potential grafts for adult recipients. However, most centers employ the right lobe of the donor for this procedure.

The preoperative evaluation of the potential living donor is an essential part of the transplant process. A thorough medical evaluation is done to ensure that there are no risk factors that would contraindicate donation. This involves ruling out major disease processes that may involve the extrahepatic systems such as cardiac, respiratory, or renal. Biochemical markers of liver function and injury such as bilirubin, transaminases, and international normalized ratio (INR) need to be performed. Viral pathogens such as hepatitis B and C need to be screened for.

Removal of the right lobe is a substantially bigger operative procedure than removal of the left lateral segment. A much larger volume of the liver is to be removed. Therefore, an important part of the preoperative evaluation is to make an accurate volume measurement of the donor's liver. The purpose of this is twofold: (1) to make sure that the recipient is receiving enough liver tissue to sustain life, and (2) to make sure that the donor has adequate residual liver volume to sustain life. For the recipient, one should target a GW/RW ratio of at least 0.8%. The donor should have at least 30% of his or her total liver volume left behind at the end of surgery.

Besides the volumetric evaluation preoperatively, many centers also routinely employ a liver biopsy for the evaluation of a potential right lobe donor. The purpose of this is to rule out steatosis, and occult diseases of the liver. Other centers biopsy on a selective basis, depending on the presence or absence of risk factors such as obesity, elevated triglycerides or cholesterol levels, and abnormal imaging studies or liver function tests.

The choice of surgical procedure for adult living-donor transplant varies from center to center, but most prefer the right lobe. Inflow is based on the right hepatic artery and right portal vein, while outflow is based on the right hepatic vein. Outflow issues tend to be more prominent with right lobe vs. left lateral segment grafts. Various methods have been tried to improve outflow for these grafts including taking the middle hepatic vein with the right lobe, and reconstructing large venous tributaries using a vascular graft.

The greatest concern with this procedure, in fact with any living-donor procedure, is the risk of death to the donor. Unfortunately, there is some risk of mortality associated with any surgical procedure, but the magnitude of risk associated with this procedure has been difficult to determine. As of January 31, 2003, 1158 adult LDLTs (ALDLTs) had been performed in the U.S. and reported to UNOS (United Network for Organ Sharing). There had been three associated donor deaths (0.26%). Of these three deaths, two (0.17%) were early in the postoperative period and hence directly related to the surgery. The third death was a suicide at 2 years postdonation and likely not related to the donation surgery. The number of deaths worldwide, however, is more difficult to determine, as there is no mandatory reporting. By some reports, there have been 14 or 15 deaths worldwide. Most centers cite a 0.5% risk of mortality associated with this procedure, though the cited rate may vary from 0.1% to 1.0% at different centers.

A number of different complications are possible, and have been reported in donors. The vast majority of these complications tend to occur in the early postoperative period (usually within 1 month postdonation). The reported incidence of complications in the donor varies in the literature, but likely is in the 10% to 20% range. The most commonly reported major complication involves the biliary system; a bile leak or stricture has been reported in roughly 5% of the donors. Other reported complications include the need for nonautologous blood, the need for a reoperation, and a major postoperative infection. Overall, the risk of complications for right-lobe donors is felt to be significantly higher compared to that for left lateral segment or left-lobe donors.

While there is no obvious benefit for donors, there are advantages for recipients of living-donor transplants. The potential waiting-list mortality associated with waiting for a deceased donor is avoided. Additionally, patients can be transplanted before they develop far advanced liver disease associated with marked overall decompensation. The disadvantage for living-donor recipients, at least for adult recipients, is that there are some data to suggest that outcomes may be inferior compared to whole-liver transplants, especially if the patients are matched for severity of liver disease. Living-donor recipients also have been noted to have a higher incidence of surgical complications posttransplant as compared with whole-liver recipients. Partial grafts have smaller vessels, more complicated biliary reconstructions, and a cut surface, all of which make for a technically more challenging procedure and a higher incidence of surgical complications. Most centers have reported a 15% to 20% incidence of early bile leaks after transplant and a 15% to 20% incidence of late biliary strictures. Those figures are significantly higher than generally reported for whole-liver recipients.

Certain subgroups of recipients especially may do worse after living-donor transplants. Critically ill adult recipients with advanced liver failure, high MELD (Model for End-Stage Liver Disease) scores, and numerous secondary complications have generally been reported to have very poor outcomes with this procedure. Such recipients have minimal functional reserve and are probably ill-equipped to manage the lower hepatocyte mass and the higher complication rate associated with partial transplants.

The recipient operation with LDLTs is not greatly different from whole-organ deceased-donor liver transplants. The hepatectomy is performed in a similar fashion, but the recipient cava should be preserved in all such cases, because the graft will generally only have a single hepatic vein for outflow. This hepatic vein is then anastomosed directly to the recipient's preserved vena cava (Figure 6.97). Outflow can be augmented by including the middle hepatic vein with the graft or by reconstructing large segment V or VIII tributaries to the middle hepatic vein using a vascular conduit. Inflow to the graft can be done by reconnecting the corresponding hepatic arterial and portal venous branches. Finally biliary reconstruction is performed either by a duct-to-duct technique or with a hepaticojejunostomy.

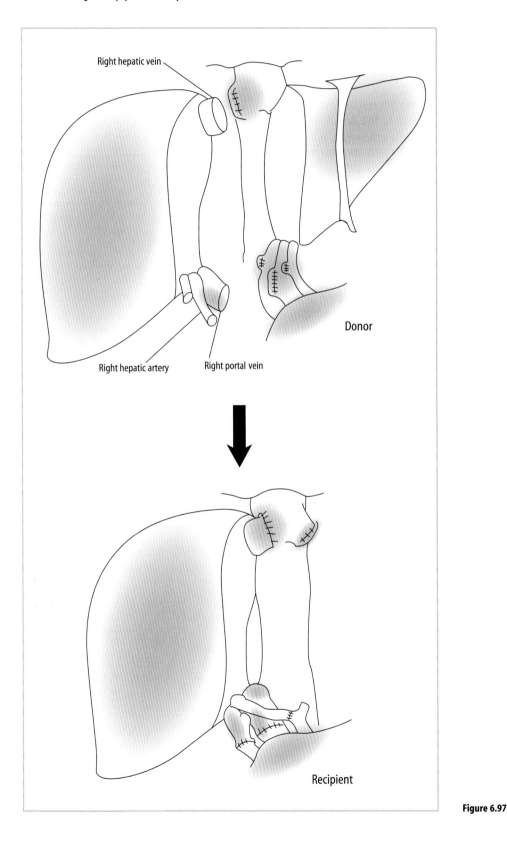

Figure 6.97

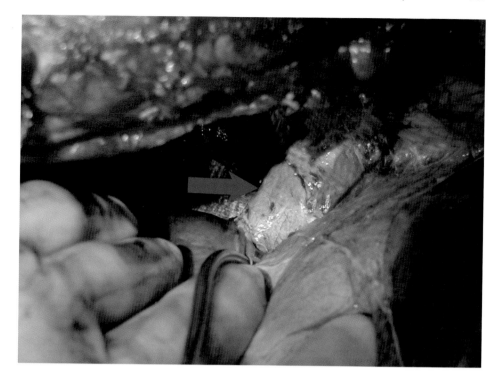

Figure 6.98

a) Donor Procedure

1. A bilateral subcostal incision is made. The falciform ligament is divided and then continued posteriorly until the anterior wall of the right hepatic vein (blue arrow) is visualized (Figure 6.98). The groove between the right and middle hepatic veins should be defined (Figure 6.99).

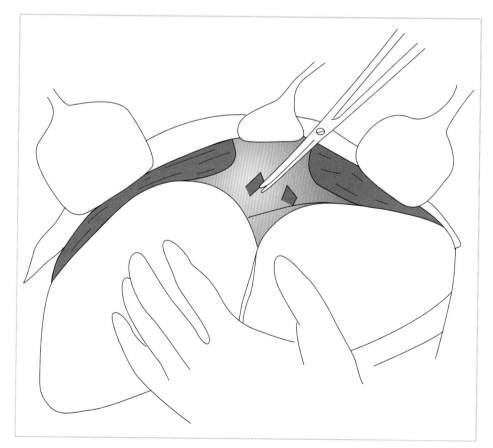

Figure 6.99

2. The right lobe of the liver is completely mobilized by division of the right triangular ligament and freeing of the bare area from the underlying retroperitoneum (Figure 6.100). The right lateral border of the retrohepatic cava should be seen.

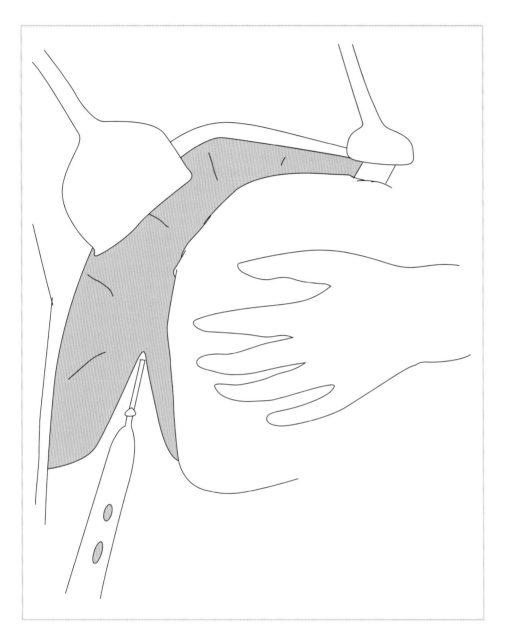

Figure 6.100

3. The right lobe is mobilized from the retrohepatic cava itself by dividing the short hepatic veins that drain into the cava. Any branches 5 mm or larger (yellow arrow) should be preserved for later reimplantation in the recipient (Figure 6.101).

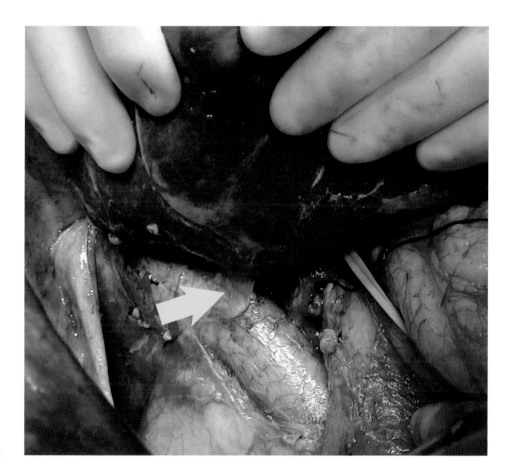

Figure 6.101

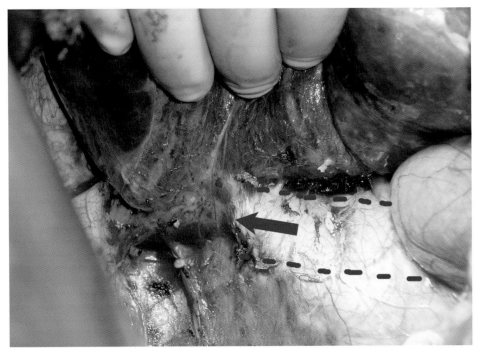

Figure 6.102

4. The undersurface of the right hepatic vein marks the superior extent of the dissection. The hepatocaval ligament (blue arrow) is encountered just inferior to the right hepatic vein (Figures 6.102 and 6.103). This band of tissue attaching the posterior right lobe to the inferior vena cava (broken blue line) is variable in its composition. It may contain a sizable vein, may be composed of liver parenchyma, or may consist of just fibrous tissue. It should be divided between clamps and suture ligated in case there is a vein within it.

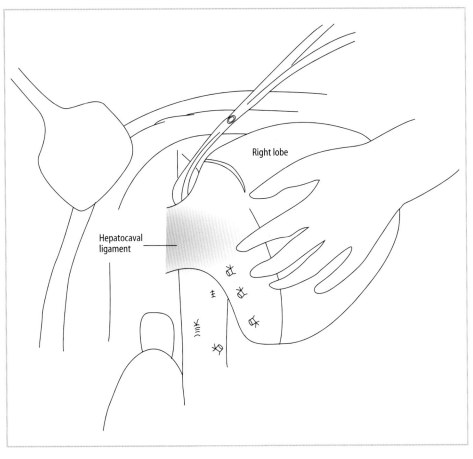

Figure 6.103

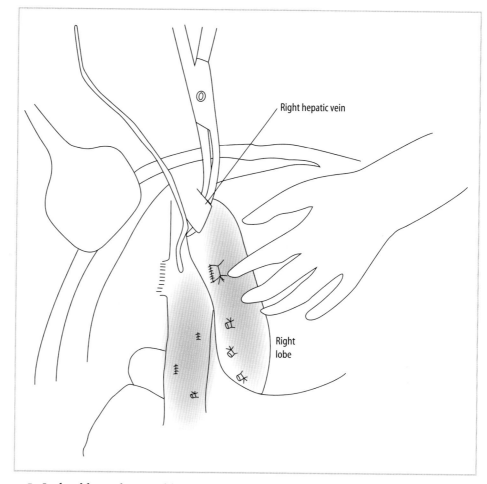

Right hepatic vein

Right lobe

Figure 6.104

5. It should now be possible to encircle the right hepatic vein (blue arrow) and pass an umbilical tape around it (Figures 6.104 and 6.105).

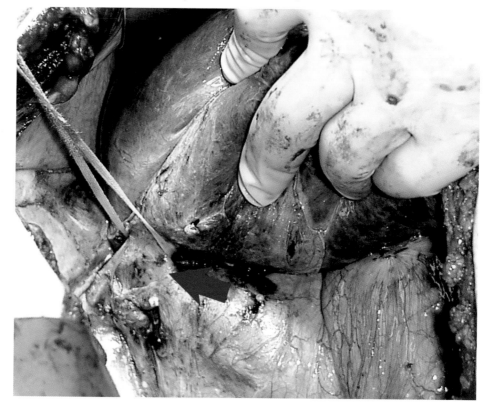

Figure 6.105

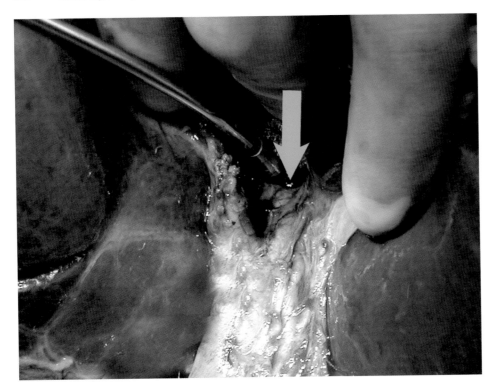

Figure 6.106

6. Attention is now turned toward the hilar dissection. A cholecystectomy is performed. The right hilar plate is taken down and the junction of the right and left hepatic ducts (green arrow) is defined (Figure 6.106).

7. The right hepatic artery (yellow arrow) is identified close to where it enters into the liver (Figure 6.107). It is then traced proximally to the point where it usually is passing behind the common bile duct (CBD) (broken green line). It usually should not be dissected much proximal to this point so as not to risk causing vascular injury to the CBD.

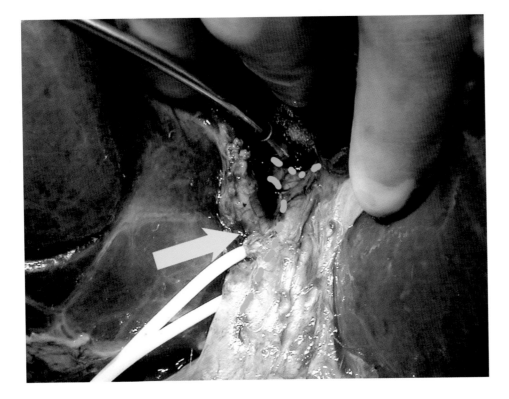

Figure 6.107

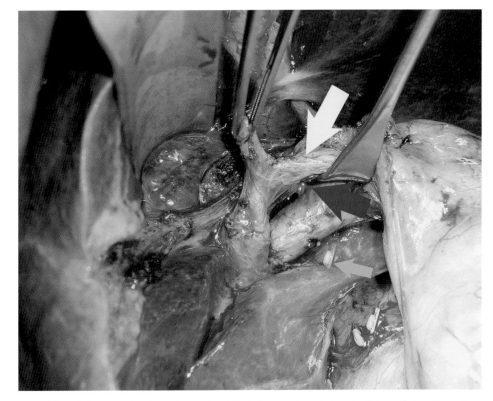

Figure 6.108

8. The right portal vein is then identified. It is easiest to locate this vein by dissecting along the posterior right edge of the hepatoduodenal ligament, behind the right hepatic artery (yellow arrow). The junction with the left portal vein (blue arrow) is clearly defined so as to not compromise the latter when the right portal vein is eventually divided (Figure 6.108). There are usually one or two small branches from the right portal vein going to the caudate lobe. It is important to divide these veins (green arrow) to maximize the length of the right portal vein.

9. With the right hepatic artery (HA) and right portal vein (PV) retracted inferiorly, the right hepatic duct (green arrow) can be encircled with a right-angle instrument and a radiologic marker of some form passed around it (Figure 6.109).

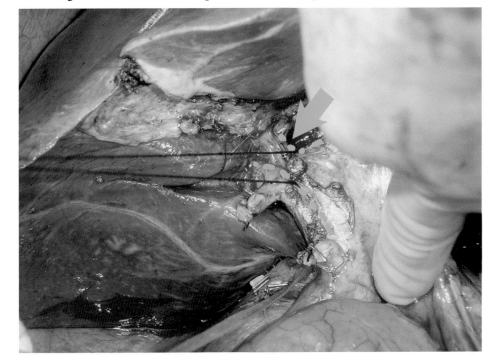

Figure 6.109

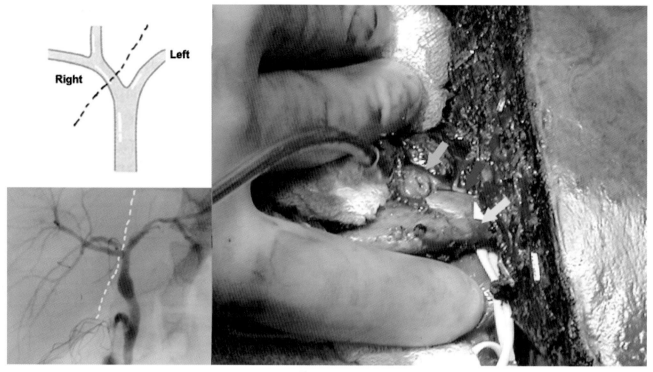

Figure 6.110

10. An intraoperative cholangiogram is now performed to delineate the biliary anatomy. In the first cholangiogram, the right anterior and posterior sectoral ducts join to form a common trunk, which then joins the left hepatic duct (Figure 6.110). This situation should result in a single bile duct (green arrow) to the right lobe graft. In the second cholangiogram, the right posterior sectoral duct drains into the left hepatic duct (Figure 6.111). This will result in two separate bile ducts (green arrows) to reanastomose in the right lobe graft.

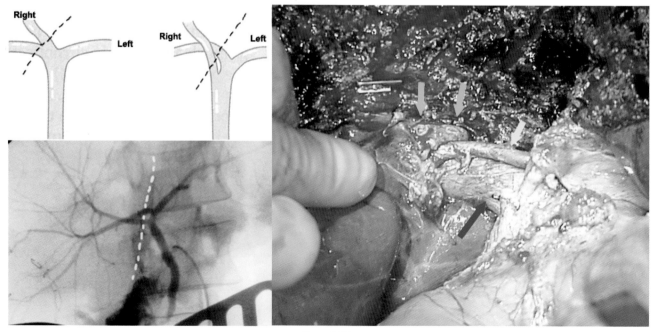

Figure 6.111

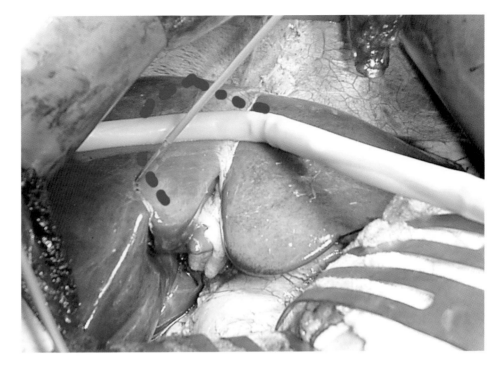

Figure 6.112

11. Intraoperative ultrasound is then performed to outline the course of the middle hepatic vein (MHV) (Figure 6.112). This is correlated with the preoperative imaging study (Figure 6.113). We prefer to perform the parenchymal transection just to the right of the MHV, leaving that structure with the donor. Others have described doing the parenchymal transection to the left of the MHV, leaving that structure with the right lobe graft.

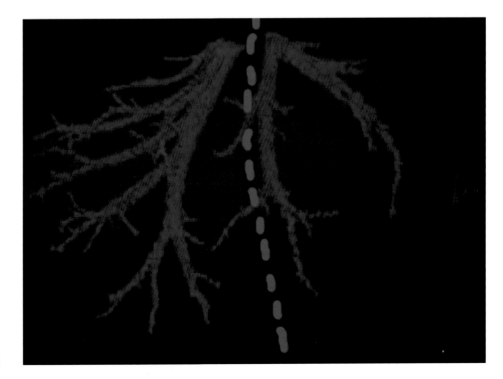

Figure 6.113

12. The ultrasound is also useful to help identify large venous tributaries draining segment V and/or VIII (yellow arrow) into the middle hepatic vein (blue arrow) (Figure 6.114). The location of these can be marked on the surface of the liver, which is useful during the parenchymal transection. If large (>4mm), these may need to be reconstructed in the recipient. (IVC, inferior vena cava; RHV, right hepatic vein.)

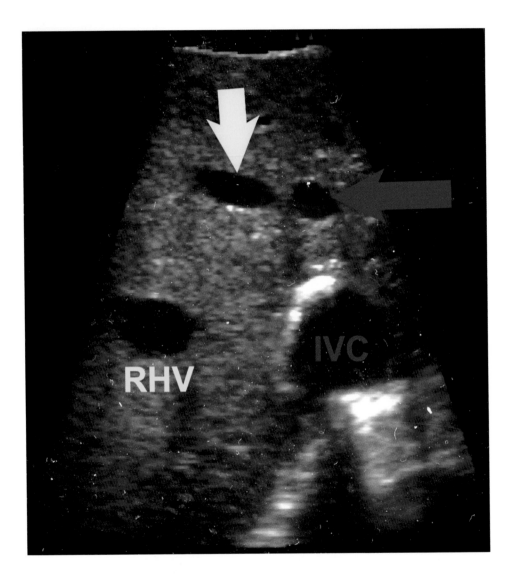

Figure 6.114

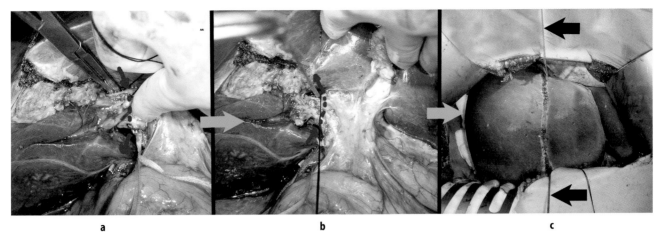

a   b   c

Figure 6.115

13. The umbilical tape previously passed around the right hepatic vein is passed around the entire right lobe (Figure 6.115a). The tape is passed inside the three right hilar structures (artery, vein, and hepatic duct) (blue arrows) (Figure 6.115b). The two ends of the umbilical tape can then be pulled up (black arrows), acting as a sling that helps to direct the line of parenchymal transection (Figure 6.115c). This is known as the "hanging" technique (Figure 6.116).

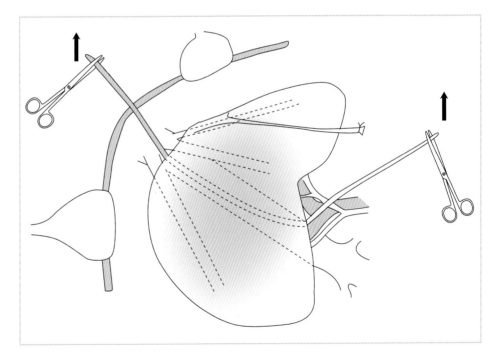

Figure 6.116

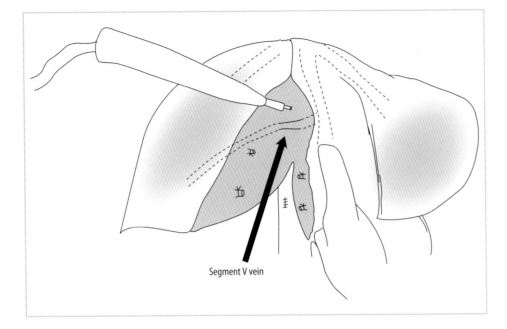

Segment V vein

Figure 6.117

14. During the parenchymal transection, it is helpful to keep the central venous pressure in the donor low, so as to minimize bleeding. When any large tributaries (>4 mm) draining into the middle hepatic vein are encountered (blue arrow), they can be divided and tagged for later reimplantation in the recipient (Figures 6.117 and 6.118).

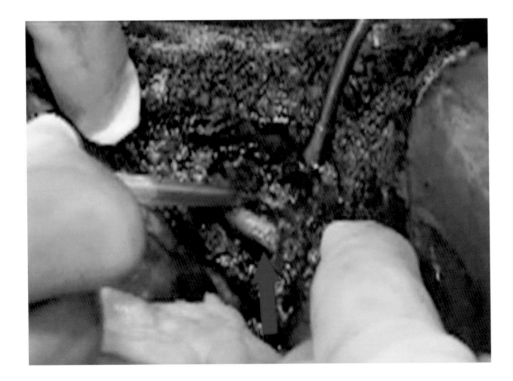

Figure 6.118

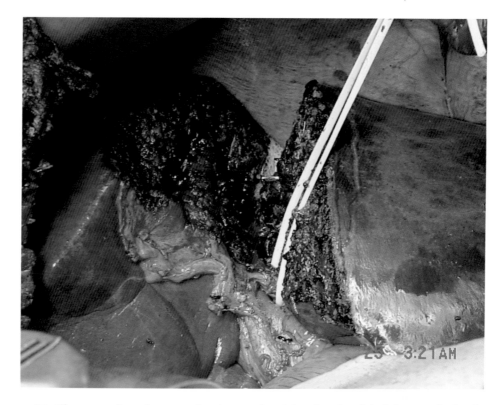

Figure 6.119

15. The parenchymal transection is completed, leaving the right lobe attached only by its vascular and biliary attachment (Figure 6.119).

16. The right hepatic duct is divided at the determined site based on the cholangiogram. The corresponding biliary stump on the left side is closed, taking care not to narrow the common hepatic duct (Figure 6.120).

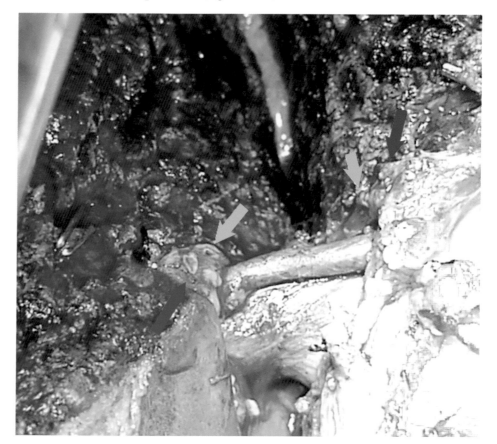

Figure 6.120

17. We prefer to wait at this point until the recipient team is ready to receive the liver. This also allows for close inspection of the two pieces of the liver to ensure that they are both adequately perfused (Figure 6.121).

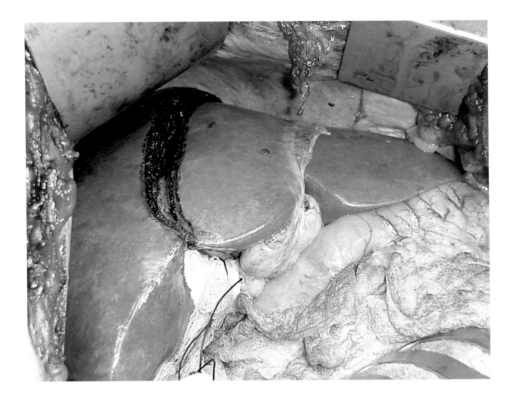

Figure 6.121

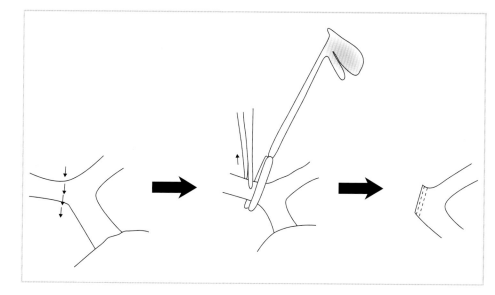

Figure 6.122

18. When the recipient team is ready, the vascular structures of the right graft are divided. The right hepatic artery is taken first with a vascular clamp. The right portal vein is divided next, either using a vascular clamp or a linear stapling device for proximal control. Regardless of how control is achieved, it is important that the stump of the right portal vein is closed in an anterior to posterior fashion, rather than a side-to-side manner. This ensures that there is no narrowing at the junction between the left and main portal veins (Figures 6.122 and 6.123).

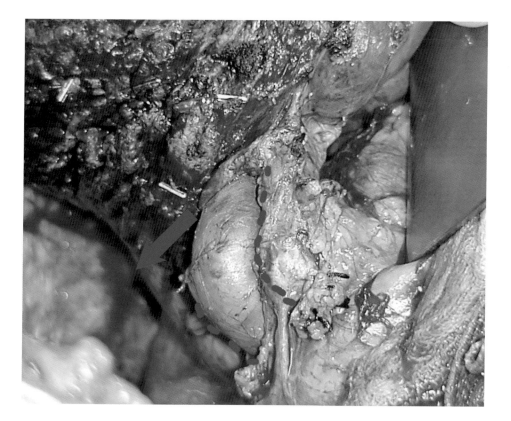

Figure 6.123

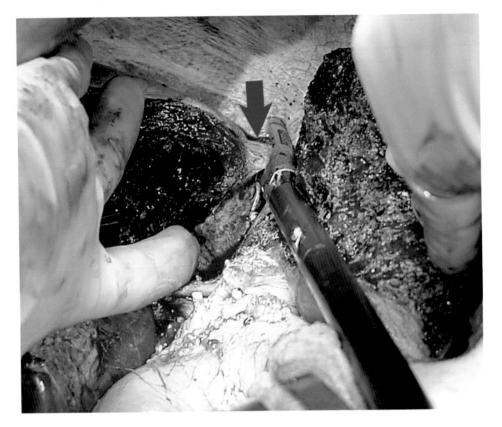

Figure 6.124

19. The right hepatic vein (blue arrow) is easiest to divide using a laparoscopic stapling device (Figures 6.124 and 6.125).

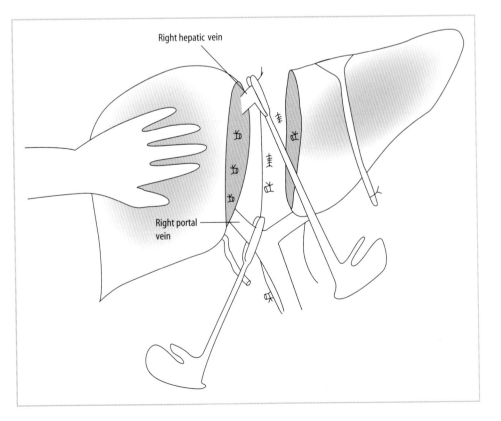

Right hepatic vein

Right portal vein

Figure 6.125

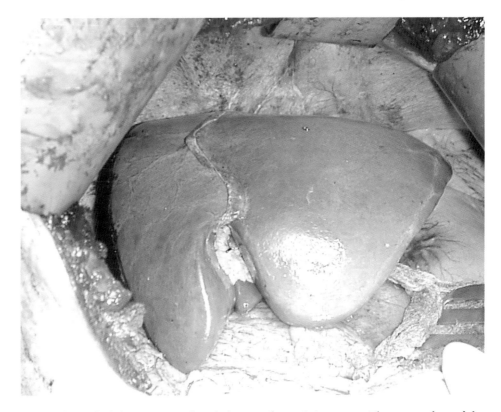

Figure 6.126

20. The right lobe is removed and given to the recipient team. The cut surface of the left lobe is carefully inspected for any evidence of bile leak or bleeding (Figure 6.126). The falciform ligament is reattached using a running suture to prevent torsion of the remaining left lobe. We prefer to leave a drain in place, but many centers do not. The incision is then closed.

b) Recipient Procedure

1. The graft is flushed with preservative solution and weighed. If there are any segment V or VIII veins that will need to be reimplanted (based on size being ≥5 mm), then a vein graft should be anastomosed onto them in an end-to-end fashion (yellow arrow) (Figure 6.127). Options include using cryopreserved vein, recipient's saphenous or superficial femoral vein, or using a segment of vein from the resected liver (such as the left portal vein). A saphenous vein graft has been used in this case.

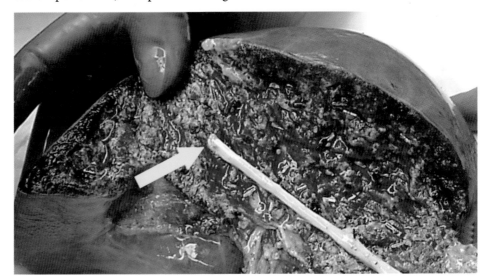

Figure 6.127

2. A standard inferior vena cava–sparing hepatectomy is done in the recipient; the liver is mobilized off the underlying cava and all short hepatic veins are divided (Figure 6.128).

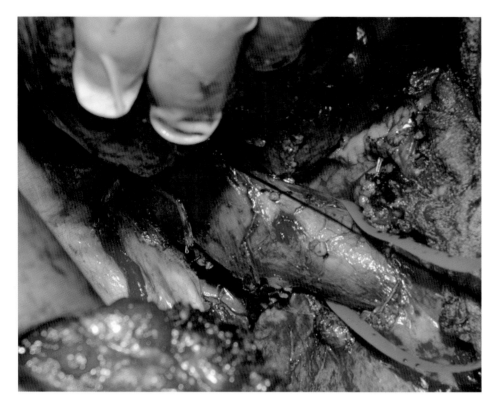

Figure 6.128

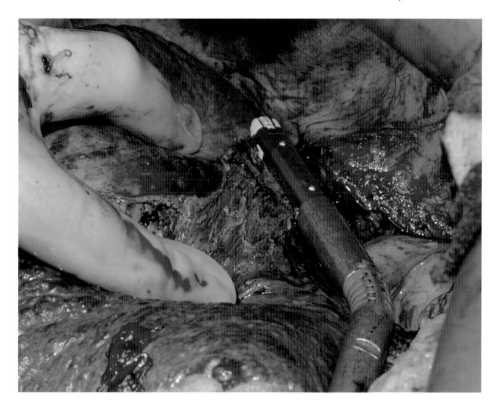

Figure 6.129

3. The orifices of the three hepatic veins are stapled shut (Figure 6.129), and the liver is removed completely (Figure 6.130).

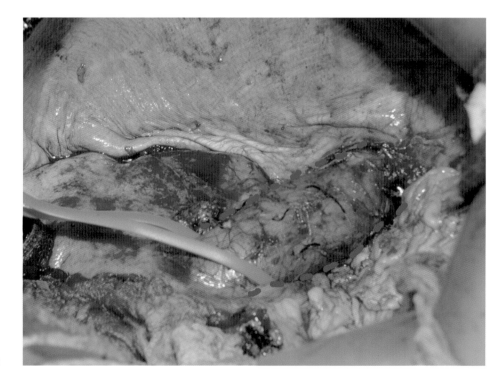

Figure 6.130

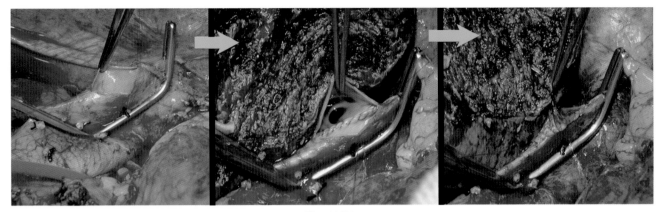

Figure 6.131

4. The donor right hepatic vein (HV) is anastomosed to a venotomy made on the anterior wall of the cava. It is important to have a nice patulous anastomosis to maximize outflow (Figure 6.131).

5. The donor right portal vein (PV) is anastomosed to the recipient main PV. The graft can now be flushed (Figure 6.132).

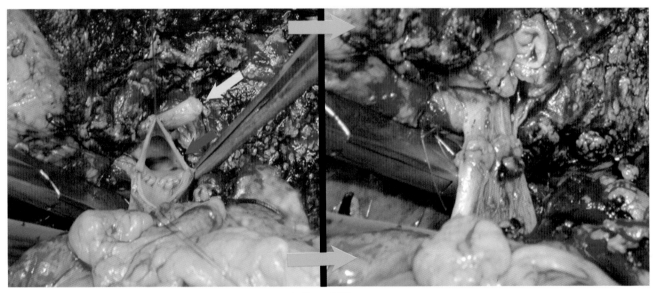

Figure 6.132

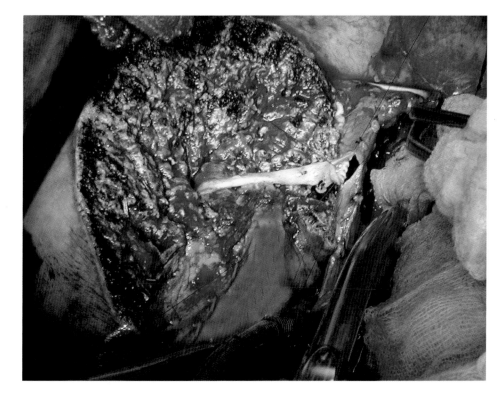

Figure 6.133

6. Any middle hepatic vein tributaries that had been reconstructed can be reimplanted. This can be done by anastomosing the end of the vein graft to the recipient cava (Figures 6.133 and 6.134).

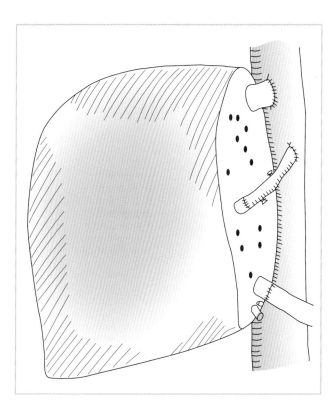

Figure 6.134

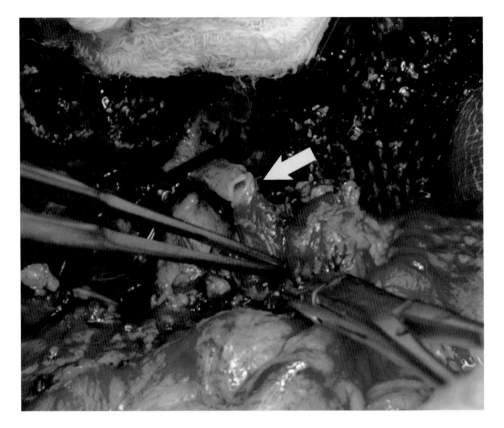

Figure 6.135

7. The donor right hepatic artery (HA) is anastomosed to the recipient right HA using fine (7.0) interrupted sutures (Figures 6.135 and 6.136).

8. Finally, the bile ducts are reconstructed. If the recipient bile duct reaches the donor bile duct without tension, a duct-to-duct anastomosis can be done (yellow arrow). Even

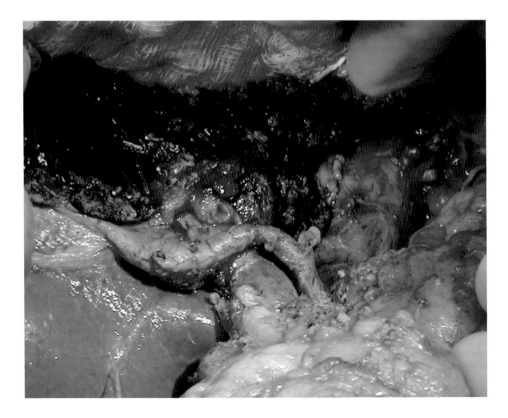

Figure 6.136

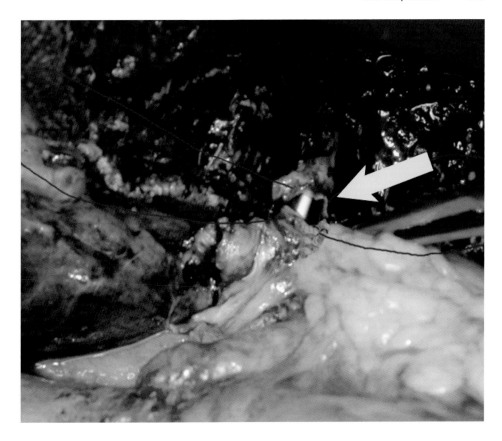

Figure 6.137

when there are two ducts in the donor graft, as long as the recipient ducts have been divided high in the hilum, a duct-to-duct anastomosis is possible to the native right and left hepatic ducts (Figure 6.137). It is helpful to perform this anastomosis over an internal stent.

9. Alternatively, a Roux-en-Y loop can be used if it is not possible to use the recipient's own ducts. Using an external biliary stent is helpful when performing this anastomosis, and allows for easy imaging afterward (Figure 6.138).

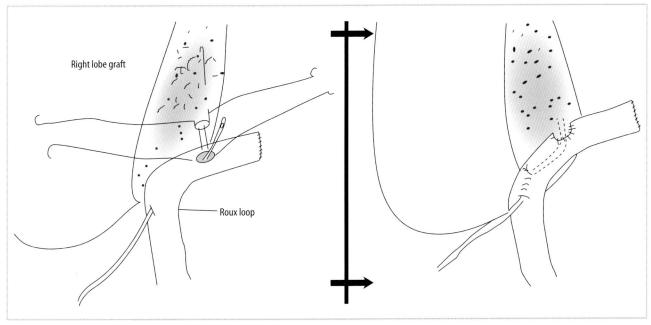

Right lobe graft

Roux loop

Figure 6.138

Surgical Complications After Liver Transplant

The incidence of surgical complications after liver transplant remains significantly higher than that after kidney transplant. This is not surprising given the increased complexity and magnitude of the operative procedure and, often, the more critical condition of the recipients. Most surgical complications occur early posttransplant, usually within the first few weeks.

Risk factors vary depending on the exact complication, but generally partial-liver transplants (i.e., living-donor and deceased-donor splits) have a higher technical complication rate than whole-liver transplants. Recipients who are significantly debilitated at the time of their transplant and critically ill, also tend to have increased complications postoperatively, especially infection related. While numerous potential complications are possible after transplant, surgical complications related directly to the operation most commonly include postoperative hemorrhage and problems with either the vascular or the biliary anastomoses. Common complications include the following:

a) Hemorrhage

Bleeding is common in the postoperative period and is usually multifactorial. It may be compounded by an underlying coagulopathy resulting from deficits in coagulation, fibrinolysis, and platelet function. Blood loss should be monitored via the abdominal drains; hemoglobin and central venous pressure should be measured serially. If bleeding persists despite correction of coagulation deficiencies, an exploratory relaparotomy should be performed.

b) Hepatic Artery Complications

The incidence of hepatic arterial vascular complications is reportedly 5% to 10%. Thrombosis is the most common early event; stenosis and pseudoaneurysm formation occur later. Hepatic artery thrombosis (HAT) has a reported incidence of about 3% in adults and about 5% to 10% in children. Partial-liver transplant recipients have a higher incidence than whole-liver recipients. After HAT, liver recipients may be asymptomatic, or they may develop severe liver failure secondary to extensive necrosis. Doppler ultrasound evaluation is the initial investigation of choice, with more than 90% sensitivity and specificity. Urgent exploration with thrombectomy and revision of the anastomosis are indicated; if the diagnosis is made early, up to 70% of grafts can be salvaged. If hepatic necrosis is extensive, a retransplant is indicated. A HAT also may present in a less dramatic fashion. Thrombosis may render the common bile duct ischemic, resulting in a localized or diffuse bile leak from the anastomosis, or a more chronic, diffuse biliary stricture.

c) Portal Vein Complications

Thrombosis of the portal vein is far less frequent compared to its arterial counterpart. Liver dysfunction, tense ascites, and variceal bleeding may occur. Doppler evaluation should establish the diagnosis. If thrombosis is diagnosed early, operative thrombectomy and revision of the anastomosis may be successful. If thrombosis occurs late, liver function is usually preserved, due to the presence of collaterals; a retransplant is then unnecessary, and attention is diverted toward relieving the left-sided portal hypertension.

d) Biliary Complications

Biliary complications continue to be significant, occurring in 15% to 35% of liver transplants. Such complications manifest either as leaks or as obstructions. Again, partial-liver transplant recipients seem to be at higher risk, for both leaks and strictures. Leaks tend to occur early postoperatively and often require surgical repair, while obstructions usually occur later and can be managed with radiologic or endoscopic techniques. Clinical symptoms of a bile leak include fever, abdominal pain, and peritoneal irritation. Ultrasound may demonstrate a fluid collection; cholangiography is required for diagnosis. Some leaks may be successfully managed by endoscopic placement of a biliary stent. If the leak does not respond to stent placement or if the patient is systemically ill, a relaparotomy is warranted.

Biliary stricture occurs later in the postoperative period and is most common at the anastomotic site, likely related to local ischemia. Strictures usually manifest as cholangitis, cholestasis, or both processes. Initial treatment involves balloon dilatation or stent placement across the site of stricture, or both. If these initial options fail, surgical revision is required.

e) Wound Complications

Common problems related to the wound are infection, hematoma, and seroma. Wound hematomas can result from the presence of huge collateral veins in the abdominal wall. Wound infections usually present after postoperative day 5. Treatment consists of opening the wound, changing the dressings, and allowing healing by secondary intention. If significant cellulitis or systemic symptoms are present, intravenous (IV) antibiotics should be administered. Late wound complications generally consist of incisional hernias, which may present at any time after transplant. Repair is warranted if the patient is symptomatic.

f) Primary Nonfunction

Primary nonfunction is a devastating complication, and the attendant mortality rate is >80% without a retransplant. By definition, this syndrome results from poor or no hepatic function from the time of the transplant procedure. The incidence in most centers is about 3% to 5%. Donor factors associated with primary nonfunction include advanced age, increased fat content of the donor liver, longer donor hospital stay before organ procurement, prolonged cold ischemia time, and reduced-size grafts. Conditions that may mimic primary nonfunction must be ruled out, such as HAT, accelerated acute rejection, and severe infection. Intravenous prostaglandin E_1 has some useful effect and should be administered to recipients with suspected primary nonfunction. They should be listed for an urgent retransplant.

Similar to primary nonfunction is small-for-size syndrome, seen in recipients of partial-liver transplants. Presentation is with liver dysfunction, manifesting as cholestasis, coagulopathy, and failure to thrive. It is believed that portal hyperperfusion causes damage to the relatively small graft. Some studies have suggested that splenic artery ligation or portal shunts may be beneficial in this scenario, but experience is limited.

Selected Readings

Bismuth H. Surgical anatomy and anatomical surgery of the liver. World J Surg 1982;6:3–9.

Brown R Jr, Russo M, Lai M, et al. A survey of liver transplantation from living adult donors in the United States. N Engl J Med 348(9):818–825.

Brown A, Williams R. Long-term postoperative care. In: Maddrey WC, Schiff ER, Sorrell MF, eds. Transplantation of the Liver. Lippincott Williams & Wilkins, 2001.

Couinaud C. Le Foie: Etudes Anatomiques et Chirurgicales. Paris: Masson, 1957.

Everson GT, Kam I. Immediate postoperative care. In: Maddrey WC, Schiff ER, Sorrell MF, eds. Transplantation of the Liver. Philadelphia: Lippincott Williams & Wilkins, 2001.

Fan ST, Lo CM, Liu CL. Technical REF1inement in adult-to-adult living donor liver transplantation using right lobe graft. Ann Surg 2000;231(1):126–131.

Humar A, Gruessner R. Critical care of the liver transplant recipient. In: Intensive Care Medicine, 4th ed. Rippe JM, Irwin RS, Fink MP, Cerra FB, eds. Philadelphia: Lippincott-Raven, 1998.

Icoz G, Kilic M, Zeytunlu M, et al. Biliary reconstructions and complications encountered in 50 consecutive right-lobe living donor liver transplantations. Liver Transplant 2003;9(6):575–580.

Kim-Schluger L, Florman S, Schiano T, et al. Quality of life after lobectomy for adult liver transplantation. Transplantation 73(10):1593–1597.

Kiuchi T, Inomata Y, Uemoto S, et al. Living-donor liver transplantation in Kyoto. Clin Transplant 1997;191–198.

Lee T, et al. Split-liver transplantation using the left lateral segment: a collaborative sharing experience between two distant centers. Am J Transplant 2005;5:1646–1651.

Marcos A, Fisher RA, Ham JM, et al. Right lobe living donor liver transplantation. Transplantation 1999; 68(6):798–803.

Nashan B, Lueck R, Becker T, Schlitt MH, Grannas G, Klempnauer J. Outcome of split liver transplantation using ex-situ or in-situ splits from cadaver donors. Joint meeting of the International Liver Transplantation Society, European Liver Transplantation Association, and Liver Intensive Care Group of Europe, Berlin, Germany, July 11–13, 2001.

Neuhaus P, Blumhardt G, Bechstein WO, Steffen R, Platz KP, Keck H. Technique and results of biliary reconstruction using side-to-side choledococholedochostomy in 300 orthotopic liver transplants. Ann Surg 1994;219(4):426–434.

Renz JF, Busuttil RW. Adult-to-adult living-donor liver transplantation: a critical analysis. Semin Liver Dis 2000;20(4):411–424.

Reyes J, Gerber D, Mazariegos GV, et al. Split-liver transplantation: a comparison of ex vivo and in situ techniques. J Pediatr Surg 2000;35:283–289; discussion 289–290.

Rogiers X, Malago M, Gawad K, et al. In situ splitting of cadaveric livers. The ultimate expansion of a limited donor pool. Ann Surg 1996;224:331–334.

Shah SA, Grant DR, Greig PD, et al. Analysis and outcomes of right lobe hepatectomy in 101 consecutive living donors. Am J Transplant 2005;5(11):2764–2769.

Strong RW, Lynch SV, Ong TN, et al. Successful liver transplantation from a living donor to her son. N Engl J Med 1990;322:1505–1507.

Surman OS. The ethics of partial liver donation. N Engl J Med 346(14):1038.

Trotter J, Talamantes M, McClure M, et al. Right hepatic lobe donation for living donor liver transplantation: impact on donor quality of life. Liver Transplant 7(6):485–493.

Trotter JF, Wachs M, Everson GT, Kam I. Adult-to-adult transplantation of the right hepatic lobe from a living donor. N Engl J Med 2002;346(14):1074–1082.

Umeshita K, Fujiwara K, Kiyosawa K, et al. Japanese Liver Transplantation Society. Operative morbidity of living liver donors in Japan. Lancet 2003;362(9385):687–690.

Wachs ME, Bak TE, Karrer FM, et al. Adult living donor liver transplantation using a right hepatic lobe. Transplantation 1998;66,1313–1316.

Washburn K, et al. Split-liver transplantation: results of statewide usage of the right trisegmental graft. Am J Transplant 2005;5:1652–1659.

Wiesner RH. Current indications, contraindications, and timing for liver transplantation. In: Busutill RW, Klintmalm GB, eds. Transplantation of the Liver. Philadelphia: WB Saunders, 1996.

Yersiz H, et al. One-hundred in situ split-liver transplantations: a single center experience. Ann Surg 2003; 238(4):496–505.

Zimmerman MA, Trotter JF. Living donor liver transplantation in patients with hepatitis C. Liver Transplant 9(11): S52–S57.

7

Intestinal and Multivisceral Transplantation

Thomas M. Fishbein and Cal S. Matsumoto

Isolated Intestine Transplant
a) Donor Procedure
b) Back-Table Procedure
c) Recipient Procedure
Combined Liver–Intestine Transplant
a) Donor Procedure
b) Back-Table Procedure
c) Recipient Procedure
Multivisceral Transplant
a) Donor Procedure
b) Recipient Procedure
Living-Donor Small-Bowel Transplant
a) Surgical Procedure
Perioperative Management

Intestinal transplantation has evolved from an experimental procedure with limited success to standard of care for patients with intestinal and parenteral nutrition failure, achieving outcomes commensurate with other solid-organ transplants.[1,2] Paramount to achieving the success of intestinal and multivisceral organ transplant procedures has been the refinement of donor organ procurement and transplantation techniques.[3] Early graft failures and deaths due to technical and donor-related complications have been minimized using the techniques described here, leaving the current challenge largely of optimizing immunologic and infection management strategies.[4,5] Techniques depicted here are those of choice in our experience, while mention is made of alternative techniques that may be preferred by others. Because patients requiring intestinal transplantation often present with multiple organ failures and require multiorgan transplantation, modification of these techniques may be required on an individual basis. Addition of renal allotransplantation, inclusion of the colon in a small-bowel or multivisceral graft, and modified multivisceral transplantation with preservation of the native liver are some of the common modifications. Intimate description of all possible techniques is beyond the scope of the chapter.

The three most common types of allografts involving the small intestine are isolated intestinal transplantation, combined liver–small bowel transplantation, and multivisceral transplantation. These are described in turn, detailing our commonly preferred methods for both donor and recipient surgical techniques.

Isolated Intestine Transplant

a) Donor Procedure

1. The standard sternum to pubis incision is made, taking care not to injure the bowel upon entering the abdomen. On many occasions, due to either the nature of injury or the preoperative state of the donor, the intestine may be dilated or edematous and may closely abut the abdominal wall. A nasogastric tube should decompress the stomach and upper gastrointestinal tract. We additionally prefer to decontaminate the allograft through instillation of antibiotics into the lumen through the indwelling nasogastric tube. Immediately upon entering the abdomen, another dose of selective gut decontaminant may be administered, and passed through the pylorus into the small intestinal graft.

A broad Kocher and Cattell maneuver are each performed, and the aorta and inferior vena cava are exposed behind the intestinal mesentery up to the superior mesenteric artery (Figure 7.1).

2. The ligament of Treitz is broadly mobilized from the retroperitoneum and aorta, mobilizing the distal duodenum and proximal jejunum. The abdominal aorta is encircled distally for eventual aortic cannulation and flush. The gastrocolic omentum is

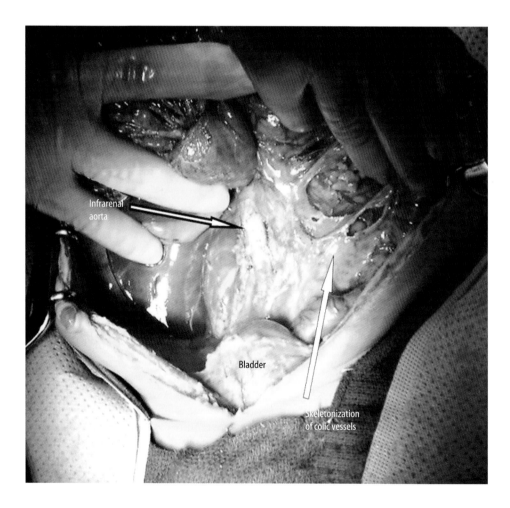

Figure 7.1

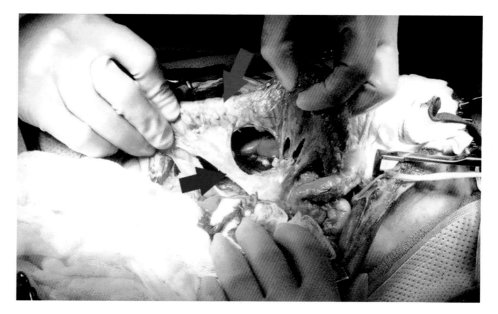

Figure 7.2

divided, and the left colon is mobilized (red arrow) (Figure 7.2). The mesentery of the colon is then dissected, exposing right, middle and left colic vessels. Exposure of the colic vessels (blue arrow) facilitates rapid removal of the colon immediately prior to heparinization and cannulation.

3. A medial visceral rotation mobilizes the tail of the pancreas (yellow arrow) with the spleen (blue arrow), exposing the left side of the aorta and origin of the mesenteric vessels (Figure 7.3). As with standard pancreas procurement, the pylorus is transected with a linear stapler, leaving sufficient length to invert the staple line with another layer of suture. The stomach is rotated laterally out of the abdominal field after ligation of the left gastric artery, separation of the stomach from the greater omentum, and division of the short gastric vessels to the spleen. The use of the inferior mesenteric vein (IMV) for flush during intestinal procurement is discouraged, as high flow and pressure in the IMV flush may decrease intestinal outflow through the superior mesenteric vein. In multivisceral graft procurement, care must be taken to avoid injury to the left gastric artery, while attachments of the stomach to the colon via the greater omentum are still divided.

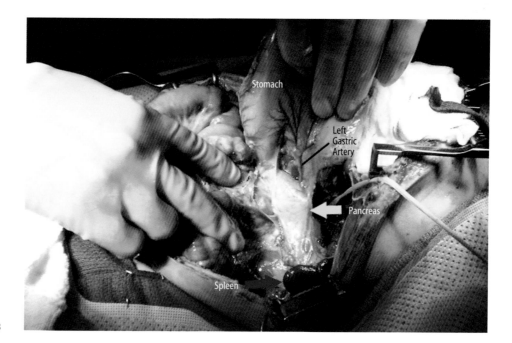

Figure 7.3

4. The liver graft dissection is performed in the standard manner, previously described in this atlas. Once there is satisfactory dissection by all participating procurement teams (heart, lung, liver, pancreas), and *prior* to administration of systemic anticoagulants, the small intestine luminal contents are manually propulsed in an antegrade fashion from the pylorus to the ileocecal valve. Since the bowel is a hollow viscus, air left in the organ may allow more rapid rewarming during cold preservation. Care must be taken while manually advancing luminal contents to prevent serosal injury of the sometimes fragile intestine. This maneuver decompresses the small intestine of both air and liquids and advances the luminal contents into the colon, allowing the ileocecal valve to prevent reflux. This should be the final maneuver performed prior to heparinization and aortic cannulation.

Once the small intestine is decompressed, the bowel is transected at the distal ileum and sigmoid. The colonic mesenteric vessels (blue arrow), which had been previously dissected, are ligated and transected, and the colon is rapidly removed from the cadaver (Figure 7.4). Vascular transection of the colon should be performed last to prevent drainage from an ischemic colon into the liver.

5. The donor cannulation, cross-clamping, flushing, thoracic venting, and topical cooling are performed in the standard manner. A laparotomy pad should protect the intestine from direct exposure to ice slush, as this may cause subserosal hematomas. Immediately prior to cross-clamping, the small intestine mesentery must be examined closely to ensure that there is no unintended volvulus. This will ensure adequate flush to both the intestine and liver portal system.

6. The liver is removed first, with transection of the portal vein at the level of the coronary vein, and transaction of the splenic artery. As in standard pancreas procurement, the splenic artery is always tagged with a fine suture for later identification. Our preference is to remove the pancreas and intestine graft en bloc, and separate the pancreas from the intestine at the backtable dissection. This technique ensures rapid organ retrieval from the cadaver after flush and allows for identification and ligation of individual proximal jejunal and duodenal mesenteric vessels in a controlled environment. Using this technique, both the pancreas and intestine grafts can be removed quickly from the cadaver by simply transecting the superior mesenteric artery at its aortic origin with or without a Carrel patch, as preferred by the pancreas surgeon.

7. Division of the base of the small intestine mesentery just below the inferior pancreaticoduodenal arcade may be performed in situ in a stable donor, although we usually avoid it due to prolongation of the donor procedure. In this case, the middle colic vessels

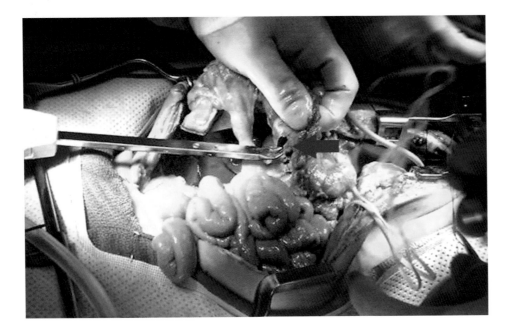

Figure 7.4

are divided, and the ligament of Treitz is widely mobilized from over the aorta and the inferior margin of the pancreas. The mesentery may be isolated by placing the entire small bowel over a moist laparotomy pad after removal of the colon. The jejunum may be divided with a stapling device approximately 10 cm distal to the ligament, and the superior mesenteric vein is identified laterally in the mesentery. Fine ligation of all lymphatic structures is performed, isolating the superior mesenteric vein and artery. The artery will usually give off a proximal jejunal arcade that requires division. Additionally, care must be taken not to injure the main jejunal vein draining the proximal allograft, as this usually runs posterior to the artery, joining the ileal vein to form the superior mesenteric high in the mesentery.

The isolated intestine donor operation historically precluded the use of the pancreas from the same donor; however, with close coordination between liver, pancreas, and intestinal procurement teams, successful procurement of all of these individual organs can be safely achieved.[10] The notable exception is the case in which the donor has a replaced right hepatic artery arising low on the superior mesenteric artery.

b) Back-Table Procedure

1. In the event that the pancreas is not being transplanted, the back-table dissection begins at the level of the portal vein. Stay sutures are placed on the portal vein and cuff of superior mesenteric artery (Figure 7.5)

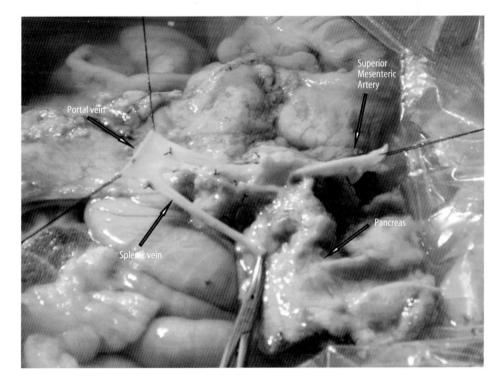

Figure 7.5

2. The portal vein dissection begins at the level of transection. Small pancreatic venous tributaries are identified and ligated. Care should be taken to preserve the splenic vein (Figure 7.6), as this provides a useful conduit for flush of preservation solution from the allograft at the time of reperfusion. (SMV, superior mesenteric vein; IMV, inferior mesenteric vein.)

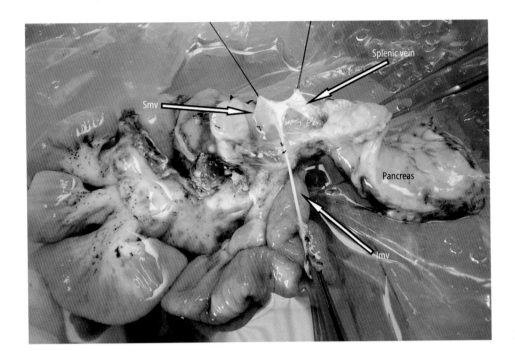

Figure 7.6

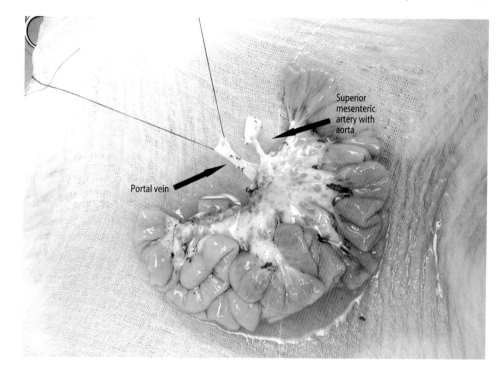

Figure 7.7

3. During separation of the intestinal graft from the pancreas, the jejunum is first transected, and the small and numerous jejunal mesenteric vessels are ligated. The finished graft should have a well-developed portal vein and superior mesenteric artery (SMA) for implantation (Figures 7.7 and 7.8).

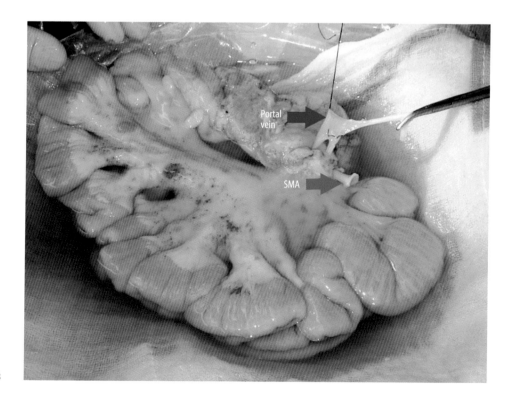

Figure 7.8

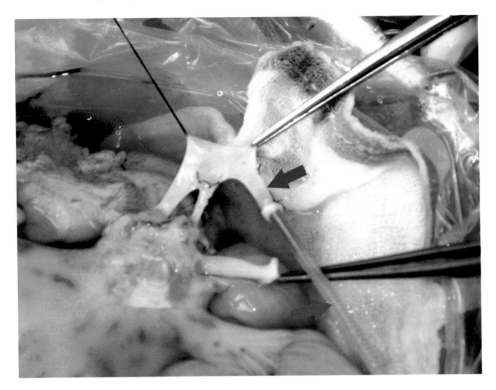

Figure 7.9

4. To facilitate the graft blood flush, a small cannula may be placed in the splenic vein (blue arrow) for ease in flush measurement. We prefer the use of a Sundt carotid endarterectomy shunt (red arrow), which is used to allow egress of the preservation solution prior to opening the venous clamp (Figure 7.9). The shunt is then removed, venous outflow clamp opened, and the splenic stump ligated.

5. If the pancreas is also to be transplanted as a whole-organ allograft, the mesentery is isolated upon a moist lap pad, and the mesenteric vessels are isolated below the inferior pancreaticoduodenal artery and vein, which provide necessary flow to the pancreas allograft. The middle colic vessels and first jejunal arcade usually must be ligated. Care should be taken not to injure the major jejunal vein, which usually courses behind the superior mesenteric artery to join the ileocolic vein high in the base of the small bowel mesentery. Small vascular clamps are placed on the superior mesenteric artery and vein after the flush, and these vessels are transected. The pancreatic side is individually oversewn with fine nonabsorbable suture and the bowel graft is again flushed on the back table. The pancreas and liver are then removed in the usual fashion. In the event that an aberrant right hepatic artery or aberrant common hepatic artery is encountered from the SMA, care must be taken to avoid injury to these vessels and the SMA must be divided distal to the origin of the aberrant vessel. When this is encountered, good-quality iliac or common femoral artery and vein extension grafts are required for implantation of the small bowel graft.

c) Recipient Procedure

Isolated intestinal transplantation is usually described by the technique of vascular reconstruction used for venous drainage, being either "mesenteric/portal" or "systemic." The surgical approach is determined by the underlying recipient intestinal disease, the health of the recipient's liver, and anatomic considerations that may influence the surgeon.[11] This is usually accomplished through a generous midline incision, although in babies less than 10 kg we sometimes prefer a transverse incision if one has previously been made.

We prefer to use mesenteric drainage for patients in whom the native small bowel is in place and will be removed at the time of transplantation. In cases of extreme short bowel, the superior mesenteric vessels carry little flow, are usually quite small and may not accommodate sufficient blood supply for the transplanted bowel; in these cases we usually prefer systemic vascular reconstruction.

Mesenteric Vascular Reconstruction

1. For candidates receiving an isolated intestinal allograft for functional disorders (infantile diarrhea or motility disorder), the native small bowel is usually in place. In this instance, blood flow through the mesenteric vessels is preserved, and they are of adequate caliber and quality for supply to the graft. Implantation, therefore, can be performed using these vessels prepared in the same manner as for isolated intestinal donor procurement. The jejunum is divided 10 to 20 cm distal to the ligament of Treitz, which is broadly mobilized. The arcade to the proximal jejunum is preserved. The recipient bowel is suspended by the root of the mesentery after disconnection at the proximal jejunum and colon, enabling fine dissection of the mesenteric root (yellow arrow), and isolation of the superior mesenteric artery and vein (Figure 7.10).

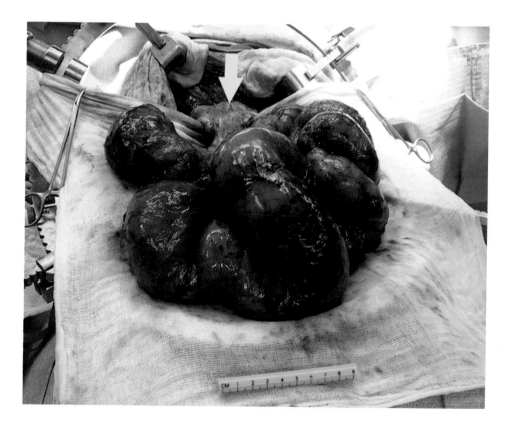

Figure 7.10

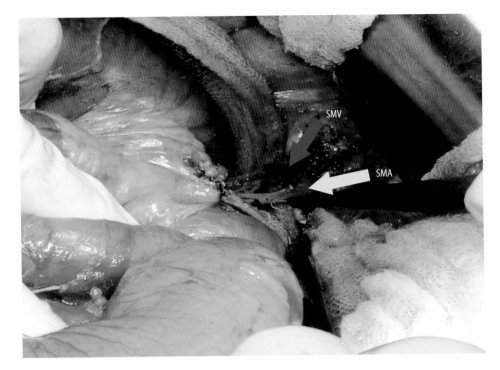

Figure 7.11

2. If the colon is intact, the middle colic vessels are ligated, the right and transverse colon mobilized, and the left transverse or descending colon divided. We always mobilize or remove the splenic flexure of the colon to assure endoscopic access to the ileum from below after closure of the stoma. The superior mesenteric vein (SMV, blue arrow) is located lateral to the superior mesenteric artery (SMA, yellow arrow) (Figure 7.11). Dissection of the base of the mesentery is undertaken to skeletonize these vessels. These tissues should all be ligated to avoid lymphatic or chylous ascites after transplantation.[12]

3. Small vascular clamps may be used to control the superior mesenteric artery (SMA) and vein (SMV), dividing them distally and preserving long cuffs for anastomosis (Figure 7.12). The proximal native jejunum should be preserved with the proximal jejunal arcade of the SMA for anastomosis to the donor jejunum.

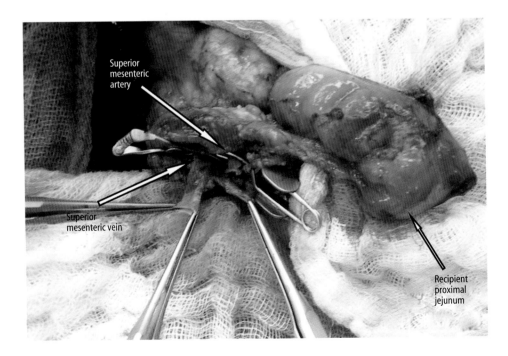

Figure 7.12

4. In some cases, placement of iliac or femoral arterial and venous conduits onto the graft vessels will be required (Figure 7.13). We have found that this facilitates transplantation when the pancreas has been procured for transplantation, as the graft mesenteric vessels will be shorter. They are best sewn in place prior to bringing the allograft into the field for implantation. Usually, either a short portion of external iliac or superficial femoral artery and vein are of appropriate caliber for anastomosis to the superior mesenteric vessels. The weight of the small bowel allograft may lead to tension over the duodenal sweep and predispose the graft to settle inferiorly toward the pelvis, so when using mesenteric reconstruction, attention should be paid to leaving generous length on the mesenteric vessels. Again, the main SMV should be used above the confluence of jejunal and ileal branches, which usually is quite close to the duodenal sweep.

In patients with short-bowel syndrome, the superior mesenteric vein sometimes cannot be exposed, as the base of the mesentery contracts after multiple prior resections. The venous anastomosis may be performed to the lateral wall of the portal vein in piggyback fashion, dissecting this vein free from the posterior porta hepatis, and placing an extension graft of iliac vein onto this in the end-to-side fashion.[13] We have only rarely employed this technique, and we discourage its routine use, as outcomes with systemic drainage are equivalent and accomplished with greater ease. However, it may be useful in cases of inferior vena cava thrombosis, where the alternative is placement of a venous extension graft on the suprarenal inferior vena cava, discussed below.

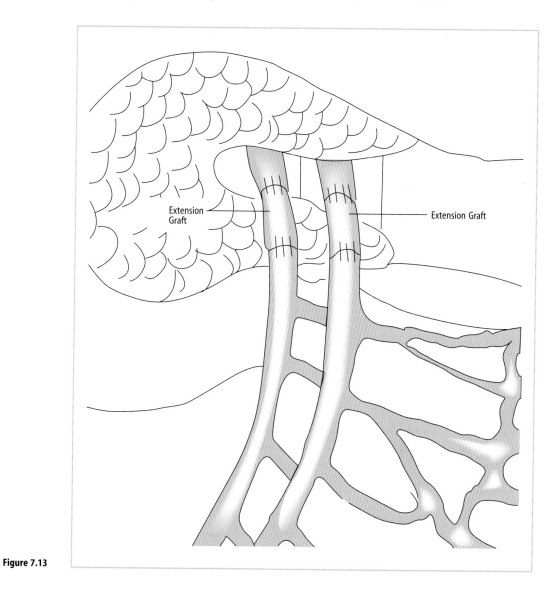

Figure 7.13

5. The bowel is then brought to the field after extension grafts are placed on the recipient vessels, and the base of the mesentery placed in a transverse plane aligning the donor and recipient vessels. The assistant is best positioned with a cold moist lap pad to both flatten the base of the mesentery as well as prevent bowel loops from entering the field, giving upward traction on the bowel allograft during anastomosis. The vessels are anastomosed end to end (Figure 7.14).

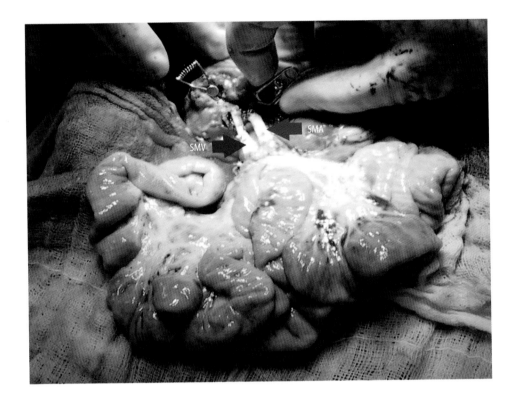

Figure 7.14

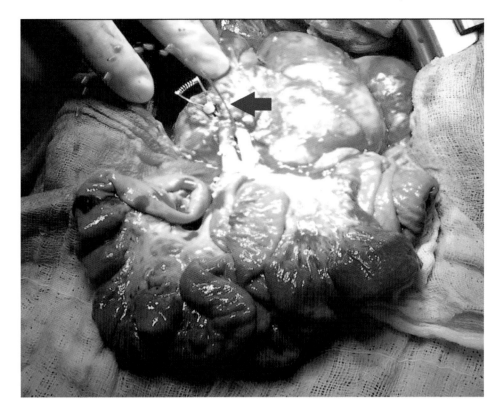

Figure 7.15

6. Reperfusion is then accomplished without heparinization. Upon reperfusion, blood and preservation solution is flushed out (blue arrow) prior to removal of the superior mesenteric vein clamp (Figure 7.15). This is facilitated by the previously placed cannula in the graft splenic vein, or through the superior mesenteric vein anastomosis.

7. The superior mesenteric vein clamp is then removed and venous return is reestablished (blue arrow, Figure 7.16).

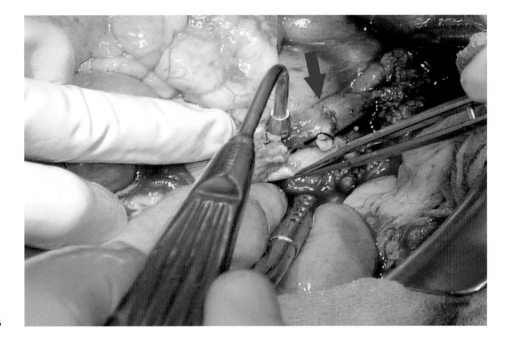

Figure 7.16

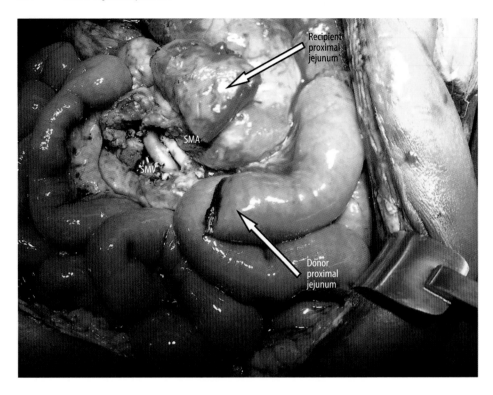

Figure 7.17

8. Fixation of the base of the mesentery transversely and without kinking of the vessels is critical to avoid volvulus or traction on the mesenteric vessels (Figure 7.17).

Systemic Vascular Reconstruction

This technique is more commonly employed for patients with short-bowel syndrome, particularly those with total or near-total loss of jejunum and ileum. In this disease state, the mesenteric vessels are often small in caliber, lacking good inflow. However, this is not always the case, and when a smaller donor with commensurately small vessels is being used, mesenteric drainage may still be used.

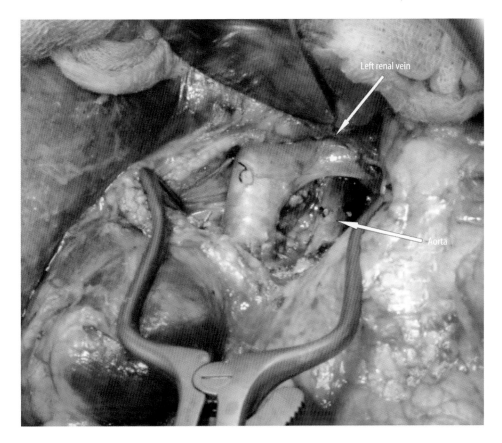

Figure 7.18

1. The recipient operation requires exposure of the infrarenal aorta for anastomosis of the arterial graft (Figure 7.18). The limits of dissection include the left renal vein above, and the inferior mesenteric artery below.

2. The inferior vena cava and aorta are clamped in preparation for systemic vascular anastomosis (Figure 7.19). The dissection may proceed below the inferior mesenteric artery, and this vessel controlled with a fine clip during anastomosis.

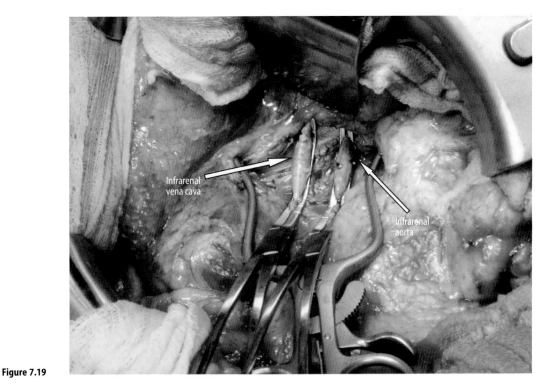

Figure 7.19

3. The arterial graft must be performed in a tension-free manner, as the weight of the bowel filled with secretions can lead to traction from the aorta to the pelvis or lead to decreased flow and thrombosis. The venous anastomosis is end-to-side to the anterior wall of the vena cava, as with a portocaval shunt (Figure 7.20). This is best accomplished after removal of an ellipse of vena cava to avoid narrowing. We prefer aortic inflow and caval drainage for patients who have demonstrated significant liver cholestasis, fibrosis, or ultrashort-bowel syndrome.[14] It is easy to accomplish, and in cases where intestinal transplantation is indicated due to reversible progressive liver disease, avoids drainage of the bowel graft into the possibly high-pressure portal circulation. The bowel graft is again oriented with the transverse mesentery parallel to the plane of the retroperitoneum, and sewn either directly to the aorta and vena cava, or as is our preference, to short extension grafts already placed to these vessels. Prior placement of extension grafts routinely makes implantation easy, not allowing loops of allograft small intestine to obscure the field of anastomosis. The mesentery is then fixed to the retroperitoneum to avoid internal hernia, volvulus, or traction on the vessels, care being taken to avoid the ureters. Systemic drainage has not been shown to yield inferior nutritional results, as some had initially predicted.[10,15,16]

4. Another technique is required when systemic drainage is being used in a patient with thrombosis of the inferior vena cava. This is not infrequently encountered, due to multiple femoral accesses for parenteral nutrition. In this case, ligation and division of a few low caudate veins allows placement of an extension graft of iliac or femoral vein on the suprarenal vena cava. This is accomplished with placement of a partially occluding clamp, removal of an ellipse of anterior caval wall, and placement of an extension graft. The graft is tunneled behind the mobilized duodenum and head of pancreas, to lie next to the infrarenal aortic anastomosis. We have found this easier to accomplish than piggyback drainage to the portal vein.

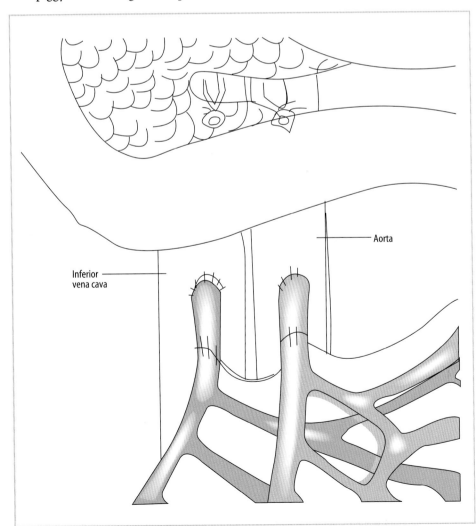

Figure 7.20

5. Enteral continuity is established proximally and distally in conjunction with an ileostomy, using either a loop-diverting ileostomy or a proximal ileocolostomy in a "chimney" fashion to provide access for surveillance allograft biopsy (Figure 7.21). These stomas also allow future ileostomy closure to be performed without a full laparotomy. Placement of tubes for intestinal access can be accomplished with gastric, jejunal, or combined tubes. These are placed to avoid prolonged need for nasogastric suction and facilitate early feeding.

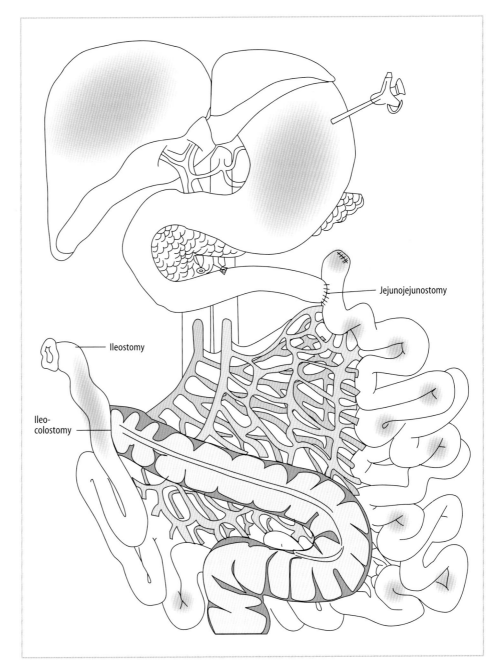

Figure 7.21

Combined Liver–Intestine Transplant

a) Donor Procedure

1. Donor management and operation begin as for isolated intestinal transplantation.[17] The gallbladder is incised and the biliary tract is flushed with saline. After broad Cattell and Kocher maneuvers, the tail of the pancreas and spleen are mobilized from the retroperitoneum, exposing the left lateral aspect of the aorta. Care is taken to avoid injury of the superior mesenteric vessels or the celiac axis (Figure 7.22).

The ligament of Treitz is widely mobilized. The proximal duodenum is then dissected at the level of the pylorus and divided with a stapling device. Care must be taken during this process to inspect the gastrohepatic ligament to avoid injury to an aberrant left hepatic artery if it is present.

2. After advancement of intraluminal contents distally, removal of the colon and systemic heparinization, the flush is performed with only aortic cannulation. Suprahepatic caval venting is performed.

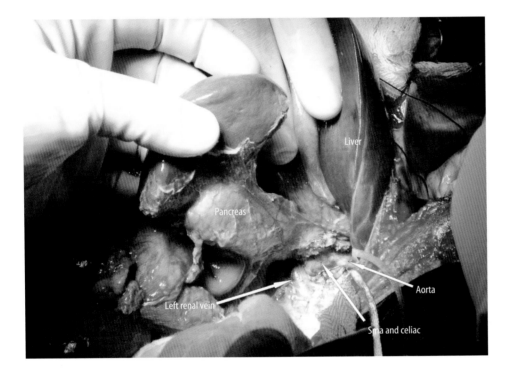

Figure 7.22

3. By retracting medially the spleen, pancreas and the small bowel in a cold lap pad, a Carrel patch or circumferential segment of aorta can then easily be taken, containing the origins of the celiac and superior mesenteric arteries. The plane is anterolateral on the left side of the aorta, and there is usually extensive mesenteric nervous plexus present in this tissue. Once this is divided, the aortic patch or segment can be clearly divided. Care must be taken not to injure the takeoff of renal arteries. If the kidneys are not being used (which is often the case with small pediatric donors), the entire aorta may be removed with the graft. We remove the entire aorta from iliac bifurcation to proximal descending aorta in the small pediatric donor; this requires the diaphragm to be split at the time of extraction. Then, the entire pancreas, spleen, small intestine and liver are removed *en-bloc* with intact inferior vena cava and duodenum (Figure 7.23).

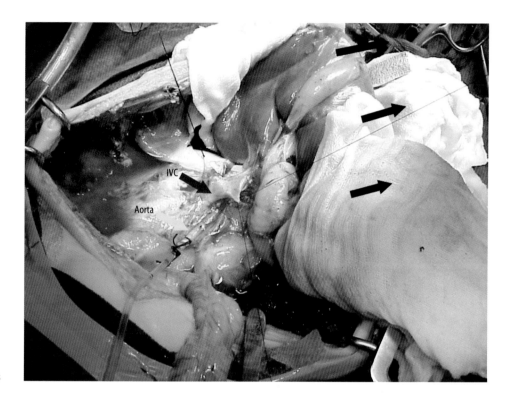

Figure 7.23

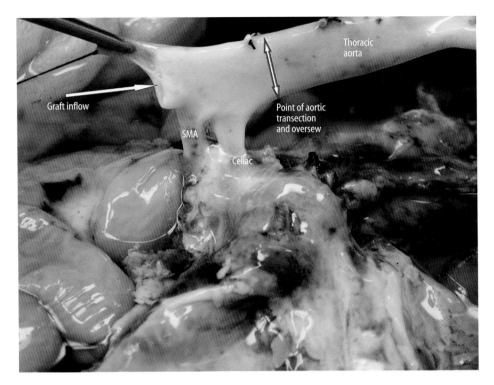

Figure 7.24

b) Back-Table Procedure

1. The back-table procedure requires cleaning of mesenteric and celiac plexus with ligation of vascular tissues surrounding these vessels. The celiac axis and superior mesenteric artery are exposed. Eventually the supraceliac aorta will be transected and oversewn (Figure 7.24). The thoracic aorta will then be used as a conduit from the native infrarenal aorta in a reversed interposition fashion.

2. The splenic vein and artery are dissected from the pancreas (Figure 7.25).

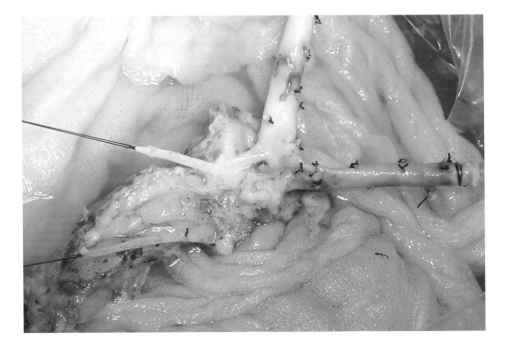

Figure 7.25

3. The pancreas is transected just to the left of the mesenteric vessels, and the splenic vein stump is used to flush preservation solution from the bowel before being ligated. It is important to oversew or staple the pancreatic remnant, reducing the pancreas gland and leading to a graft with intact duodenum with the pancreatic head. We prefer the use of a vascular stapling device for the pancreas (Figure 7.26). This technique is particularly suited to small pediatric donors in whom the pancreas is of sufficient size to warrant reduction.

4. The splenic artery must be ligated, but the gastroduodenal and inferior pancreaticoduodenal arteries are preserved, feeding the head of pancreas and duodenum to be transplanted with the allograft. If the pancreas is diminutive, no reduction is necessary. In infant donors, the small caliber of the aorta at the level of the SMA and celiac artery makes aortic inflow to the graft preferable. This can be performed using the supraceliac, infrarenal, or a transposed donor thoracic aortic segment as a conduit to the distal donor aorta (see figures in recipient procedure, below). The vena cava of the graft is then prepared as for isolated liver transplantation. The cut edge of the mesentery is evaluated closely and any small branches are sutured to avoid development of a hematoma in the mesentery. The vena cava of the liver should be prepared in the standard fashion.

The adult donor usually contains a larger pancreas gland, and this is more prone to leak if reduced. The entire pancreas may be transplanted with the liver–bowel allograft in order to facilitate use of the duodenal preservation technique. Alternatively, noncomposite transplantation of the orthotopic or piggyback liver and systemic or mesenteric isolated bowel implantation may be chosen, after removal of these two organs from the multiorgan en-bloc cluster that has been procured.

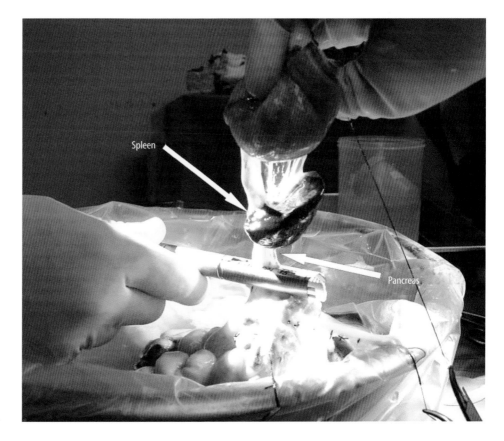

Figure 7.26

c) Recipient Procedure

1. This is most commonly accomplished using an en-bloc allograft with duodenal preservation. This technique allows for transplantation without disruption of the biliary system and hepatic arterial branches, and may be advantageous in small pediatric patients with tiny vascular and biliary structures that are otherwise easily injured.[11,12,18] The recipient is explored through a midline incision with bilateral subcostal extension, usually placed lower on the abdominal wall than for liver transplantation to provide improved lower abdominal exposure. Most patients will have prior incisions, and individualizing the opening may be required. Children have often undergone prior supraumbilical transverse incisions, which may be utilized.

2. Initial dissection of the liver hilum allows ligation of the hepatic artery and common bile duct. The portal vein is then skeletonized and the infrahepatic vena cava is isolated for construction of a portacaval shunt. Thereafter, the liver is dissected from the cava as for piggyback liver transplantation.

3. The infrarenal or supraceliac aorta is then exposed for anastomosis. Particularly among patients whose disease was inflammatory (i.e., necrotizing enterocolitis) adhesions may be dense and vascular, and care must be taken to avoid significant bleeding during this phase of the operation. Mobilization of the recipient duodenum is important to gain exposure of the infrarenal aorta. An aortic extension graft (either donor thoracic aorta or a bifurcation iliac artery graft) can now be placed on the recipient infrarenal aorta to facilitate inflow to the graft. Alternatively, some prefer to use supraceliac aorta, with direct anastomosis of the donor supraceliac aorta. This is easiest to expose during the anhepatic phase. We have found that smooth bloodless preparation of the site of graft arterial inflow prior to liver explantation is critical to a short warm ischemic implantation procedure and overall technical success.

4. The hepatic veins can now be clamped and the native liver is removed, maintaining long cuffs for anastomosis. Because the native foregut is preserved, a portocaval shunt must be performed to provide venous outflow for these organs after the composite liver–bowel graft is transplanted.[13,19] An end-to-side portocaval shunt is constructed most efficiently during the anhepatic phase (Figure 7.27).

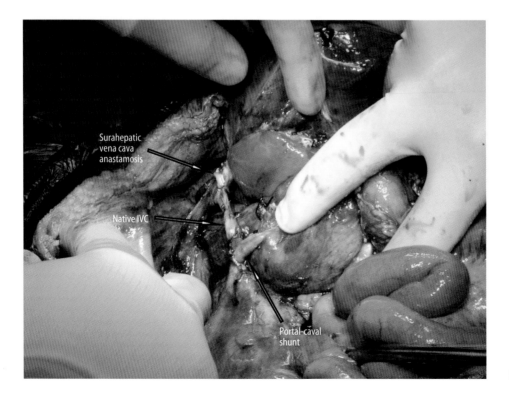

Figure 7.27

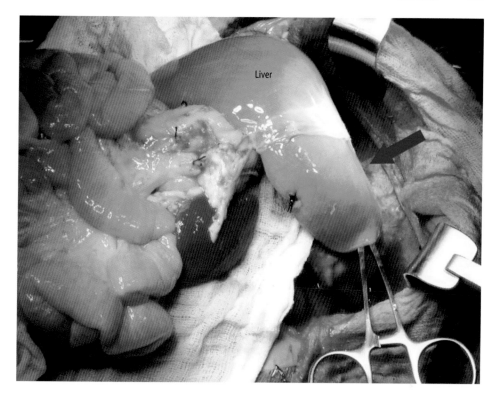

Figure 7.28

5. With relief of the portal hypertension, the adhesions from multiple prior operations can be lysed, taking care to avoid enterotomy, which otherwise may be disastrous. The graft is brought to the table and the suprahepatic caval anastomosis (blue arrow) is performed as in piggyback liver transplantation (Figures 7.28 and 7.29).

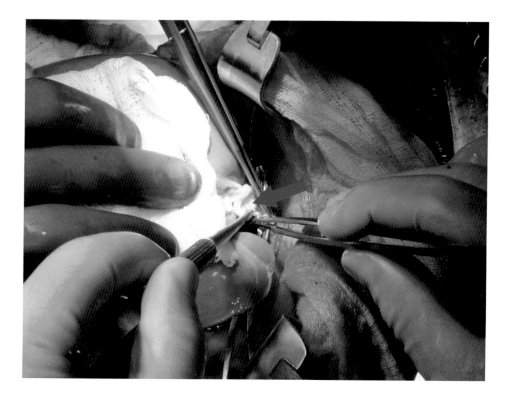

Figure 7.29

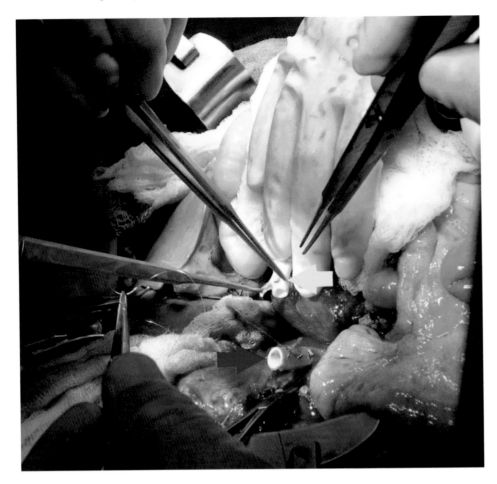

Figure 7.30

6. The Carrel patch or SMA/celiac complex (yellow arrow) can now be anastomosed either directly to the aorta or more commonly to an interposition conduit of donor thoracic aorta (blue arrow) (Figures 7.30 and 7.31) or bifurcating iliac artery.

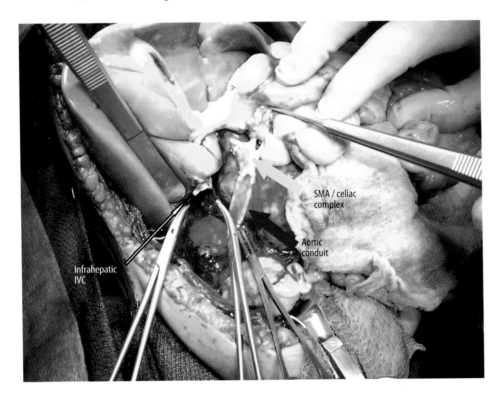

Figure 7.31

7. The stump of the splenic vein may be used to vent preservation solution, and if this is planned, the surgeon should isolate and prepare the splenic vein orifice during the back-table procedure (prior to transection of the pancreas).[20] Cholecystectomy is performed in the usual fashion.

8. Enteral continuity is reestablished with jejunojejunostomy after removal of most of the proximal recipient small bowel, anastomosis being performed distal to the ligament of Treitz of the allograft. Distal anastomosis is accomplished as with isolated intestinal allografting (Figure 7.32).

9. In some cases, it may be preferable to place separate liver and intestinal allografts, rather than employing the en-bloc allograft technique.[21] Severe portal hypertension and dense adhesions may make the aortic exposure required for combined transplantation difficult. Placement of the liver prior to aortic exposure can facilitate transplantation when faced with this difficulty. The piggyback liver transplant is performed, and the isolated intestinal transplant procedure with systemic drainage is then performed.

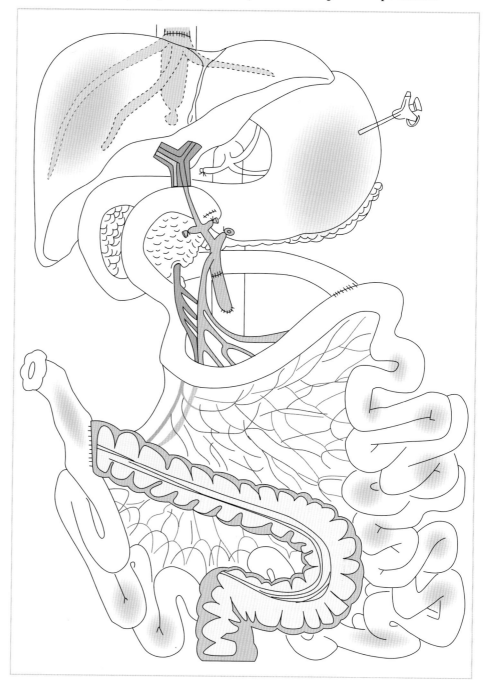

Figure 7.32

Multivisceral Transplant

a) Donor Procedure

1. Donor procurement is fundamentally the same as in the liver–intestine procurement except that variable amounts of the stomach or colon are preserved with the graft. Recipients with disorders of motility and gastric dysfunction may benefit from inclusion of the stomach in the allograft. Recipients with severe chronic pancreatitis usually require inclusion of the entire pancreas. Tumors of the mesentery sometimes require removal of the entire gastroduodenal complex, and patients suffering familial adenomatous polyposis sometimes have gastric, duodenal, or periampullary polyps requiring removal. Some children may rarely require concomitant renal transplantation. In this case, one or both pediatric kidneys can be kept in continuity with the allograft, with either the distal or the thoracic allograft aorta used for inflow. The renal arteries and veins are not disrupted from their connections to the aorta and vena cava. The fundamental technical alterations are preservation of the left gastric artery, careful preservation of the gastroepiploic arcade when removing the greater omentum (Figure 7.33), and enteric division of the gastroesophageal junction, rather than the pylorus or jejunum.

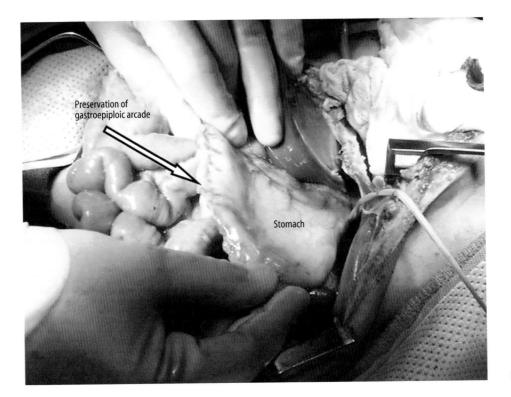

Figure 7.33

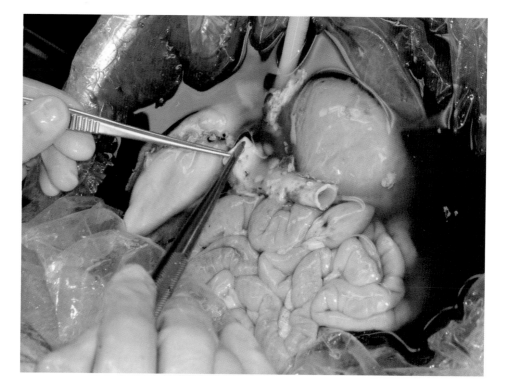

Figure 7.34

2. The abdominal viscera are then removed en bloc with the vena cava and the same Carrel patch or intact aorta (Figure 7.34), as would be the case with liver–intestine procurement.

b) Recipient Procedure

1. This transplant procedure is different from the previously described ones in that the entire splanchnic circulation with accompanying organs is removed; no portocaval shunt or bypass is therefore necessary. The pancreas and spleen, the root of the intestinal mesentery, the stomach, and the liver are removed together, preserving vena cava continuity. Thus, the recipient operation is similar to the multivisceral donor operation itself. The procedure begins with mobilization of the liver from the retrohepatic vena cava to allow piggyback placement of the allograft. No portal dissection is required.

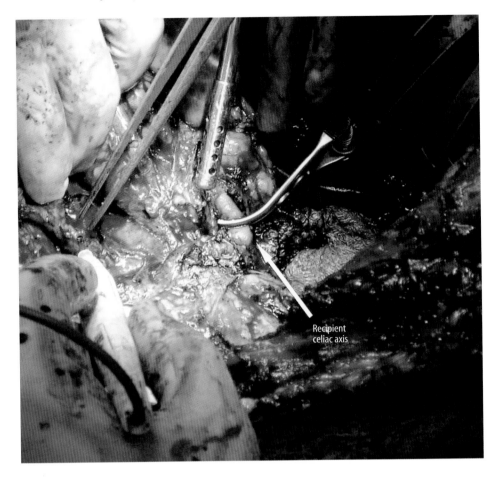

Recipient
celiac axis

Figure 7.35

2. Next, the proximal stomach is isolated, allowing for division with a stapling device, preserving the gastroesophageal junction in the recipient, with descending blood supply from the esophagus. This exposes the supraceliac aorta, sometimes allowing the celiac to be identified. However, this is most easily found proceeding from the left with a medial visceral rotation, leading to isolation of the base of the celiac and superior mesenteric arteries from the anterolateral left approach (Figure 7.35). Cattell and Kocher maneuvers (if the colon is intact) expose the right side of the superior mesenteric artery, and mobilization of the entire base of the intestinal mesentery.

3. The left colon is divided, taking care to preserve the left colic artery and inferior mesenteric arteries, as no collateral flow from the superior mesenteric artery will exist after exenteration. Vascular clamps can then be placed on the base of the celiac and superior mesenteric arteries and they may be transected. This step leaves the patient functionally anhepatic, so preparation to remove the organs prior to this step is critical. The hepatic veins are clamped and divided. The stomach, pancreas, spleen, small bowel, right colon, and liver are removed together, preserving the inferior vena cava for piggyback allograft implantation.

4. The hepatic venous piggyback anastomosis is usually performed first, aligning the graft in proper position.

5. Inflow must be brought to both the celiac and superior mesenteric arteries. Two inflow vascular anastomoses may be used, using the native celiac and superior mesenteric arteries end-to-end with the same donor structures (our preferred method), using an iliac bifurcating graft to these vessels from either the supraceliac or infrarenal aorta after ligation of the native vessels, or through a single anastomosis of infrarenal aorta of the donor allogaft end to side to the infrarenal aorta of the recipient (Figure 7.36).

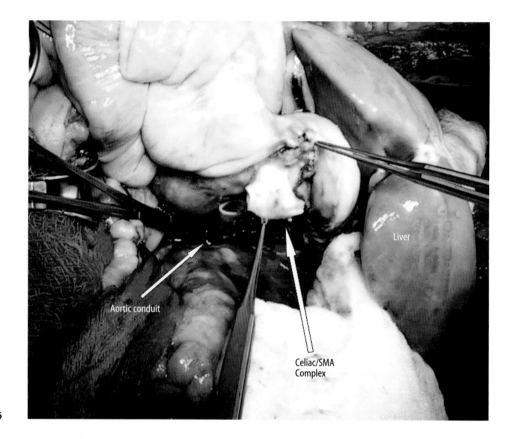

Figure 7.36

6. Preservation of a cuff of native stomach allows for a two-layer gastrogastric anastomosis, rather than an esophagogastric anastomosis. We have encountered no anastomotic leakage with this technique.[22] Pyloroplasty is required to provide gastric emptying of the denervated stomach. Distal enteral continuity is reestablished with ileostomy construction and colon anastomosis as described above (Figures 7.37 and 7.38).

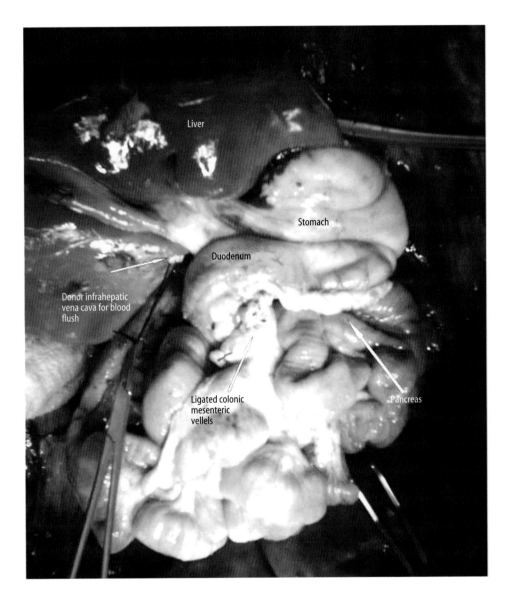

Figure 7.37

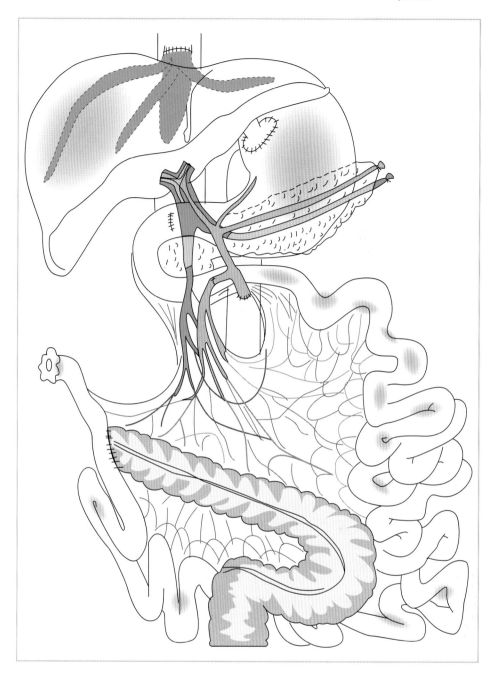

Figure 7.38

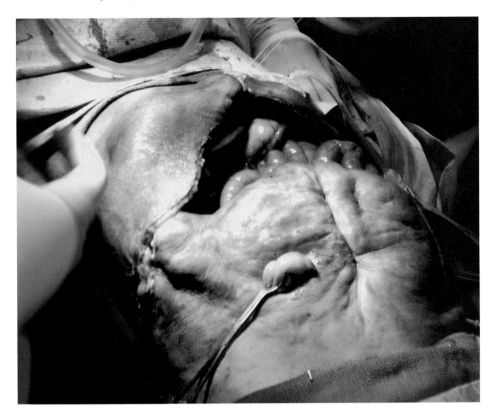

Figure 7.39

7. Transplantation of the stomach may result in either gastric stasis or mild dumping, and some form of gastric decompression tube is mandatory, usually with a combined gastrostomy-jejunostomy tube to allow early feeding into the graft jejunum. Drains are placed in case of the development of chylous ascites that may emanate from the graft after a fat-containing diet is resumed (Figure 7.39).

Living-Donor Small-Bowel Transplant

Very few small-bowel transplants have been done to date utilizing living donors. Less than 50 cases have been reported to the International Intestinal Transplant Registry. Primarily this is because the results with deceased donors are satisfactory, and the issues with organ shortage are not as great as with liver or kidney transplant. Nonetheless, the mortality list on the waiting list is high, especially in pediatric patients. Use of living donors has the potential advantages of lowering waiting time, reducing preservation injury, and allowing for better human leukocyte antigen (HLA) matching.[25–28]

Various segments of bowel have been reported to have been used for such transplants, but the most experience is with a long segment of the donor terminal ileum as the graft for the recipient. In this scenario, approximately 150 to 200 cm of distal ileum is used. The graft inflow is based on the distal part of the superior mesenteric artery (SMA); graft outflow is based on the corresponding part of the superior mesenteric vein (SMV).

As with all living-donor transplants, donor selection is a critical part of the process. Potential donors should be ABO blood group compatible and carefully evaluated for possible cardiopulmonary risk factors. The medical evaluation is not too dissimilar to the evaluation for a potential kidney donor. Specific to the potential small-bowel donor is radiologic imaging to evaluate the anatomy of the superior mesenteric vessels. This can be done with conventional selective mesenteric angiogram. However, this is an invasive test with some potential risk. The same information can be obtained with a good-quality computed tomography (CT) angiogram with three-dimensional reconstructions.

a) Surgical Procedure

1. A midline incision is made and the abdominal cavity is explored. The first important step is to measure the length of bowel and mark the portion to be removed (Figure 7.40). The last 20 to 30 cm of terminal ileum, including the ileocecal valve, should be preserved in the donor. Therefore, starting at the ileocecal valve, 20 cm is measured proximally and the bowel is marked here, which represents the distal margin of resection. The bowel is then marked 150 to 200 cm proximal to this, which represents the proximal resection margin. One should also ensure that at least 60% of the total small-bowel length will be left in the recipient.

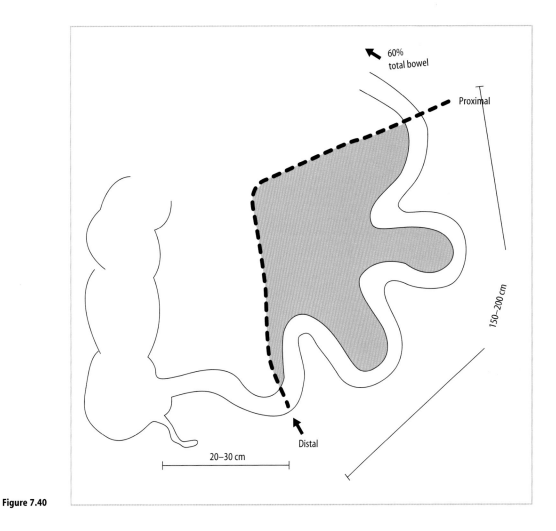

Figure 7.40

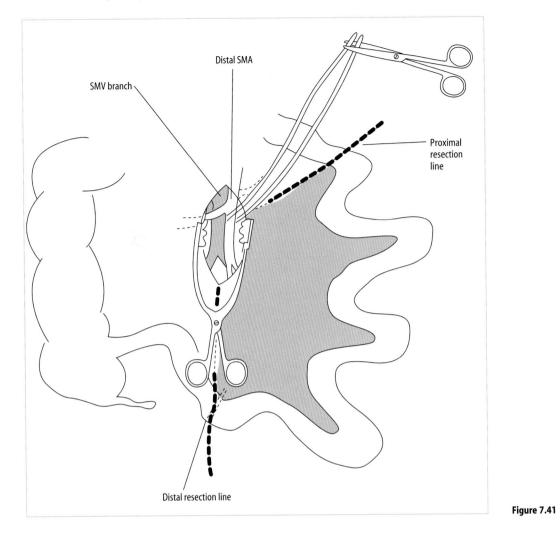

SMV branch

Distal SMA

Proximal resection line

Distal resection line

Figure 7.41

2. Using transillumination and palpation, the distal branch of the SMA is identified, and dissected free for 2 to 3 cm. Care should be taken to ensure that this is distal to the major branches of the SMA that supply the jejunum, proximal ileum, and right colon. The corresponding portion of the superior mesenteric vein is identified next to the artery and dissected free for a similar length (Figure 7.41).

3. Next, the mesentery of the bowel to be removed is scored and divided. This is done in a V-shaped fashion, with the apex corresponding to the mobilized portion of the SMA and SMV, and the two ends corresponding to the proximal and distal resection margins (Figure 7.42).

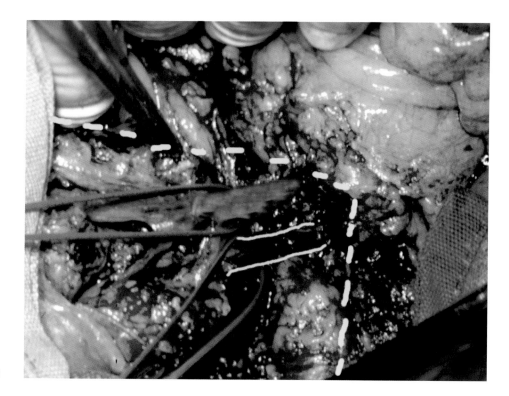

Figure 7.42

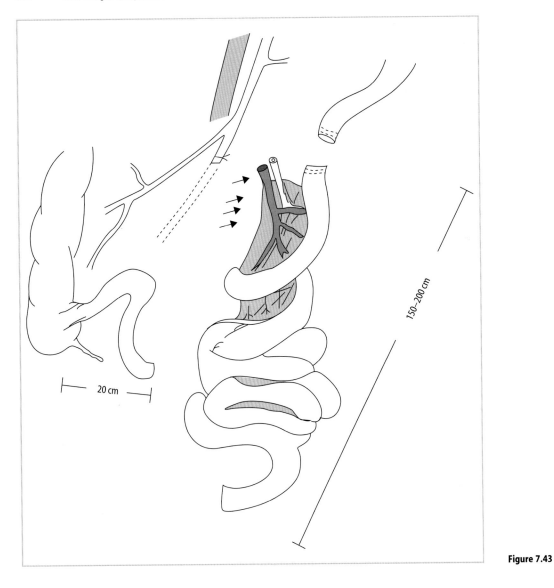

20 cm

150–200 cm

Figure 7.43

4. The bowel is divided proximally and distally. The vessels are divided after application of vascular clamps. The graft is removed and flushed (Figure 7.43).

5. The two divided ends of the bowel are reapproximated either with a stapler or in a hand-sewn fashion to create an end-to-end anastomosis (Figure 7.44). The defect in the mesentery is closed, followed by closure of the incision.

6. The recipient operation first involves isolation of the vessels to be used for inflow and outflow of the graft. The infrarenal aorta and inferior vena cava are most commonly used. End-to-side anastomoses are performed for the vein and artery of the graft (Figure

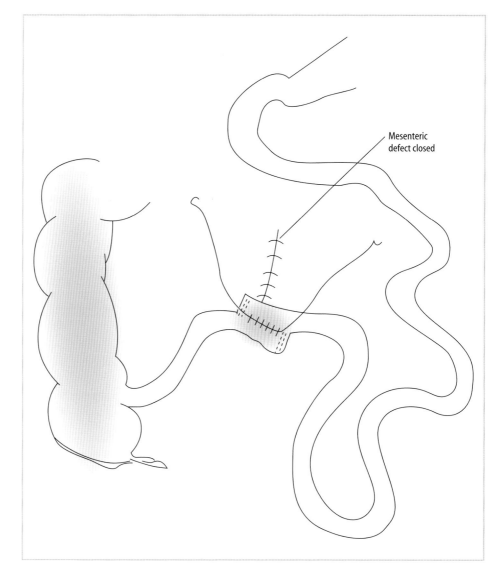

Mesenteric
defect closed

Figure 7.44

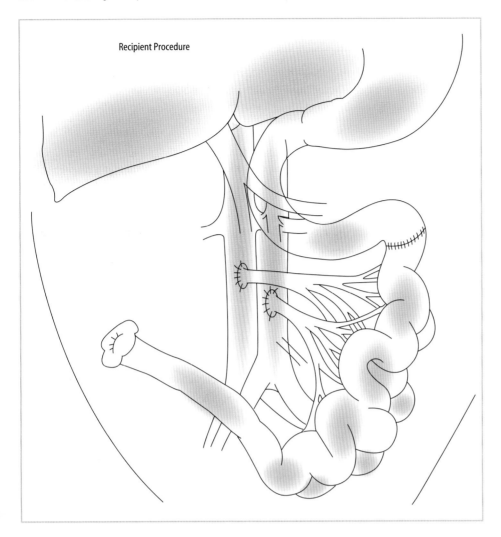

Recipient Procedure

Figure 7.45

7.45). Once the bowel is reperfused, intestinal continuity is restored by anastomosing the proximal end to the recipient remnant bowel. The distal end is usually brought out as an ileostomy.

Perioperative Management

Patients require intensive care immediately after transplant. They generally remain intubated in the early postoperative period, although isolated intestinal transplant patients may be extubated early. In the first 24 hours, the transplanted intestine usually produces minimal stool, but third-space losses can be significant, requiring aggressive hydration. If kidneys are transplanted with the graft, the urine output should be replaced on an hourly basis accordingly. Finally, pulmonary artery catheter pressures or transthoracic echocardiography may be employed to help guide fluid management at the discretion of the critical care team. The intestinal vasculature is sensitive to vasoconstrictive agents, particularly α-adrenergic agents, and they should be avoided. Sepsis syndrome that requires intervention usually indicates the need for reoperation due to vascular compromise or perforation. Because the graft is exteriorized with an ileostomy, blood flow to the graft may be assessed with Doppler flow at the bedside, rather than ultrasound duplex, which is made difficult by overlying bowel gas. A bedside nurse may employ a fetal Doppler hourly to assure good waveform as would be done for a vascularized free flap.

Electrolyte imbalances should be corrected aggressively with intravenous delivery. The transplanted bowel after the first few days may exhibit calcium and magnesium malabsorption with high ileostomy outputs, although this usually does not develop until after the institution of enteral nutrition. Water, sodium, and bicarbonate may be lost in large quantities with high ileostomy outputs. This may lead to a characteristic metabolic acidosis, requiring sodium bicarbonate added to the intravenous or enteral formula for correction. Hypomagnesemia potentiates tacrolimus-related neurotoxicity and should be avoided.

Intravenous broad-spectrum antibiotics should be continued early after transplantation or until the first biopsy confirms mucosal integrity of the transplanted bowel. Some patients will have lost the right of domain of the abdominal cavity and will return to the intensive care unit closed with a prosthetic mesh. Although we carefully match donor and recipient sizes, at times abdominal lavage and staged closure is necessary. A dedicated line for parenteral nutrition should be maintained during the intensive care unit stay, as the average time to the achievement of complete enteral nutrition after intestinal transplantation is approximately 1 month.[1,11] We generally institute feeding 5 days after transplantation if no reoperation is planned, and early graft function is adequate, judged by initiation of stomal output.

Conclusion

Intestinal transplantation is a very technically demanding field, requiring intimate knowledge of advanced techniques in both liver transplantation and gastrointestinal surgery. Some degree of individualization of procedures is required, based on each recipient's gastrointestinal anatomy, function, and vascular complications of parenteral nutrition. Appropriate technical and logistical planning will minimize unnecessary complications and keep ischemic times short, and have helped attain the current acceptable outcomes.

References

1. Grant D, Abu-Elmagd K, Reyes J, et al. 2003 report of the intestine transplant registry: a new era has dawned. Ann Surg 2005;241(4):607–613.
2. The Intestinal Transplant Registry. http://www.intestinaltransplant.org/.
3. Fishbein TM, Gondolesi GE, Kaufman SS. Intestinal transplantation for gut failure. Gastroenterology 2003;124(6):1615–1628.
4. Fishbein TM. The current state of intestinal transplantation. Transplantation 2004;27:78(2):175–178.
5. Fishbein TM, Matsumoto CS. Regimens for intestinal transplant immunosuppression. Curr Opin Organ Transplant 2005;10:12–123.
6. Abu-Elmagd K, Fung JJ, Bueno J, et al. Logistics and techniques for procurement of intestinal, pancreatic, and hepatic grafts from the same donor. Ann Surg.
7. Fishbein TM, Kaufman SS, Florman SS, et al. Isolated intestinal transplantation: proof of clinical efficacy. Transplantation 2003;76(4):636–640.
8. Reyes J, Bueno J, Kocoshis S, et al. Current status of intestinal transplantation in children. J Pediatr Surg 1998;33(2):243–254.
9. Tzakis A, Toso S, Reyes J, et al. Piggyback orthotopic intestinal transplantation. Surg Gynecol Obstet 1991;172(216):605–609.
10. Berney T, Kato T, Nishida S, et al. Portal versus systemic venous drainage of small bowel allografts: comparative assessment of survival, function, rejection and bacterial translocation. J Am Coll Surg 2002;195:804–813.
11. Bueno J, Abu-Elmagd K, Mazariegos G, et al. Composite liver-small bowel allografts with preservation of donor duodenum and hepatic biliary system in children. J Pediatr Surg 2000;35(2):291–196.
12. Kato T, Romero R, Verzaro R, et al. Inclusion of entire pancreas in the composite liver and intestinal graft in pediatric intestinal transplantation. Pediatr Transplant 1999;3:210–214.
13. Grant D, Wall W, Mimeault R, et al. Successful small bowel/liver transplantation. Lancet 1990;335:181–184.
14. Fishbein T, Schiano T, Jaffe D, et al. Isolated intestinal transplantation in adults with nonreconstructible GI tracts. Transplant Proc 2000;32(6):1231–1232.
15. Shaffer D, Diflo T, Love W, et al. Immunological and metabolic effects of caval versus portal drainage in small bowel transplantation. Surgery 1988;104:518–524.

16. Reyes J, Mazariegos GV, Bond G, et al. Pediatric intestinal transplantation: historical notes, principles and controversies. Pediatr Transplant 2002;6:193–207.

17. Sindhi R, Fox IJ, Hefron T, et al. Procurement and preparation of human isolated small intestinal grafts for transplantation. Transplantation 1995;60:771–773.

18. Sudan D, Iyer K, Deroover A, et al. A new technique for combined liver/small intestinal transplantation. Transplantation 2001;72(11):1846–1848.

19. Starzl T, Rowe M, Todo S, et al. Transplantation of multiple abdominal viscera. JAMA 1989;261:1449–1457.

20. Fishbein T, Facciuto M, Harpaz N, et al. A simple blood flush technique and mannitol promote homodynamic stability and avoid reperfusion injury in isolated intestinal transplantation. Transplant Proc 2000; 32:1313–1314.

21. Fishbein TM, Florman SS, Gondolesi GE, et al. Noncomposite simultaneous liver and intestinal transplantation. Transplantation 2003;27:75(4):564–565.

22. Kato T, Tzakis A, Selvaggi G, et al. Surgical techniques used in intestinal transplantation. Curr Opin Organ Transplant 2004;9(2):207–213.

23. Buchman AL, Scolapio J, Fryer J. AGA technical review on short bowel syndrome and intestinal transplantation. Gastroenterology 2003;124(4):1111–1134.

24. Reyes J, Mazariegos GV, Bond GM, et al. Pediatric intestinal transplantation: historical notes, principles and controversies. Pediatr Transplantant 2002;6(3):193–207.

25. Kato T, Ruiz P, Thompson JF, et al. Intestinal and multivisceral transplantation. World J Surg 2002;26(2).

26. Benedetti E, Baum C, Cicalese L, et al. Progressive functional adaptation of segmental bowel graft from living related donor. Transplantation 2001;71(4):569–571.

27. Gruessner RW, Sharp HL. Living-related intestinal transplantation: first report of a standardized surgical technique. Transplantation 1997;64(11):1605–1607.

28. Testa G, Holterman M, John E, Kecskes S, Abcarian H, Benedetti E. Combined living donor liver/small bowel transplantation. Transplantation 2005;79(10):1401–1404.

Index

Page numbers followed by f indicate figures.
Large page ranges indicate main discussions.

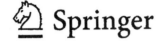

Springer